A Manual of Clinical Refraction

A Manual of Clinical Refraction

Previously Known as Clinical Refraction Guide

THIRD EDITION

Ajay Kumar Bhootra
B Optom DOS FAO FOAI FCLI ICLEP FIACLE (Australia)
Diploma in Sportvision (UK)
Ex-CEO and Dean
Krishnalaya School of Optometry
Kolkata, West Bengal, India

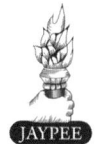

JAYPEE BROTHERS MEDICAL PUBLISHERS
The Health Sciences Publisher
New Delhi | London

Jaypee Brothers Medical Publishers (P) Ltd

Headquarters
Jaypee Brothers Medical Publishers (P) Ltd.
EMCA House
23/23-B, Ansari Road, Daryaganj
New Delhi 110 002, India
Landline: +91-11-23272143, +91-11-23272703
+91-11-23282021, +91-11-23245672
E-mail: jaypee@jaypeebrothers.com

Corporate Office
Jaypee Brothers Medical Publishers (P) Ltd.
4838/24, Ansari Road, Daryaganj
New Delhi 110 002, India
Phone: +91-11-43574357
Fax: +91-11-43574314
E-mail: jaypee@jaypeebrothers.com

Overseas Office
JP Medical Ltd.
83, Victoria Street, London
SW1H 0HW (UK)
Phone: +44-20 3170 8910
Fax: +44(0)20 3008 6180
E-mail: info@jpmedpub.com

Website: www.jaypeebrothers.com
Website: www.jaypeedigital.com
© 2025, Jaypee Brothers Medical Publishers

The views and opinions expressed in this book are solely those of the original contributor(s)/author(s) and do not necessarily represent those of editor(s) and publisher of the book.

All rights reserved. No part of this publication may be reproduced, stored or transmitted in any form or by any means, electronic, mechanical, photocopying, recording or otherwise, without the prior permission in writing of the publishers.

All brand names and product names used in this book are trade names, service marks, trademarks or registered trademarks of their respective owners. The publisher is not associated with any product or vendor mentioned in this book.

Medical knowledge and practice change constantly. This book is designed to provide accurate, authoritative information about the subject matter in question. However, readers are advised to check the most current information available on procedures included and check information from the manufacturer of each product to be administered, to verify the recommended dose, formula, method and duration of administration, adverse effects and contraindications. It is the responsibility of the practitioner to take all appropriate safety precautions. Neither the publisher nor the author(s)/editor(s) assume any liability for any injury and/or damage to persons or property arising from or related to use of material in this book.

This book is sold on the understanding that the publisher is not engaged in providing professional medical services. If such advice or services are required, the services of a competent medical professional should be sought.

Every effort has been made where necessary to contact holders of copyright to obtain permission to reproduce copyright material. If any have been inadvertently overlooked, the publisher will be pleased to make the necessary arrangements at the first opportunity.

Inquiries for bulk sales may be solicited at: jaypee@jaypeebrothers.com

A Manual of Clinical Refraction

First Edition: 2013
Second Edition: 2019
Third Edition: **2025**

ISBN: 978-93-5696-723-6

Printed in India at Sterling Graphics Pvt. Ltd.

Dedicated to

Late Sri Krishna Kumar Binani, my mentor, guide, and inspirer. His enduring influence has profoundly shaped my personality and played a pivotal role in my journey. I owe much of what I am today to his invaluable guidance, and even in his absence, his memory remains a source of inspiration

and

The tireless pursuit of knowledge, the spirit of collaboration, and an unwavering commitment to excellence. To all those who embark on the path of understanding clinical refraction, may this book illuminate their journey of exploration and learning.

May this contribution further advance the field and foster a deeper appreciation for the intricate interplay between science, technology, and the human experience.

PREFACE TO THE THIRD EDITION

Greetings to all aspiring and practicing optometrists and eye care practitioners!

I penned this preface during a memorable trip to Singapore, celebrating my son's promotion. Witnessing his growth and success brought immense joy as a father. Amidst the celebration, I found inspiration in motivational books and decided to channel my revived passion for writing into this preface.

Clinical refraction has always been a burning passion—an intriguing challenge, a puzzle to solve, and a constant source of fascination. Each case offered an opportunity to explore, learn, and evolve.

One guiding philosophy shaped my practice: the question, "Why did I do what I did?" This introspective approach transformed routine corrections into thoughtful explorations, fostering a thinking power that allowed me to view the procedure from different angles.

Asking "Why" led to another crucial question: "How will I do it again?" This process was not about settling into a routine but a continuous refinement of technique, seeking improvement and excellence. This introspective journey, fueled by questions—why, what, and how—became the foundation of my values in clinical refraction.

After years of navigating the landscape of clinical refraction, I am convinced that these questions are not just the foundation but the pillars that help someone to learn the intricate science of this procedure.

Clinical refraction is both an art and a science—a process of determining an individual's refractive error through tests, tailoring a lens prescription for optimal retinal imagery. Various methods are employed, adaptable based on factors like age and medical history. The clinician's role is to choose the right methods to assess visual function and refractive error, enhancing the patient's visual acuity.

I often say that a good practice of clinical refraction requires an engineering brain. Just as an engineer optimizes a machine for peak performance, clinical refraction is the systematic fine-tuning of refractive correction. Precision is paramount, with each diopter adjustment akin to a fine-tuning process for optimal vision accuracy. Like engineers rely on feedback loops, clinicians encourage patients to provide feedback, ensuring the correction aligns with their subjective visual experience.

This fusion of art, science, and engineering makes clinical refraction fascinating.

How have I organized this book?
This thoughtfully crafted book seamlessly merges theoretical knowledge, practical insights, and clinical wisdom, catering to both seasoned practitioners and aspiring professionals.

Starting with a dedicated focus on grasping the fundamentals, the initial chapters meticulously explain each essential component vital to the clinical refraction process. Emphasis is placed on every element, recognizing their significance—often overlooked but crucial. This approach lays the groundwork for a comprehensive understanding, ensuring a smooth and enjoyable learning experience. The structured progression aids in seamlessly transitioning to the practical aspects of clinical refraction.

Continuing, the book explores various clinical tests, procedures, and associated tools and equipment. Descriptions of unusual tests add an element of surprise with their simplicity, fostering an engaging learning experience. The core of the book introduces a symphony of topics, covering the fundamentals of refraction procedures, intricacies of vision, and vision correction. This orchestration includes diagnostic techniques and the latest advancements in refractive technologies, guiding readers through the symphonic process of assessing and enhancing visual acuity.

The final chapters delve into specific cases and situations requiring a different thought process. Practical examples enhance problem-solving skills, offering a hands-on and pragmatic approach to applying knowledge. Throughout these pages, you encounter a symphony of topics, from fundamentals to the intricacies of vision and correction. Alongside technical brilliance, there is an emphasis on the human touch—understanding each patient's unique visual needs and tailoring the approach accordingly.

The book concludes with a harmonious blend of theoretical depth, practical application, and personal insights, leaving readers well-equipped to navigate the intricate world of vision correction with confidence and proficiency.

Lastly, a glimpse into my personality: while perceived as reserved by others, a deeper exploration reveals my profound passion for learning and my openness to share knowledge and experiences. You may know more about me at *www.ajaykrbhootra.com.*

Ajay Kumar Bhootra

PREFACE TO THE FIRST EDITION

Over the last 30 years, a lot of technological advancements have occurred in the field of optometry and ophthalmology. The progress has provided many equipment and instruments to perform the clinical refraction to elicit various refractive errors. Many textbooks have focused on the different aspects of the whole procedure. Several multivolume books detailing the procedure have been written. Yet, there remains a need for a handbook which can serve as a reference guide.

The idea of *Clinical Refraction Guide* has been conceived to fill this gap and to create a source, which is readily available with the eyecare practitioners in their bag. The book is designed to have the relevant texts so that the reader can assess the key information quickly. The majority of the chapters also follow the sequential steps of the whole procedure. Meticulous planning has been done to design the contents and put them into different chapters.

The book has two sections: Section I explains the basic clinical procedures used for routine refraction and Section II deals with retinoscopy procedure. Retinoscope is one of the most wonderful and simple instruments used for ocular examination as the clinical procedure. Retinoscopy is an art that cannot be learned through books. It needs a long practice either on schematic eye or on patients to really master the art. I have tried to arrange the basic information as to the use and application of the retinoscope in a very small package, so that an individual can turn over its pages to look for the assistance.

The book has been compiled in a very simple language so that it serves as a reference guide in the clinic as well as in the classes. The readers must take the help of other textbooks available on the subject to get into the depth. I hope, it serves the purpose for which it has been written. I would also like to welcome your suggestions to improve it in further edition.

Ajay Kumar Bhootra

ACKNOWLEDGMENTS

I am sincerely grateful to express my appreciation for the invaluable support and collaboration. I received during the creation of this book. I extend my heartfelt thanks to Mr SK Lohia of Modern Surgical, Kolkata, West Bengal, India; Tatjana Heidorn of Heine Optotechnik GmbH & Co. KG, and Mr Saleem Bhalla, the country manager of Heine Optotechnik GmbH & Co. KG. Their generous contributions, both in text material and images, played a pivotal role in bringing this book to fruition.

I would like to express my gratitude to Ms Swarnali Pal for capturing the photographs essential for this book.

I wish to acknowledge their unwavering support, without which this endeavor would not have been possible. Their support to advancing knowledge in this field has significantly enriched the content of this book.

I am also indebted to the Jaypee Brothers Medical Publisher (P) Ltd.—Shri Jitendar P Vij (Group Chairman), Mr Ankit Vij (Managing Director), Mr MS Mani (Group President), Dr Madhu Choudhary (Director—Educational Publishing), Ms Pooja Bhandari [Director-Production (Books and Journals)], Dr Upma Tomar (Sr Development Editor), Mr Ajay Kumar Sharma [DGM (Books and Journals)], Ms Sunita Katla (Executive Assistant to Group Chairman and Publishing Manager), Ms Samina Khan (Executive Assistant to Director-Educational Publishing), Mr Vijay Kumar Bhatia (Manager-Production), Ms Seema Dogra (Cover Visualizer), Ms Neha Verma (Graphic Designer—Cover), Ms Uma Adhikari (Indesign Operator), Ms Geeta Barik (Proofreader), and Mr Sanjeev Kumar (Graphic Designer), who involved in the production process.

CONTENTS

1. **Eye**   1
   - Parts of the Eye   3
   - Accessory Organs of the Eyeball   9
   - Ocular Muscles   12
   - Ocular Glands   16
   - Axial Length   18

2. **Vision and Visual Function**   22
   - Vision and Visual Perception   22
   - Different Facets of Visual Perception   25
   - Classification of Vision   29
   - Components of Vision   32
   - Binocular Vision   39
   - Monocular Vision   42
   - Dominant Eye   43
   - Visual Field   50
   - Visual Angle   52
   - Depth of Field and Depth of Focus   54

3. **Visual Symptoms**   57
   - Causes of Visual Symptoms   57
   - Common Visual Symptoms   60
   - Optical Correction of Visual Symptoms   66

4. **Retinal Image**   71
   - Retinal Image: Foundation of Vision   71
   - Chromatic Aberration   74
   - Monochromatic Aberrations   76
   - Rationale for Higher Order Aberration   80

5. **Refractive Error**   84
   - Myopia   85
   - Hypermetropia   86
   - Regular Astigmatism   90
   - Pathological Hypermetropia   93
   - Pathological Myopia   94
   - Irregular Astigmatism   94
   - Presbyopia   95

Contents

6. Fundamentals of Clinical Refraction — 99
- Laws of Clinical Refraction 100
- Goal of Clinical Refraction 106
- Cardinal Principle of Clinical Refraction 107
- Clinical Refraction: An Intellectual Process 111
- Methods of Clinical Refraction 117
- Correction of Refractive Error 122
- Trial Framing 124

7. Trial Lens Set — 128
- Spherical and Cylinder Trial Lenses 128
- Prism 129
- Pinhole Disc 130
- Stenopeic Slit 130
- Red and Green Filter 131
- Maddox Rod 132
- Occluder 132
- Trial Frame 133

8. Visual Acuity Test — 136
- Objectives of Visual Acuity Test 136
- Factors Affecting Visual Acuity 137
- Implications of Visual Acuity Test 140
- Limitations of Visual Acuity Test 140
- Designation of Visual Acuity 141
- Visual Acuity Test Charts 146
- Snellen's Test Chart 147
- Visual Acuity Test Chart Formats 154
- Clinical Assessment of Visual Acuity 157
- Uncorrected Visual Acuity 157
- Near Visual Acuity 159

9. History Taking and Entrance Tests — 165
- History Taking 165
- Scripting an Effective Case History for Refraction 168
- Baseline Data Assimilation 172

10. Objective Methods of Refraction — 187
- Objective Refraction 187
- Retinoscopy 187

- Autorefractometer 210
- Keratometry 215
- Assimilation of Initial Data and Goal Setting 217

11. Subjective Methods of Refraction — 220
- Subjective Refraction 220
- Challenges Faced During Subjective Refraction 222
- Methods of Subjective Refraction 224
- Delayed Subjective Refraction 233
- Determination of Near Addition 235
- Jackson Cross-cylinder Test 237
- Refraction Using Stenopeic Slit 239

12. Refinement Tests — 243
- Duochrome Test for Spherical 243
- Tests for Binocular Balancing 245

13. Prescribing and Counseling — 249
- Prescribing Considerations 250
- Factors that Influence Prescribing Decision 256
- Fundamental Rule for Prescribing Correction 261
- Counseling 267

14. Refraction in Myopia — 275
- Classification of Myopia 276
- Treatment of Myopia 277

15. Refraction in Hypermetropia — 281
- Correction of Hypermetropia 282
- Subjective Refraction in Hypermetropia 288

16. Refraction in Astigmatism — 290
- Symptoms 290
- Treatment 291
- Tests for Astigmatic Correction 292

17. Refraction in Presbyopia — 295
- Symptoms 296
- Correction of Presbyopia 297
- Test for Near Addition 298
- Premature Onset of Presbyopia 303

Contents

18. Refraction in Anisometropia — 305
- Symptoms 306
- Vision in Anisometropia 306
- Correction in Anisometropia 307

19. Refraction in Aphakia — 309
- Vision in Aphakia 309
- Correction in Aphakia 310

20. Pediatric Refraction — 312
- Development of Vision 313
- Emmetropization 314
- Amblyopia and Strabismus 316
- Retinopathy of Prematurity 317
- Measuring Refractive Error in Children 318
- Prescribing Refractive Correction in Children 325

21. The Geriatric Refraction — 332
- Aging Changes in Eyes 333
- Aging Changes in Visual Functions 336
- Measuring Refractive Error 340
- Prescribing Correction 347

22. Refraction for Sports Athletes — 352
- Importance of Good Refraction in Sports 353
- Consideration for Prescribing Correction 356

23. Refraction in Nonadaptation Cases — 359
- Importance of Effective Handling 359
- Psychological Condition of Patient 360
- Goal of Re-evaluating Refraction in Cases of Nonadaptation 360
- Flow of Re-evaluating the Refraction 361

Bibliography — *367*

Index — *369*

PLATE 1

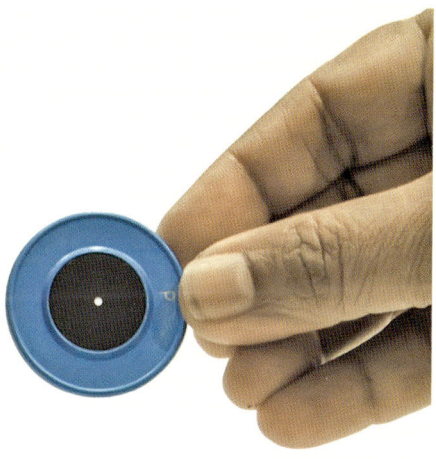

Fig. 7.3: Pinhole disc.

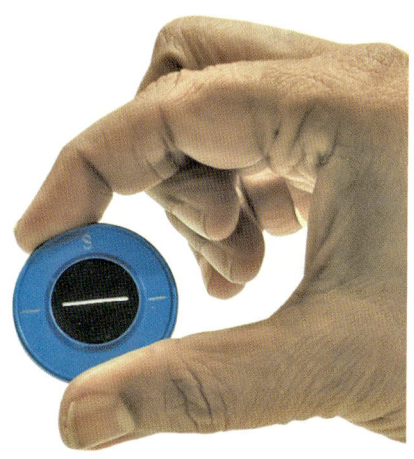

Fig. 7.4: Stenopeic slit.

PLATE 2

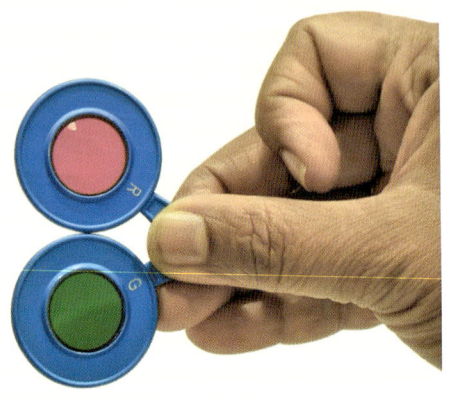

Fig. 7.5: Red and green filter.

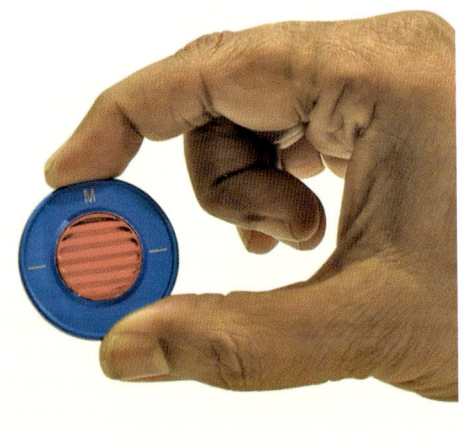

Fig. 7.6: Maddox rod.

CHAPTER 1

Eye

CHAPTER OUTLINE

- Parts of the Eye
- Accessory Organs of the Eyeball
- Ocular Muscles
- Ocular Glands
- Axial Length

Eyes are small but they provide us with what is being considered to be the most important sense—vision. Vision is one of the most important senses, enabling us to navigate, recognize faces, read, and appreciate the beauty of our surroundings. The complexity and precision of the eye's structure and function are fascinating, and they underscore the significance of eye health and the importance of regular eye care. The human eye is composed of several tissues. While some of them are supportive tissues, others like retina and optic nerve are light sensitive. There are some refracting tissues also that help focus light onto the retina. **Table 1.1** shows the various components of eye grouped into three main categories based on their functions.

Table 1.1: Components of eye categorized in three different groups.

Refractive components	Supportive components	Protective components
Cornea	Sclera	Eyelids
Crytalline lens	Choroid	Eyelashes
Aqueous	Ciliary body	Conjunctiva
Vitreous	Ciliary processes	Lacrimal gland
	Zonules	Lacrimal apparatus
	Vitreous	

Chapter 1: Eye

Each group of organs plays a vital role in maintaining the health and proper functioning of the eye. The refractive organs focus light onto the retina, the supportive organs provide structural integrity and nourishment, and the protective organs shield the eye from external elements and help maintain a healthy environment for optimal vision.

The eye is actually a closed optical system. It is an adaptive optical system. Visible rays from a point object enter the eye through the pupil. But they do not focus as a point image because of diffraction and also because of light scattering through the ocular medium. They form a circle of least confusion, also called the blur circle. The circle of least confusion is a term used in optics to describe a specific point where the image formed by a lens is most sharply focused. This circle of least confusion can be moved anteriorly or posteriorly during clinical refraction. The size, shape, and position of the circle of least confusion vary directly in proportion to the refractive status of the eye and the refractive power of the lens placed before the eye. Visual acuity is related to the size and the axial position of the circle of least confusion with respect to the retina. The outer limiting membrane of the retina is the effective plane at which best focus should be achieved in order to obtain maximum visual acuity. The finer the circle of least confusion and the closer it is to the outer limiting membrane of the retina, where it is formed, the better the visual acuity.

Retina and fundus are often used interchangeably. While the retina is a thin layer of tissue at the back of the eye that contains specialized cells called photoreceptors, which are responsible for detecting light and transmitting visual information to the brain, the fundus refers to the interior surface of the eye that is visible through the pupil. It includes the retina, the optic disc, and the blood vessels that supply blood to the retina. When an ophthalmologist examines the fundus of the eye, they are looking at the back of the eye, including the retina. The main difference between the retina and the fundus is that the retina is a specific layer of tissue in the eye, while the fundus is a broader term that refers to the interior surface of the eye visible through the pupil, including the retina. A healthy fundus has a bright red or orange color due to the presence of pigment cells in the retina. The optic disc, which is the area where the optic nerve exits the eye, is a pale yellow color, and the surrounding retina is a healthy pink color. A healthy eye is important for maintaining good vision because it is responsible for capturing light and sending visual signals to the brain.

PARTS OF THE EYE

The eye has many parts as shown in **Figure 1.1**.

There are three chambers as shown in **Flowchart 1.1**.

The anterior chamber is the space between cornea and iris. The posterior chamber is the narrow space between iris and the lens of the eye. It lies behind the peripheral portion of the iris. The vitreous chamber is the large chamber located behind the lens and in front of optic nerve. Both the anterior and posterior chambers are the part of the anterior segment of the eye.

The eye sits in a protective bony socket called the orbit. Six extraocular muscles in the orbit are attached to the eye. The extraocular muscles are attached to the white part of the eye called the sclera and they move the eye up and down, side to side, and rotate the eye.

Sclera

Sclera is a strong layer of tissue that looks white in color and is opaque (**Fig. 1.2**). It covers nearly 80% of surface of the eyeball, around the cornea. The sclera is relatively inactive metabolically. The main

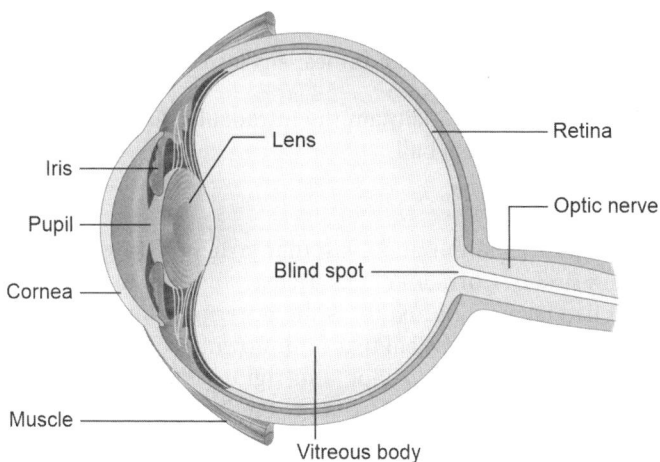

Fig. 1.1: Parts of the eye.

Flowchart 1.1: Three chambers of eye.

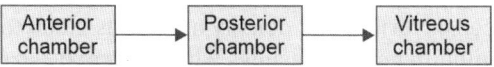

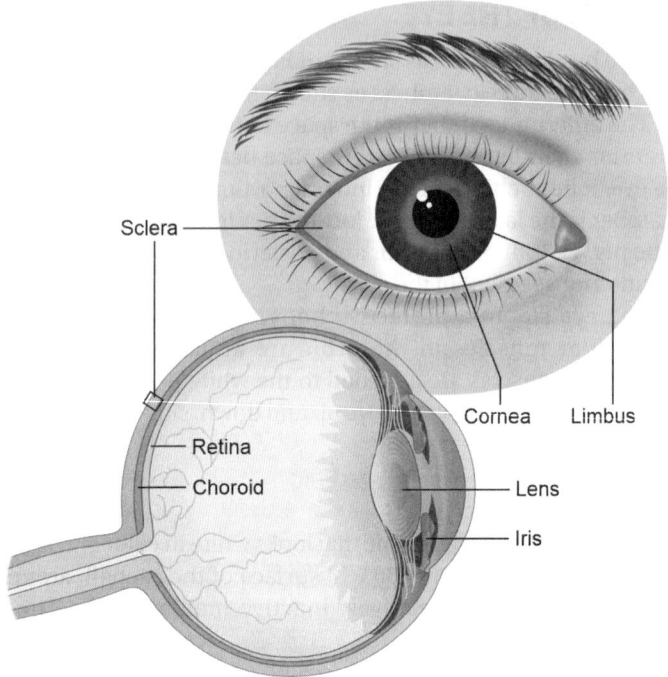

Fig. 1.2: Sclera, cornea, lens, iris, limbus.

function of sclera is to maintain the intraocular pressure of the eye and the shape of the eyeball.

Cornea

Cornea is a transparent and avascular structure **(Fig. 1.2)**. It is a refracting tissue. Cornea acts as a clear window to the eye. It is made of five layers. Epithelium is the outermost layer. It helps the adherence of the precorneal tear film. Bowman's membrane is the 2nd layer that maintains shape and rigidity of the cornea. If it is damaged, it results in scar. Stroma is the 3rd layer and is also the thickest layer. 90% of corneal thickness is stroma. It is highly regular cellular structure packed with collagen fibrils, which confers both strength and transparency. Descemet's membrane bounds the stroma posteriorly. It is very resistant to trauma, infection and other pathological processes. Endothelium is the 5th layer, consists of flat polygonal cells. Normal cell density at birth is 4,000 to 5,000 cells per square millimeter that declines with aging at 0.3–0.6% per year.

Endothelium is the area of high metabolic activity. It contains the pump mechanism that maintains the water balance and is involved in active secretion and protein synthesis.

Limbus

The limbus surrounds the cornea and forms the border between the cornea and sclera (**Fig. 1.2**). Limbus contains the pathways of aqueous humor outflow. It is also the site of surgical incisions for cataract and glaucoma.

Aqueous humor

The aqueous humor is a thin, transparent fluid, made up of 99.9% water and the other 0.1% consists of sugars, vitamins, proteins and other nutrients. It is continuously produced by the ciliary body, the production of which is balanced by drainage at an equal rate. A small variation in the production or outflow of the aqueous humor is significant, as it has a large influence on intraocular pressure. Aqueous nourishes the cornea and the lens.

Iris

Iris is the anterior most part of the uveal tract (**Fig. 1.2**). It forms the colored, visible part of the eye in front of the lens that contains the pupil in the center. The average diameter of iris is 12 mm. It looks smooth with naked eyes but presents radial and circular furrows and folds when seen under magnification. The color of the iris represents the color of the eyes which is the result of variation in the amount of melanin, a pigment found in the front of the iris. More pigments give brown iris and lack of pigments gives blue iris. Some pigments give green iris. The main function of the iris is to provide protection to the eye from microorganisms.

Pupil

Pupil is an aperture that lies in the center of the iris. It controls the amount of light entering into the eyes. The shape of the pupil is almost circular in normal people. However, irregularities in pupil shape are noticed in many pathological conditions. The size of the pupil is relatively small at birth, largest during adolescence and gradually becomes smaller with increasing age. Normal pupil size in adults varies from 2-4 mm in diameter in bright light to 4-8 mm in the dark. The pupils are generally equal in size. Both pupils constrict when the light is shown in one eye. Constriction of pupil to which light is shown is called 'Direct light reflex' and constriction of an other pupil is called 'Consensual light reflex'. In normal subjects both direct and consensual light reflex are almost always same in time, course and magnitude. Constriction and dilation of pupil size also affect the amount of chromatic and spherical aberration in the retinal image.

Ciliary Body

Ciliary body is the forward continuation of the choroid at ora serrata, connecting the choroid to the iris. It is roughly a triangular structure which lines the interior of the sclera behind the limbus. The main function of ciliary body is to change the shape of the lens when the eye focuses. It also makes the fluid that fills the space between cornea and iris. It also maintains lens zonules for the purpose of anchoring the lens in place. Functionally, it has two structures components—ciliary process and ciliary muscles.

Zonules

Zonules or Zonule of Zinn are the series of fibers connecting the ciliary body and lens of the eye, suspending the lens in place behind the iris and the pupil. The primary function of zonules is to stabilize the lens and allow accommodation to occur. The attachment of the zonular fibers to the lens capsule is superficial with few fibers penetrating into the capsule to form a mechanical or chemical union.

Lens

Lens is a transparent biconvex structure that lies behind the pupil. It is enclosed in a thin transparent capsule and is held in position by the zonules arising from ciliary body. It is an avascular structure that also lacks innervation. The size, shape and weight of the lens continue to increase throughout the life. It is colorless in young and turns into yellow in adults and gray in old age. Cataract develops when the lens becomes cloudy. Lens is a refracting tissue and it helps to refract incoming light and focus them onto the retina. The crystalline lens has a gradient refractive index, with a refractive index of 1.385 near the poles and a higher refractive index of 1.406 at the center of the nucleus. The refractive index also shows increasing tendency with the advancement of age.

Conjunctiva

Conjunctiva is a modified mucous membrane that covers the inner surface of the eyelids and is reflected onto the anterior surface of the globe. It is highly vascular tissue. It is a supportive tissue and its main function is to protect the globe. A number of well-differentiated small glands are found in conjunctiva.

Choroid

Choroid is the highly vascular middle layer of the eye between the retina and the sclera **(Fig. 1.3)**. It is a supportive tissue. It contains a pigment that absorbs excess light. Choroid contains many tiny blood vessels and has the vital role of nourishing the retina.

Retina

Retina is a light-sensitive layer that lines the interior of the eye. It is composed of light sensitive cells known as rods and cones. It appears purplish-red and turns to opaque white after the death of the person. The retina captures the light that enters the eye through pupil and helps translate it into the images. Photoreceptor cells in the retina react to light and change light energy into an electrical signal.

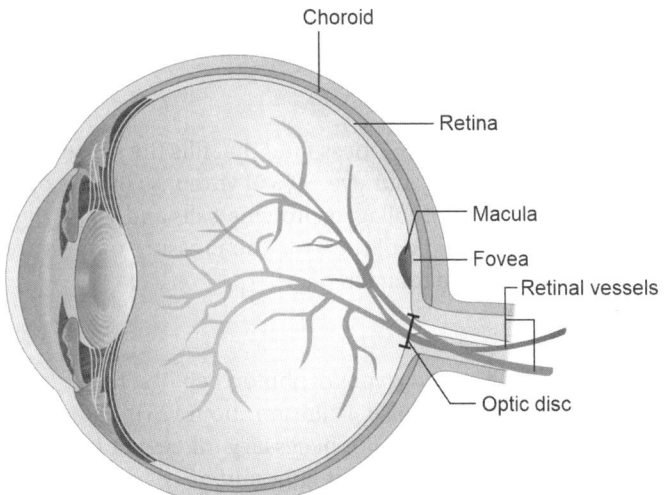

Fig. 1.3: Choroid, retina, macula, fovea, optic disc.

Macula

A yellow spot of approximately 5.5 mm in diameter on the retina at the back of the eye which surrounds the fovea. Macula corresponds to approximately 15% of the visual field. Photopic and color vision are the primary function of macula.

Fovea

Fovea is like a small indentation at the center of the macula, where there is a great concentration of cone cells **(Fig. 1.3)**. When the eye is directed at an object, the part of the image that is focused on the fovea is the image most accurately registered by the brain.

Optic Disc

When the eye is examined, the visible portion of the optic nerve, found on the retina, is the optic disc **(Fig. 1.3)**. It is identified as the start of the optic nerve where messages from cone and rod cells leave the eye via nerve fibers to the optic center of the brain. This area is also known as the 'blind spot'.

Optic Nerve

Optic nerve leaves the eye at the optic disc and transfers all the visual information to the brain to create visual image. Damage to an optic nerve can be the reason for vision loss in one or both eyes.

Vitreous Humor

Vitreous humor is a clear, colorless fluid that fills the space between the lens and the retina of your eye. 99% of vitreous consists of water and the rest is a mixture of collagen, proteins, salts and sugars. It helps it to hold 'spherical' shape of the eye. The pressure of the vitreous humor helps to keep the retina in place.

Rods and Cones

Rods and cones cells are two types of photoreceptors. They transform light energy into visual impulse. There are about 125 million rods and 6–7 million cone cells. Rods are necessary for seeing in dim light. Cone cells function best in bright light and are essential for acute vision. It is thought that there are three types of cones, each sensitive to the wavelength of a different primary color—red, green or blue. Other colors are seen as combinations of these primary colors.

ACCESSORY ORGANS OF THE EYEBALL

The accessory organs of eye are the structures that surround and protect the eyeball **(Fig. 1.4)**. They include the extraocular muscles, the eyebrows, the eyelashes, the eyelids, the lacrimal apparatus and the orbit. Since the extraocular muscles play very important role in pathophysiology of the eye and work in tandem with other ocular muscles of the eye, we will discuss while discussing ocular muscles.

Orbit

The orbit is an anatomical space in the skulls in which the eyeball is situated. Besides, orbital fat, nerves and vessels are situated in

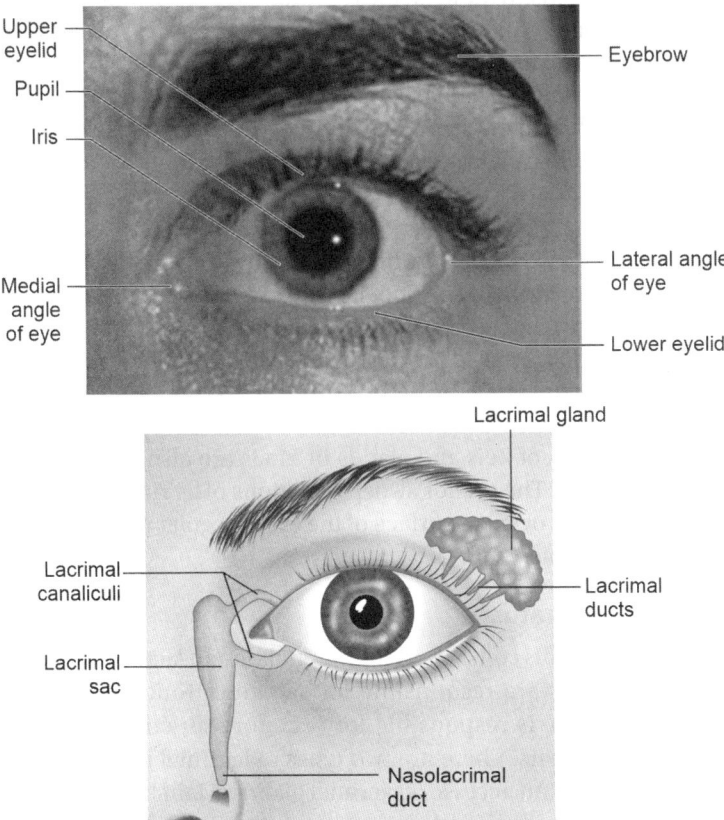

Fig. 1.4: Accessory organs of the eye.

the orbit. Although orbit is a bony structure, it can fracture because of blunt trauma to the eye, usually caused by sports injuries and accidents.

Eyebrows

Eyebrows are thick, short hairs above the eye. Eyebrows follow the shape of the lower margin of the brow ridges. The main function of eyebrows is to prevent sweat, water, and other debris from falling down into the eye socket.

Eyelashes

The eyelashes are short and stout hair arranged in two or three rows. They are very sensitive and tactile receptors. The upper lid eyelashes are approximately 100–150 and are directed upwards. Lower eyelid lashes are approximately 20% less than that in upper eyelid and are turned downwards, such that when the lids are closed, the upper and lower lashes do not interlace. They regenerate within a span of nearly 10 weeks and are usually replaced after every 4–5 months.

Eyelids

The eyelids are two moveable folds of skin covering the orbital cavity and the anterior eyeball. The upper eyelid extends up to the eyebrows and the lower eyelid merges with the skin of the cheek. The edges of the either eyelid are called lid margin, the two lid margins meet at the medial and lateral angles called the canthi. The Meibomian glands or tarsal glands lie within the eyelid and secrete the lipid part of the tear film. Glands of Zeis and glands of Molls are also found on the margin of eyelid. The eyelids sweep secretions of lacrimal apparatus and other glands over the surface of the eye at regular interval by the process of blinking.

Lacrimal Apparatus

Lacrimal apparatus consists of lacrimal glands and lacrimal passage. Lacrimal glands are responsible for secretory function and the lacrimal passage is responsible for excretory function. Lacrimal glands release tears. There are two types of lacrimal glands—main lacrimal glands and accessory lacrimal glands. Main lacrimal gland is located in the upper and outer part of the eye socket in a fossa. The main glands secrete tears only when it receives a nerve impulse like in case of eye irritation, crying, etc. It is responsible for reflex secretion. Accessory lacrimal glands, also known as glands of Krause and glands of Wolfring are situated within the conjunctival tissues of fornices. They secret, throughout the day and form the basal secretion and maintain the normal amount of tears on the surface of conjunctiva.

The tear film covers the ocular surface and is essential for:
- Protecting the eye from the environment,
- Lubricating the ocular surface,
- Maintaining a smooth surface for light refraction, and
- Preserving the health of the conjunctiva and the cornea.

The tear film is thought to be having three layers—mucin, aqueous and lipid.

Mucin is the inner most layer and plays a vital role in the stability of tear film. Aqueous is the middle layer that constitutes the main bulk of tear thickness. It washes away the debris and noxious irritants and contains antibacterial substances like lysozyme and betalysin. Lipid layer is the outermost layer that prevents the overflow of tears and tears evaporation.

Lacrimal passage, also known as drainage system consists of four important parts:
1. Lacrimal puncta,
2. Lacrimal canaliculi
3. Lacrimal sac, and
4. Nasolacrimal duct.

Each eyelid has one punctum that sends the tears to lacrimal canals, known as canaliculi. Lacrimal canaliculi are the curve shaped structure that convey tears to lacrimal sac which is a hollow space from where nasolacrimal duct carries the tears into the inferior meatus of the nasal cavity.

OCULAR MUSCLES

The eye muscles are integral to its function and motion. These muscles are either external muscles or internal muscles. Any deficit in the muscles or the nerves innervating these muscles can result in functional impairment of the involved structures. **Flowchart 1.2** shows the different types of ocular muscles:

Flowchart 1.2: Internal and external ocular muscles.

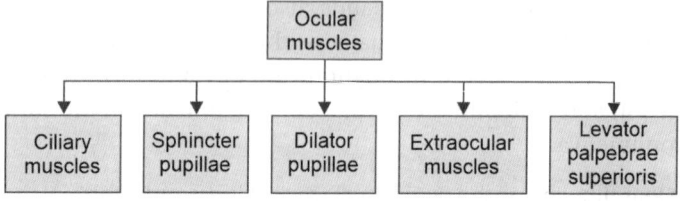

Extraocular Muscles (Fig. 1.5)

Extraocular muscles are attached to the globe by broad, flat thin insertions and at the back of the eye in the annulus of Zinn. The only muscle which is not attached in the annulus area is the inferior oblique which is attached nasally at the anterior floor of the orbit.

There are six extraocular muscles that stabilize and move the eyes. These muscles are shown in **Flowchart 1.3**.

These six muscles control the movement of the eyes, allowing us to look up, down, left, right, and move the eyes in circular motions. These muscles are responsible for maintaining proper alignment of the eyes, so that they point in the same direction and work together as a team to create a single, stable image. If the EOMs are not functioning properly, it can cause a variety of vision problems, including

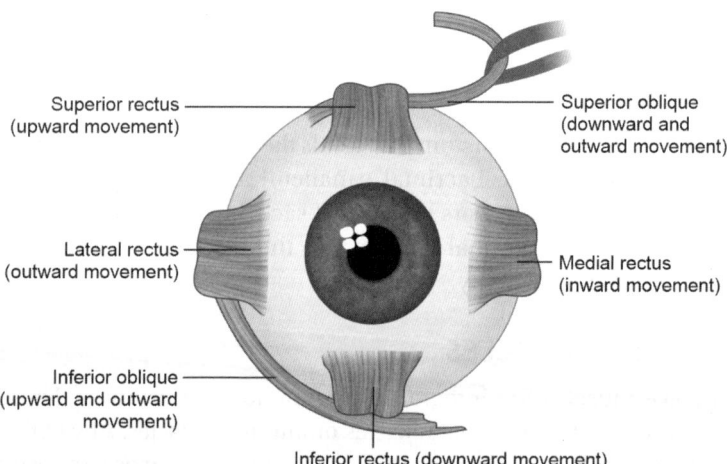

Fig. 1.5: Extraocular muscles.

Flowchart 1.3: Six extraocular muscles.

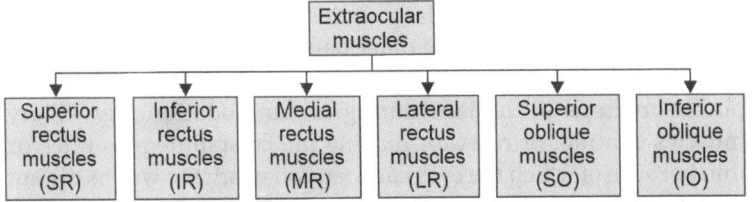

strabismus, diplopia, nystagmus, asthenopia and reduced visual acuity. There are several factors that can lead to poor functioning of extraocular muscles.

- Neurological conditions that affect the nerves that control the extraocular muscles such as a stroke, multiple sclerosis, or a brain tumor.
- Eye muscle diseases: Certain eye diseases, such as myasthenia gravis, can weaken the extraocular muscles and cause vision problems.
- Eye infections, such as conjunctivitis, can cause inflammation and affect the movement of the EOMs.
- Trauma to the head or eye can damage the EOMs and cause vision problems.
- Aging makes the EOMs less flexible that results in reduced ability of EOM's to move the eyes accurately.
- Uncorrected or poorly corrected nearsightedness, farsightedness, or astigmatism can strain the EOMs and cause visual discomfort or fatigue.
- Tumors in or near the eye can press on the EOMs and affect their movement.

The EOMs work together as a team to maintain proper alignment of the eyes and create a single stable image. Therefore, proper function of the EOMs is essential for clear and accurate vision.

Extraocular muscles are among the fastest muscles in the body. The speed and precision of extraocular muscles is unsurpassed anywhere in the body. Extraocular muscles are richly supplied with blood vessels which may be the reason for their prolonged resistance to fatigue.

Chapter 1: Eye

Ciliary Muscles

Ciliary muscles are intraocular muscles of the eye (**Fig 1.6**). Ciliary muscle lines the anterior and outer part of the ciliary body. It holds the lens with the suspensory ligaments and also adjusts the optical power or shape of the lens during accommodation. The ciliary muscles contract or relax for making the crystalline lens thick or thin because of which the eyes can focus on nearby as well as distant objects on the retina.

When the ciliary muscles contract, they cause the ciliary body to move forward, which in turn reduces the tension on the suspensory ligaments that attach to the lens. This allows the lens to become thicker and more rounded, which increases its refractive power and allows for clear near vision. When the ciliary muscles relax, the tension on the suspensory ligaments increases, causing the lens to become thinner and flatter, which reduces its refractive power and allows for clear distance vision.

The ciliary muscles are innervated by the parasympathetic nervous system, which is responsible for their contraction. They are also affected by aging, with their function decreasing over time,

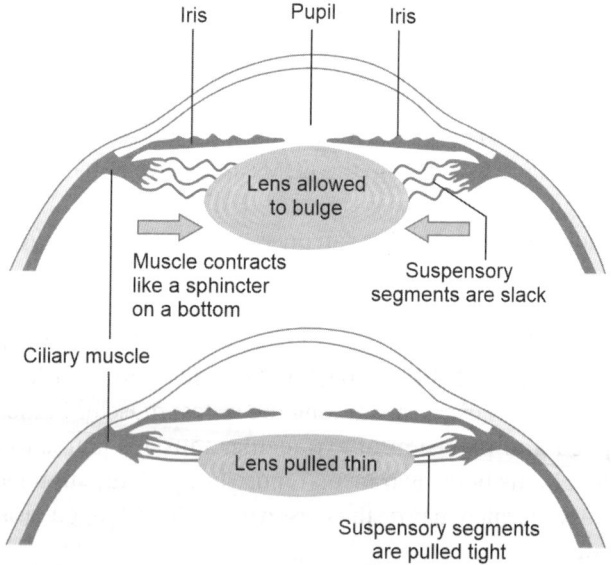

Fig. 1.6: Ciliary muscles.

which can lead to a decrease in the eye's ability to accommodate and a need for corrective lenses or other interventions.

Sphincter Pupillae and Dilator Pupillae (Fig. 1.7)

The sphincter pupillae and dilator pupillae regulate the size of the pupil that allows light to enter the eye. Like ciliary muscles the sphincter pupillae and dilator pupillae are also composed of smooth muscle. The sphincter pupillae encircles the pupil that constricts the pupil. It is controlled by the parasympathetic nervous system, which is responsible for regulating many involuntary bodily functions.

The dilator muscle is arranged radially and dilates the pupil. It is controlled by the sympathetic nervous system, which is responsible for the body's fight or flight response.

The size of the pupil can be influenced by a variety of factors, such as the amount of light entering the eye, the level of arousal or excitement in the body, and certain drugs or medications. By regulating the size of the pupil, the sphincter pupillae and dilator pupillae help to control the amount of light entering the eye and maintain visual clarity.

Levator Palpebrae Superioris (Fig. 1.8)

The levator palpebrae superioris muscle is located in the upper eyelid. It is responsible for lifting the eyelid. It is a thin, ribbon-like muscle that originates from the lesser wing of the sphenoid bone and extends up into the eyelid.

The levator palpebrae superioris is controlled by the oculomotor nerve, also known as cranial nerve III. This nerve sends signals to the muscle, causing it to contract and lift the eyelid. The muscle also works in conjunction with other muscles in the eye, such as the orbicularis

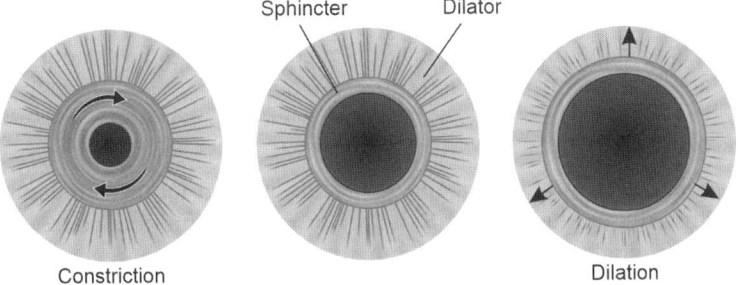

Fig. 1.7: The sphincter pupillae and dilator pupillae.

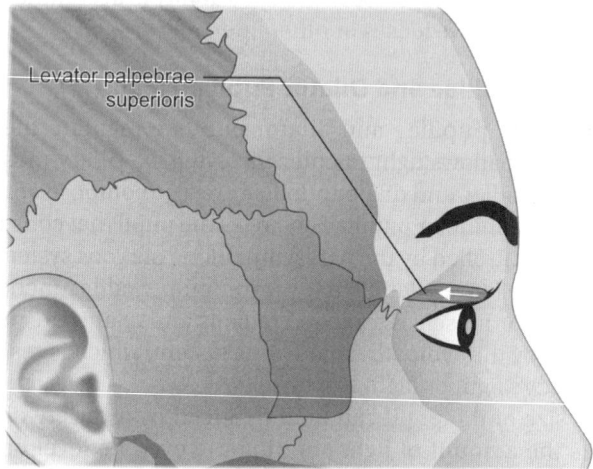

Fig. 1.8: Levator palpebrae superioris muscle.

oculi muscle, to allow for precise control of eye movements and facial expressions.

The levator palpebrae superioris can be affected by a variety of conditions, such as ptosis or Horner's syndrome. These conditions can cause the muscle to become weaker or paralyzed, resulting in difficulty opening the eye or a drooping appearance of the eyelid.

OCULAR GLANDS

Glands are important organs, and they are located throughout the body. Glands produce and release substances that perform certain unique functions. The ocular surface has different glands. They produce different components of tears. The largest single gland is the lacrimal gland that lies in the temporal orbit and produces aqueous tears. The other ocular glands are given here.

Goblet Cells

Goblet cells are unicellular mucous glands. They are found abundantly within the epithelium of all the regions of the conjunctiva except the marginal mucocutaneous junction and limbal conjunctiva. The density of goblet cells is higher in children and young adults than in the older population. The main function of ocular goblet cells is to produce and secrete mucus, a gel-like substance that plays several important roles in maintaining the health and function of the eye. The mucin secreted by goblet cells lubricates and protects the epithelial cells of the conjunctiva and the cornea and ensures the stability of the tear film by lowering the surface tension. Mucus produced by ocular goblet cells also helps to protect the eye from foreign particles, such as dust, dirt, and other irritants. The mucus traps these particles and prevents them from reaching the sensitive tissues of the eye. The mucus produced by goblet cells also contains antibodies and enzymes that help fight off pathogens and other harmful microorganisms that can cause infections.

Meibomian Glands

The meibomian glands are modified sweat glands present in the posterior part of stroma of the tarsal plates **(Fig. 1.9)**. They are arranged in a single row vertically parallel to each other numbering about 20–30 in each lid. Opening of the meibomian glands are arranged in a single row, on the lid margin between the grayline and the posterior border of the lid. These glands secret oil that is an important part of the eye's tears. The oily layer is the outside of the tear film that prevents evaporation of tear and allows smooth movements of eyelids over the globe. A number of eye problems can involve the meibomian glands.

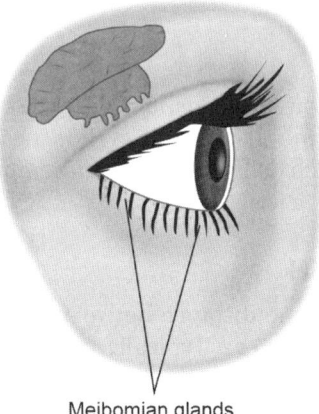

Meibomian glands

Fig. 1.9: Meibomian glands.

These include:
- ❖ Blepharitis
- ❖ Dry eye
- ❖ Sjögren's syndrome

Glands of Wolfring

The glands of Wolfring are located on the inside surface of your eyelids in the conjunctiva. They are named after August Wolfring, a 19th-century Austrian anatomist who first described them. These glands help make the watery layer of the tear film that helps to lubricate and protect the surface of the eye. This secretion, which is rich in electrolytes and proteins, helps to maintain the proper pH balance of the tear film and prevent the growth of bacteria and other microorganisms.

Glands of Krause

The gland of Krause is a small, accessory lacrimal gland located in the conjunctiva of the eye, near the upper outer corner of the eye. It functions to produce tears, which help to keep the eye lubricated and protect it from foreign particles.

Glands of Zeis

These are also modified sebaceous glands. They are attached directly to the eyelash follicle. Secretion from the Zeis gland prevents the eyelashes from becoming dry and brittle. It also contributes towards the oily layer of the tear film.

Glands of Moll

These are modified sweat glands, located in the eyelids. They are also known as the apocrine glands of the eyelid. These glands function to produce sweat, which helps to regulate the temperature of the eyelid and surrounding area.

AXIAL LENGTH

The axial length is the distance between the front of the eye to the back portion of the eye. Typically, axial length increases from typically 16.8 mm in infancy to 23.6 mm in adults. The expected change in an emmetropic child under the age of 8 years is 0.20 mm/

year. However, it varies between race, age and baseline refractive error. Axial length changes earlier than the change in refractive error. 1 mm change in axial length is taken to be changing the prescription by 2.00 D/2.50 D increase or 1.00 D of change in myopia is roughly taken to be equivalent to 0.30 mm increase in axial length.

MULTIPLE CHOICE QUESTIONS

1. **Which of the following structures determines the amount of light entering the eye?**
   a. Cornea
   b. Pupil
   c. Fovea
   d. Optic disc

2. **Which of the following is responsible for the change in focal length of an eye lens to focus the image of the object onto the retina?**
   a. Pupil
   b. Ciliary muscles
   c. Retina
   d. Choroid

3. **What is the number of blood vessels that can be seen in human cornea?**
   a. 0
   b. 10
   c. 100
   d. 72

4. **What is the average center thickness of the human cornea?**
   a. 0.52 mm
   b. 0.59 mm
   c. 0.49 mm
   d. 0.60 mm

5. **What is conjunctiva?**
   a. A transparent membrane and is modified skin that is closely adherent to the sclera.
   b. A fibrous, protective, outer layer of the eye containing collagen and elastic fiber
   c. A visible border between the cornea and the white part of the human eye.
   d. None of the above.

6. "Also known as the white of the eye, is the opaque, fibrous, protective, outer layer of the eye containing collagen and elastic fiber." What is it?
   a. Sclera
   b. Cornea
   c. Choroid
   d. None of the above
7. "It is the transparent front part of the eye that covers the iris, pupil, and anterior chamber. It contributes most of the eye's focusing power and refractive power of the eye." What is it?
   a. Sclera
   b. Cornea
   c. Choroid
   d. None of the above
8. Where are rod and cone cells located in the eye?
   a. Organ of Corti
   b. Retina
   c. Choroid
   d. Cornea
9. Where do we find the fovea within the eye?
   a. Iris
   b. Crystalline lens
   c. Retina
   d. Organ of Corti
10. Which of the following is the relay station between the retina and the visual cortex?
    a. The optic chiasm
    b. The superior colliculus
    c. The lateral geniculate nucleus of the thalamus
    d. The vestibular nucleus
11. The reason we cannot see light that falls on the blind spot is:
    a. Photoreceptor cells in that region of the retina are light adapted.
    b. Photoreceptor cells in that region of the retina are dark adapted.
    c. Photoreceptor cells in that region of the retina are covered by blood vessels.
    d. None of the above.
12. Which of the following is known as refracting tissue of the eye?
    a. Retina
    b. Optic nerve
    c. Choroid
    d. Cornea

ANSWER KEY

1. b	2. b	3. a	4. a	5. a	6. a	7. b	8. b
9. c	10. c	11. d	12. d				

SELF-PRACTICE QUESTIONS

1. How does pupil size influence vision?
2. How does the tear film affect efficient visual functioning?
3. How do ocular muscles contribute to the whole mechanism of vision?

CHAPTER 2

Vision and Visual Function

CHAPTER OUTLINE

- Vision and Visual Perception
- Different Facets of Visual Perception
- Classification of Vision
- Components of Vision
- Binocular Vision
- Monocular Vision
- Dominant Eye
- Visual Field
- Visual Angle
- Depth of Focus and Depth of Field

VISION AND VISUAL PERCEPTION

Vision is the ability to take in information through the eyes and derive meaning from it. It implies taking the information and initiating the appropriate response. The two eyes capture the image and transmit it to the brain, where the two images are fused together, interpreted, and integrated as a three-dimensional phenomenon. The brain then sends the message down the spinal cords to the arms or legs muscles, telling them to move.

The process of vision is a self-directed process and can be explained in the broader framework by **Flowchart 2.1**.

With both eyes open, the process of vision starts when the attention is directed towards an object in the environment and ends

Flowchart 2.1: Process of vision.

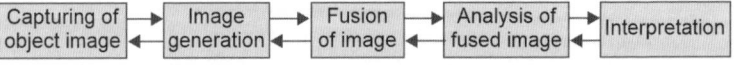

Chapter 2: Vision and Visual Function

with the formation of an image on the retina, which is sent to the brain in the form of electrical signals via the optic nerve for visual perception.

Visual perception is the process by which the brain interprets and makes sense of the visual information that it receives from the eyes. **Flowchart 2.2** describes broader stages that are involved in the process of visual perception.

Transduction is the process by which the eyes convert light into electrical signals which are sent to the brain through optic nerves, the process is called transmission. The brain does the job of initial processing of visual signals as transmitted including the identification of basic features such as color, brightness, and shape. It also organizes the visual information into coherent patterns and objects, based on past experiences, context, and expectations. Finally, it also interprets the same. The interpretation of the visual information involves making sense out of it, including the identification of objects, recognition of patterns, and understanding of spatial relationships.

Visual perception is a highly complex process that involves multiple brain regions and is influenced by a variety of factors, including attention, motivation, experience, and context. It is a dynamic process that constantly adapts to the changing visual environment and can be influenced by a variety of factors, such as lighting, contrast, and distance. Therefore, visual perception is not simply a passive process of receiving and decoding visual information, but an active process of constructing and interpreting the visual world.

Visual perception occurs in the brain's cerebral cortex; the electrochemical signals reach there by traveling through the optic nerve and the thalamus. The brain receives, interprets and acts upon the visual stimuli. Though the retinal image is the basis of visual perception, what we perceive does not entirely depend on retinal image alone. It is a complex integration of light sense, form sense, sense of contrast and color sense.

However, how the brain translates the signals to perceive the qualities of a scene and object into color, location, movement, shape, size and texture is still less understood. The important element of

Flowchart 2.2: Stages of visual perception.

Transduction → Transmission → Initial processing → Organization → Interpretation visual perception is that what people see is not simply a translation of retinal stimuli. A great deal of cerebral editing takes place. Some information is wholly or partially suppressed or interpreted so as to conform to previous experience. Thus, visual perception of the world is based on past experiences and stored information. Sensory receptors receive information from the environment, which is then combined with previously stored information about the world which we have built up as a result of experience and a conclusion is reached on the basis of stored information about what is out there. It can be demonstrated by **Flowchart 2.3**.

Visual perception is vital in cognitive processing. Visual perception is the process of absorbing environment inputs, interpreting and finally initiating the motor response in reaction to environmental input. Difficulty in visual perception can cause problems with cognitive processes. There are many different cognitive processes like attention, learning, perception, memory, discrimination, etc. are all aided by visual perception.

Flowchart 2.3: Visual perception of what is seen in the environment.

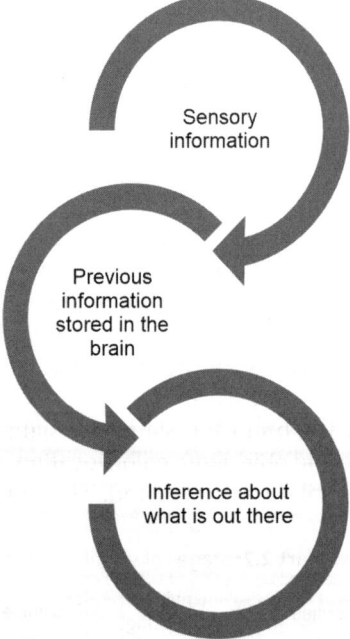

DIFFERENT FACETS OF VISUAL PERCEPTION

There are different facets of visual perception that contribute to our ability to see and understand the world around us, including:

Spatial Perception

Spatial perception refers to the ability to perceive and interpret the spatial relationships between objects in the visual field, including their position, size, shape, and orientation. It expresses the ability to be aware of oneself in space. This is a complex cognitive skill that provides an individual with an understanding that as he walks towards an object, the object will come closer to his body.

The skill makes the individual more aware of his personal space and enables him to control his movement around others. Poor spatial awareness tends to make the individual appear clumsy. He may bump into others or stand too close or too far away from the person or objects that he is interacting with. In occupations like sports a well-developed spatial awareness skill is fundamental to quick and correct reaction and balance. A child with poor spatial awareness may leave out the spaces between words, start the sentence in the middle of the page, have difficulty keeping on the line or write diagonally instead of horizontally.

Spatial awareness develops naturally early in the life when children have the ability to freely explore their environment. However, two elements of visual system—visual field and depth perception—affect spatial awareness skill of an individual.

Depth Perception

Depth perception is an important element of normal and healthy vision and is the result of good stereo vision. It is the ability of the human eye to see the object in three dimensions and allows us to form an idea about the length, width and height of the object. It also provides the ability to visually judge the relative distance between the objects and percept accurate movement in three-dimensional space. While it allows us to see the object in three-dimension it also uses previous knowledge of it to understand the world around us. It occurs unconsciously and very quickly without us ever realizing that we are using it. Depth perception allows us to move through life without bumping into things. It also allows us to determine the speed of approaching objects. This skill is important while crossing the

street. Problems with depth perception may develop when another condition is present. Some of the common conditions that may cause depth perception problems include:
- Blurred vision, typically in one eye
- People who are strabismus
- People with amblyopia often struggle with depth perception
- People who have an injured eye often have trouble with depth perception while the eye is healing.
- People with anisometropia
- Cranial nerve palsy
- Cataract affecting one eye
- Macular degeneration
- Anophthalmos absence of one eye

Color Perception

Color perception is a complex process that involves the interaction of light, the eye, and the brain. It refers to the ability to perceive and distinguish between different colors excited by different wavelengths of light. Color perception is mediated by the cone cells in the retina. So, it is better appreciated in photopic vision. There are three different types of cones—red sensitive, green sensitive and blue sensitive which work together to perform the function of color vision. Each cone cell is sensitive to a different range of wavelengths of light, which correspond to different colors. When light enters the eye, it activates the cone cells and the signals are sent to the brain via the optic nerve. The brain then interprets these signals and creates the perception of color. In dim light, all colors are seen as gray and the phenomenon is called Purkinje shift phenomenon.

Contrast Perception

Contrast detection is a crucial part of visual perception. Contrast refers to the difference in luminance or color between two adjacent regions in the visual field. The ability to detect contrast is essential for various visual tasks, such as object recognition, depth perception, and motion detection. Contrast perception is the visual process of recognizing the difference in brightness or color between an object and its background or two objects.

In the visual system, contrast detection involves the comparison of the light intensity or color of adjacent stimuli by specialized neurons in the retina and visual cortex. The neurons in the retina, called bipolar cells and ganglion cells, encode the contrast information and transmit it to the brain. In the visual cortex, neurons in the primary visual cortex and higher visual areas further process and integrate the contrast signals to form a perceptual representation of the visual scene.

Contrast sensitivity can be affected by various factors. Diffraction and ocular aberrations set the upper limit to contrast of the retinal image in a healthy eye. Refractive error, aging, lenticular changes, ocular and systemic disease can also affect the contrast of retinal image adversely. Neurological disorders can affect contrast perception in visual cortex.

Motion Perception

Motion perception refers to the ability of the brain to interpret and understand the movement of objects in the environment. It is a complex process that involves the integration of multiple sensory cues and the processing of information in the brain. Our visual system is capable of detecting and analyzing the motion of objects, which allows us to navigate our surroundings and interact with our environment.

Motion perception is based on the detection of changes in visual stimuli over time. This is achieved through a variety of mechanisms in the brain, including specialized neurons in the visual cortex that respond to movement in specific directions and at specific speeds.

One of the most important aspects of motion perception is the ability to differentiate between self-motion and the motion of objects in the environment. The brain is able to do this by comparing the motion of objects to our own movement, which provides a frame of reference for determining whether objects are moving or stationary.

Motion perception is also influenced by a number of other factors, including the lighting conditions, the distance between objects, and the presence of other visual cues such as texture and depth. For example, objects that are closer to us appear to move faster than those that are further away.

Pattern Recognition

In visual perception, pattern recognition refers to the ability of the brain to identify and categorize visual patterns, such as shapes, objects, and textures. The process of pattern recognition in visual perception involves the integration of sensory information from the eyes and the processing of that information by the brain.

Retinal cone cells play a major role in this faculty. It is, therefore, more acute at fovea. The first stage in visual pattern recognition is the detection of simple visual features, such as edges, lines, and corners. These features are then combined to form more complex visual patterns, such as shapes and objects. The brain uses both bottom-up processing, i.e., processing based on the sensory information received and top-down processing, i.e., processing based on prior knowledge and expectations to identify and categorize these visual patterns.

Visual pattern recognition is essential for many everyday tasks, such as recognizing faces, reading text, and navigating through the environment. It is also important for more complex tasks, such as driving a car or operating machinery. In addition, pattern recognition in visual perception is used in various fields, such as computer vision and image processing, where it is used to develop algorithms for tasks such as object detection and recognition.

Visual Attention

Visual attention refers to the cognitive process by which the brain selectively focuses on a particular area or feature of the visual field, while ignoring or filtering out other irrelevant information. It allows us to efficiently process and respond to relevant stimuli in our environment, while disregarding distractions.

Visual attention can be divided into two main components: bottom-up and top-down attention. Bottom-up attention is driven by the saliency of the visual stimuli, such as brightness, color, contrast, and motion. This type of attention is automatic and involuntary, and it helps us to detect and respond to important or novel stimuli in our environment.

On the other hand, top-down attention is guided by our goals, expectations, and prior knowledge. It allows us to direct our attention to specific features or objects that are relevant to the task at hand, while ignoring irrelevant distractors. Top-down attention is more flexible and can be influenced by our current mental state, motivation, and attention control.

Visual attention is a complex process that involves different brain regions and neural networks, such as the parietal and frontal lobes, the superior colliculus, and the pulvinar nucleus. It plays a crucial role in various cognitive tasks, such as perception, memory, learning, decision-making, and action planning.

These different aspects of visual perception work together to create a comprehensive understanding of the external environment around us. Any disruption or impairment in one or more of these aspects can lead to visual perceptual deficits and impact daily activities such as reading, driving, and sports.

CLASSIFICATION OF VISION

Visual function is a complex and interconnected process that involves multiple areas of the eye and brain working together, because of which it is difficult to categorize it into different groups or types. However, a categorization can be helpful based on the visual perception that they describe to study the underlying mechanisms that support them, although the proposed categorization is not mutually exclusive.

Vision can be categorized into three broad categories based upon the distance from the eye that they cover:
- Distance vision
- Near vision
- Intermediate distance vision

Further, vision can also be categorized into two broad categories based upon the location in the visual field that they cover:
- Central vision
- Peripheral vision

Vision can also be categorized into three categories based on the level of light sensitivity that they describe:
- Photopic vision
- Scotopic vision
- Mesopic vision

Distance Vision

Distance vision covers objects that are far away. Accommodation is at rest and the ciliary muscle, which controls the shape of the lens, is relaxed, allowing the lens to become flatter and thinner. This reduces the amount of light bending required to achieve a sharp image on the retina. As a result, distant objects appear clear and in focus.

The visual axes of both eyes are parallel to each other and aligned towards the object being viewed. This is known as binocular single vision, which allows for depth perception and stereoscopic vision.

During distance vision, the pupils usually remain small, typically around 2–3 millimeters in diameter, in order to optimize visual acuity and reduce the impact of aberrations. This is because a smaller pupil allows for greater depth of field, which is the range of distances that can be seen in focus at the same time.

Near Vision

Near vision covers objects that are close up. The eyes are in a state of accommodation, and the eyes increase their refractive power more and more to maintain the focus of the approaching object on the retinas. The ciliary muscles are contracted, and the lens becomes more spherical due to a lessening of tension on the zonular fibers.

Simultaneously, the angle formed between the visual axes grows increasingly larger to allow the object's images to remain on the two foveae.

The pupil also constricts, but this reaction is slower than the change in response to retinal illuminance and is sustained as long as near-vision fixation is maintained. Pupil constriction in both eyes is equal during near vision, even if vision in the two eyes differs.

Intermediate Distance Vision

Intermediate distance vision is measured at a distance which is farther than the near vision distance but closer than far distance vision. This is the distance at which most people work today, especially people working on computers.

The mechanism involved in intermediate distance vision is almost similar to that of near vision, with a little more complexity involved as eyes need to refocus from one distance to another within the range of intermediate distance vision which is more stressful.

Central Vision

Central vision is focused on the point of fixation. It refers to the ability to see fine details and distinguish objects that are located directly in front of us. When we look directly at an object, the light from the object is focused onto the fovea. Fovea contains a high density of cone cells, which are responsible for detecting fine details and color vision. Fovea is located at the center of the retina. The size of the fovea is approximately 1.5 mm in diameter. The fovea is surrounded by an area called the parafovea, which is about 2-4 mm in diameter and contains fewer cone cells but still has relatively high visual acuity. Central vision is limited to the small area of the fovea and the parafoveal region. Central vision is very important for many activities, such as reading, driving, and recognizing faces. Overall, central vision involves the precise focusing of light onto the fovea, the specialized processing of visual information in the brain, and the integration of this information with other sensory inputs to create a rich and detailed perception of the visual world.

Peripheral Vision

Peripheral vision covers the areas outside of central vision. Peripheral vision is because of the peripheral retina, which is outside the foveal and parafoveal areas. It contains a larger number of rod cells, which are more sensitive to low levels of light. Peripheral vision is less detailed, but it provides important information about the overall context of the visual scene. The brain also uses information from the surrounding areas of the retina to create a wider image of the visual scene. Peripheral vision is responsible for detecting motion, navigating the environment, and maintaining spatial awareness. The brain processes visual information differently in the peripheral visual field compared to the central visual field. For example, visual processing in the periphery is more sensitive to changes in contrast and motion, which can help us detect potential threats or changes in our environment.

Photopic Vision

Daylight vision is called photopic vision. Photopic vision is mediated by retinal cones cells, although rods cells are also active. Photopic vision is characterized by high acuity, low sensitivity to light, and good color vision. During photopic vision pupil size is small, reducing the effect of wide beam aberrations.

Scotopic Vision

Scotopic vision occurs during very low light level in the night and is mediated by rod cells. Scotopic vision exhibits high sensitivity to light, poor acuity, and no color vision. The pupil diameter is wider, increasing the effect of wide beam aberrations. An emmetrope may have a shift towards low myopia during the extremely reduced illumination. This is called 'night myopia', which is relatively of minor importance.

Mesopic Vision

Mesopic vision is the term given for the combination between photopic vision and scotopic vision in low but not quite dark lighting situation. There is a transition zone between photopic and scotopic vision when the level of illumination starts reducing. Both rods and cones are active in this range of light, with rods more dominating than cones due to lack of light. This reduces color perception.

COMPONENTS OF VISION

Vision is a complex process which involves multiple components as shown in the **Flowchart 2.4**.

Good vision goes beyond the measurement of 20/20 or 6/6 visual acuity. It also includes accommodation, vergence function, and different types of oculomotor skill. All the components work together under a feedback loop to gather, focus, capture, and process light to make sense out of vision. Deficiencies in any of these components may result in overall deficient visual performance.

Visual Acuity

Visual acuity defines the acuteness or sharpness of vision, i.e., the ability to perceive fine details. It refers to your ability to discern the shapes and details of the things you see. Visual acuity is the spatial resolving capacity of the visual system. It expresses the angular size of the object that can be just resolved by the observer.

Flowchart 2.4: Components of vision.

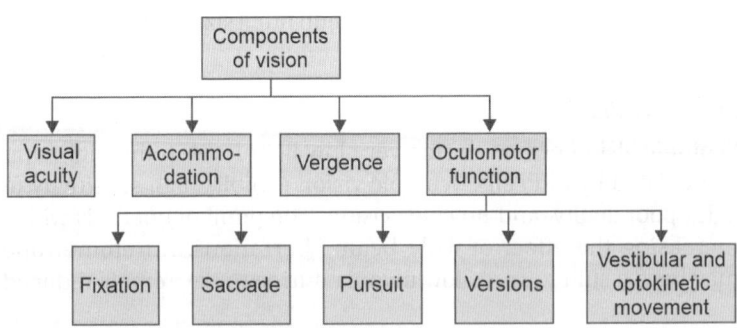

Visual acuity is also defined as a time-dependent measurement of retinal health and is specified by the date on which the eye examination took place. It is measured with the help of various eye test charts in a clinical environment. If it is measured using Snellen's chart, 20/20 or 6/6 is taken to be optimum visual acuity, denoting perfect eyesight.

Visual acuity is a measurement of central vision only. Assessment of total visual system from cornea to occipital cortex, visual acuity can be tested for both distance and near vision. Generally, individuals with good distance visual acuity tend to have good near visual acuity as well. However, this relation is not always strong and may depend on various factors such as age, and underlying ocular or visual conditions. For example, a presbyope may have good distance visual acuity but his near visual acuity may be found to be reduced. Similarly, a myope may have good near visual acuity but his distance visual acuity is reduced.

Blurring of vision caused because of defocused image as a result of refractive error, such as myopia, hypermetropia, and/or astigmatism affects the visual acuity adversely. There may be transient change in refractive error that may affect the visual acuity for a short duration due to local or systemic causes. Ciliary muscle is mostly responsible for local cause, inducing temporary hypermetropia in accommodative paralysis or temporary myopia in accommodative spasm. Diabetes and retinal detachment bring in sudden changes in refractive error. Visual acuity is also affected by eye diseases such as cataracts, glaucoma, macular degeneration, etc. Aging and amblyopia both reduce visual acuity.

Measurement of visual acuity at every presentation is important because of the following reasons:
- The measurement of visual acuity can be used as diagnostic tool.
- It is important to assess the patient's refractive state of the eye.
- It measures progression of disease.
- It forms the part of baseline data.
- It is legal requirement.

Accommodation

Accommodation is an involuntary reflex action of the eye that determines the focusing ability of the eyes. Accommodation allows the eyes to change its optical power so that it can maintain a clear image of an object as its distance varies. Accommodation is

remarkably a quick response to a stimulus. The reaction time for 'far to near' accommodation has been recorded to be approximately 0.29 second to a response time of about 0.75 second to reach the steady state. The same for 'near to far' has been approximated to be in the range of 0.35 second to 1.19 second. A healthy individual below the age of 40 years shows quick, spontaneous and effortless accommodative ability. A disorder in accommodation function can have effect on vision, for example:
- Intermittent blurring in near vision
- Delayed distance vision clarity
- Asthenopia
- Headache

Table 2.1 shows the different types of accommodative disorder.

Overall, accommodative disorder implies that the eyes are under excessive stress which can sometimes be easily helped by prescribing right spectacle lenses and/or vision therapy.

Vergence

Vergence, also known as eye teaming ability is the simultaneous movement of both the eyes in opposite directions to obtain and maintain binocular single vision. Two eyes are inset in the orbit with the help of six extraocular muscles, which control the oculomotor skills of the eye during the process of vision. To get a clear view of the world, the brain must turn the eyes so that the image of the object of regard falls on the fovea. Under normal seeing condition, the two eyes converge when the object approaches the eyes and they diverge when an object recedes. Divergence and convergence are achieved mainly with voluntary movements of the globe by the medial and lateral recti. Thus, binocular vision is possible due to

Table 2.1: Implications of accommodative disorder.	
Type of disorder	Implications
Accommodative insufficiency	Amplitude of accommodation is less than age-appropriate
Accommodative spasm	Accommodation fails to relax, making distance vision blur
Accommodative infacility	Blur distance vision after prolonged near work and vice versa
Ill-sustained accommodation	After excessive near work, near vision blurs

motor coordination of the eyes and the sensory unification of their respective views of the world. The motor function pertains to the positioning and alignment of the eyes that brings both the foveae onto the object of regard within the visual field and maintains the fixation as long as it is required. The sensory component starts with light emitted from an object is brought to a focus on the retina by each eye and is transmitted to visual cortex, where visual perception of the object in relation to the external environment is created.

The disorder in vergence function may result in one or more of the following symptoms:

- ❖ Blur vision
- ❖ Headache
- ❖ Ocular discomfort
- ❖ Fatigue
- ❖ Diplopia
- ❖ Motion sickness
- ❖ Loss of concentration during a task

Table 2.2 shows the different types of vergence function disorder.

The vergence function directly controls muscle balance. The difficulties with muscle balance at distance or near are likely to affect visual performance directly. It may also increase the possibility of visual fatigue which may be manifested in the later part of the day. Phoria can lead to altered perception of the world. If a shift occurs

Table 2.2: Implications of vergence function disorder.	
Type of disorder	Implications
Convergence insufficiency	Exophoria at near, reduced near point of convergence
Convergence excess	Esophoria at near is more than distance deviation
Divergence insufficiency	Esophoria is more at distance than at near
Divergence excess	Exophoria at distance is more than near deviation
Basic exophoria	Exophoric deviation of similar magnitude at distance and near
Basic esophoria	Esophoric deviation of similar magnitude at distance and near
Fusional vergence dysfunction	Reduced fusional vergence amplitudes
Vertical phoria	Hyper-hypophoria

in esophoric direction, perceived distance increases and the subject may see things as being smaller than they actually are. On the contrary if a shift occurs in exophoric direction, it may induce shortening of perceived distance and fixation may be broken frequently while reading that may lead to variety of problems like fatigue, headache, tension, loss of concentration, dull pain in the back of eyes and brows. Both of these tendencies can affect how people learn, interact with others and understand their surroundings. The reduced ability to control and manipulate vergence can also affect the awareness of space adversely.

Accommodation and vergence functions are in fact a coupled function. Accommodation evokes vergence changes and vergence evokes accommodative changes. The coupling is helpful because both focal and vergence distances are almost always the same no matter where the subject looks. One of the important benefits of the coupling is the increased speed of accommodation and vergence. In normal binocular vision, accommodation and vergence cooperate to place on the fovea of each eye a sharp image of the object of regard. Accommodation vergence functions have great bearing on the fundamental visual skills of fixating at the object and perceiving it as 3-dimemnsional shape. In presbyopia accommodation fails but convergence continues. The similar is observed when ciliary muscles are paralyzed by atropine. Hypermetrope continues to use his accommodation in excess of his convergence, whereas myopes have convergence in excess of accommodation.

Oculomotor functions are neuromuscular controls developed to point the visual system on the target and move it to either follow a moving target or jump from one object to another. Clear vision occurs when a precisely focused image of an object is centered on the fovea and all oculomotor functions work in harmony. The following are the components of oculomotor function that help in clear vision.

Fixation

Fixation is an important consideration during eye movement because the eye has to be static at the end of each saccade as it holds the image of object on the fovea. Fixation needs the combined involvement of all types of eye movements. This is a well-integrated sensory motor function where the muscles are in dynamic equilibrium.

Saccade

Saccades are fast and abrupt eye movement with a pause between two saccades. Saccade shifts the fixation abruptly, enabling eyes to rapidly redirect the line of sight so that the point of interest stimulates the fovea. Average saccade is 8–9-character space which is about 2% and takes about 25–30 ms. Saccades may be inaccurate in two ways:
1. **Undershoot:** The saccade is slightly short of the target, and in extreme cases, a second smaller saccade may be needed to reach the target.
2. **Overshoot:** Overshooting the target which is less common inaccuracy.

There may be several performance problems if saccadic eye movements are poor:
- The patient may complain like words are omitted or lines may be skipped.
- Frequent loss of place while reading
- "Finger reading" may indicate the need for hand support due to poor eye movements
- Head movement while reading is also a sign of poor saccades.

Smooth Pursuit

A pursuit eye movement is defined as the movement of an eye fixating a moving object. The function is to match the velocity of eye movement to target velocity. If the target velocity is too high, the pursuits break down into a jerky motion. Drugs, fatigue, emotional stress and test anxiety may adversely affect pursuit performance. Patients with poor pursuit skills may also have a history of different visual inefficiencies.

Versions

Versions are the movement that causes the eye to change the direction of gaze to a given direction **(Fig. 2.1)**. They enlarge the field of view to bring the object of attention onto the fovea. Both eyes rotate through an equal angle in the same direction. That is why they are also called conjugate eye movements. For example, dextroversion is the movement of both eyes to the right and levoversion is the movement of both eyes to the left. Version eye movements may also be made in vertical and torsional direction.

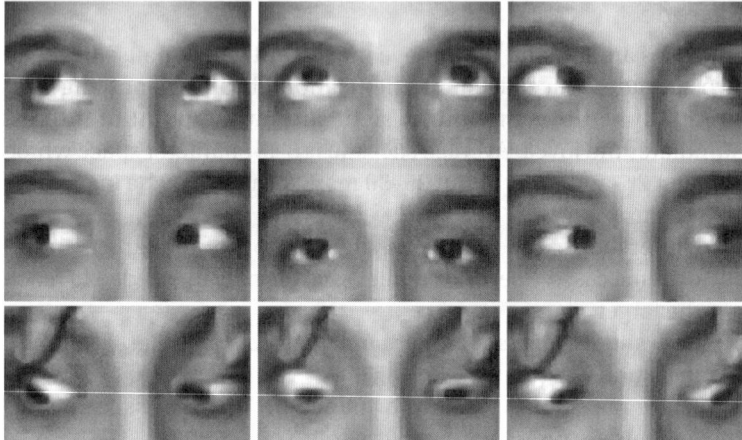

Fig. 2.1: Versions.

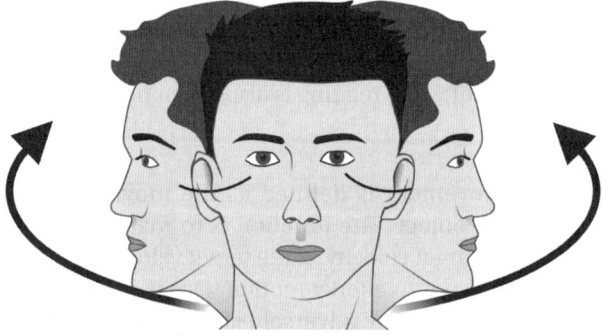

Fig. 2.2: Schematic representation of vestibular ocular movement.

Vestibulo-ocular Movement (Fig. 2.2)

The vestibular system also has immense influence on eye movements. This is used to stabilize an image on the surface of the retina during head movement. This is an orientation reflex, not requiring visual stimuli. Turning the head stimulates the vestibular organ, resulting in the turning of eyeball in the direction opposite to head turn. The vestibular system provides the sense of balance and the information about body position that allows rapid compensatory movements in response to both self-induced and externally generated forces.

BINOCULAR VISION

Binocular vision may be defined as the vision which is achieved by the co-ordinated use of both eyes so that the images which arise in each eye separately are appreciated as a single visual impression in the visual cortex. Binocular vision ability is not an innate characteristic. It is acquired gradually in the first few years of life.

It is interesting to note that even though the two eyes work together and are strictly comparable with regard to their structure, there is usually a functional difference between the eyes so that one eye tends to be dominant over the other. It can be very well noticed while lining up the two objects, the visual system relies more on the dominant eye, even though the other eye, known as non-dominant eye is open. An approximate judgment of the alignment can be made binocularly, but the binocular projection center is usually found to be nearer the dominant eye.

Binocular vision is the motor coordination of two eyes together with sensory unification of their respective image. Sensory unification employs neural processes to correct minor imperfections in ocular alignment, while motor fusion makes small physical changes in the direction of visual axes to correct minor misalignment. Sensory fusion is a neural process, motor fusion is a physical process. Sensory fusion synthesizes the retinal images from each eye or correlates together to form a single visual image, without any change in the visual direction of either eye. For this to happen, the images of the target object must fall on the corresponding or nearly corresponding points on the retina. Motor fusion requires a change in the direction of one or both eyes designed to physically create a situation where the corresponding retinal points are directed towards the same target. Thus, the sensory and motor fusion mechanism ensures the correct alignment of the eyes. If sensory fusion is prevented which is possible by occluding one eye, motor fusion will be frustrated, and a deviation of the visual axis will be the result in many patients.

If the motor fusion reflex eliminates the deviation, when the obstacle to sensory fusion is removed, the deviation is latent and is called phoria. If the fusion reflex fails to develop or is unable to function normally the deviation of the eye will be manifest and is called tropia or squint.

Flowchart 2.5: Grades of binocular vision.

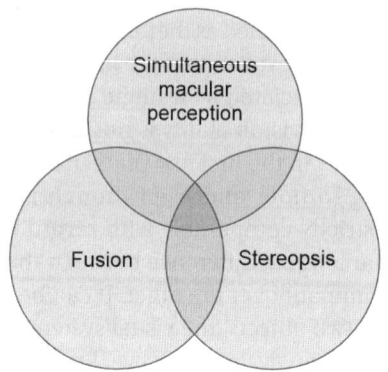

There are three grades of binocular vision as shown in **Flowchart 2.5**.

Simultaneous Macular Perception

Simultaneous macular perception is a sensory fusion and is the most elementary type of binocularity. It occurs when the visual cortex perceives separate stimuli to the two eyes at the same time. Simultaneous macular perception is not the same as superimposition. It only implies the ability to see two dissimilar objects simultaneously. Simultaneous macular perception ceases to exist when the human being suppresses the image from one eye in both eyes open condition as it happens when using monocular microscope or rifle shooting.

Fusion

Fusion implies that not just the two images are fused together, but some effort is made to maintain the fusion in spite of difficulties. It is a second grade of binocular vision and it implies a motor response is added to simplify sensory fusion. Fusion can only occur if the disparities in the images captured by both eyes are small. If the difference between the images is too great, then either double vision or suppression occurs. If an object falls within the Panum's fusional area at the corresponding points, the visual acuity will be perceived as single with depth and if the object falls outside the Panum's fusional area, the visual disparity will be too large for fusion and therefore instead of appearing as one with depth, will be perceived as double.

To get round this problem, suppression occurs which means the brain actively suppresses or ignores the image from one of the eyes. Typically, the images from the non-dominant eye are suppressed. and only the image from the dominant eye is processed by the brain, and double vision is avoided. The suppression may lead to amblyopia in children under 8 years of age.

Stereopsis

Stereopsis is the highest grade of binocularity, not only the images of the two eyes are fused but they are blended to produce a stereoscopic effect **(Fig. 2.3)**. This involves a perceptual synthesis, at a higher level.

Stereopsis is the ability to perceive space as three-dimensional through the sight difference between the right and left retinal images. The two eyes receive slightly disparate views of objects because they are separated horizontally. This disparity can be used to signal relative depth of the objects. When the brain is able to bring the two disparate images together and interpret them as one single image, fusion occurs. There has to be fusion first before we can have depth perception. During the fusion process, the two disparate images are

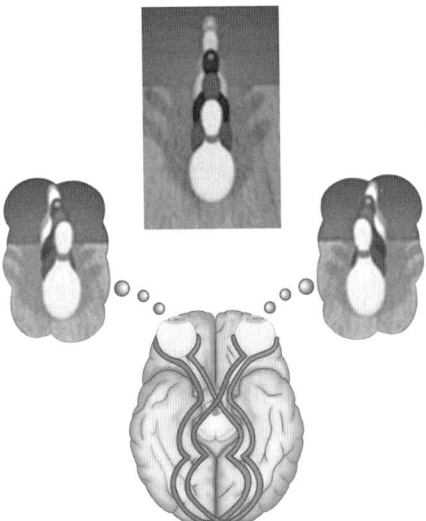

Fig. 2.3: Each eye captures its own view and the two separate images are sent on to the brain for processing. When the two images arrive simultaneously in the back of the brain, they are united into one picture.

combined into one. Similarities between the two images are matched together, and more importantly, the slight disparities are also added in. It is this that gives us the ability to perceive depth and appreciate the object in three dimensions.

It is the highly refined attainment of binocular vision and also relates to spatial judgment, i.e., how you keep yourself oriented in space. The responsiveness to disparate stimulations has its limits. There is a maximum disparity beyond which no stereoscopic effect is produced. This limiting disparity characterizes a person's stereoscopic acuity. Stereopsis is not an innate ability. Unless the binocular vision is established early in life, stereopsis cannot develop, leading to poor depth perception ability.

Stereoacuity serves as a barometer of binocular efficiency. Stereoscopic acuity depends on many factors and is greatly influenced by the method used in determining it. There are no standardized clinical stereoscopic tests comparable to visual acuity tests. Different test charts are available to measure stereoacuity. In general, the normal value of stereoacuity is taken to be 60 seconds of arc or better.

MONOCULAR VISION

Monocular vision is achieved using only one eye. Monocular vision also allows individuals to see and navigate the world, but it may lack certain attributes that binocular vision provides.

- ❖ While binocular vision provides enhanced depth perception due to the slightly different perspectives each eye offers, monocular vision relies more on other cues for depth perception. These clues may be relative size, overlapping, perspective, etc.
- ❖ Binocular vision offers a wider field of view and a larger visual field, as it combines the visual input from both eyes. Monocular vision has a narrower field of view, as it relies on the visual input from a single eye.
- ❖ Binocular visual acuity is always superior to monocular visual acuity in most cases.
- ❖ Binocular vision provides better peripheral vision, as each eye contributes to the overall field. Whereas monocular vision limits the peripheral vision as compared to binocular vision.

Despite limitations, individuals with monocular vision can lead normal lives by making use of other visual and nonvisual cues. They may learn to estimate distances through experience and may also develop a heightened awareness of their surroundings.

DOMINANT EYE

The dominant eye is an important phenomenon in the study of binocular vision. However, it is relatively a confusing area of knowledge.

The dictionary of visual science defines ocular dominance as, "The superiority of one eye over the other in some perceptual or motor task. The term is usually applied to those superiorities in function which are not based on a difference in visual acuity between the two eyes, or a dysfunction of the neuromuscular apparatus of one of the eyes". This implies that dominant eye is not necessarily an eye with superior visual acuity; still it contributes most to the visual perception.

The understanding from the definition can be explained as below:
- ❖ The dominant eye is superior either in some perceptual task or in motor task.
- ❖ The dominant eye contributes most to the visual perception.
- ❖ Visual acuity has nothing to do with ocular dominancy. An eye having a less visual acuity may also be the dominant eye.

Ocular dominancy is a complex phenomenon that involves processing of visual information in brain. The superiority may be in any of the following functions:
- ❖ The dominant eye leads in receiving the visual inputs.
- ❖ The dominant eye leads to fixation in binocular vision.
- ❖ The brain may prioritize the visual information as received by dominant eye, if presented with conflicting visual information.

Based upon the above discussion, ocular dominancy can be subdivided into three subcategories as shown in the **Flowchart 2.6**.

Flowchart 2.6: Three subcategories of ocular dominancy.

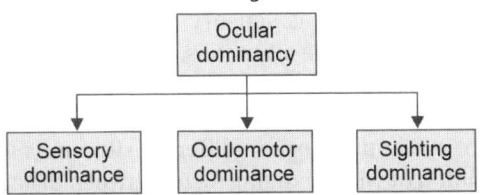

Sensory Dominance

Sensory dominance of eye refers to the dominance of one eye over another in terms of vision processing and visual perception. For example, if you are presented with conflicting visual information, your brain may prioritize visual input from one over another, leading to sensory dominance of that particular sense. Sensory dominance may occur when the visual system finds it easier to suppress one eye and favors another eye because of the difference in image clarity, color and brightness. Thus, ocular dominance refers to the preferential use of one eye when performing monocular activities. Some individuals may feel uncomfortable if their dominant eye is fractionally blurred, whereas a small residual refractive error in the non-dominant eye may not give any discomfort.

Oculomotor Dominance

Oculomotor dominance refers to the eye that is least likely to lose concentration on moving object or lose the target when the target is moving. It is difficult to measure oculomotor dominance in regular clinical practice.

Sighting Dominance

Sighting dominance refers to the phenomenon where one eye is preferred for sighting or aiming tasks. It specifically refers to the preference of one eye for aiming or aligning a target in binocular condition. The dominant eye fixates at the target and the other eye follows the dominant eye and looks at the same target at a slightly different angle, adding required depth perception. Sighting dominance is important in activities such as archery, shooting, golf, and other sports that require accurate aiming. It can also affect daily activities such as driving and reading. Determining which eye is dominant can help individuals optimize their visual performance in these activities by using the dominant eye for sighting or aiming.

It is possible to have mixed dominance where the tests reports that the patient's one eye is sensory dominant and the other is sighting dominance. In rare situations, it is also possible to have a situation where the patient does not reveal specific dominant eye. Sometimes it is also possible that the ocular dominancy switches between right eye and left eye in different situations like different lighting condition or with changing focus between distance target or intermediate distant target.

Importance of Eye Dominance

Eye dominancy is someone's innate characteristic. Human species are predominantly right eye dominant. There is a prevalence of left eye dominancy also. In some cases, the ocular dominancy may not be definite or well established, a condition commonly seen in dyslexics which might result in visual disturbances. This is frustrating because the role of dominant eye is to keep the fixation steady during the entire course of vision so that the awareness with regard to self-position in relation to the object of regard can be maintained. A stable dominant eye is very important to hold the visual system steady at the fixating target. If there is a dominancy conflict, then often attention jumps several words or lines and hence affects comprehension, leading to binocular instability. It is, therefore, important that natural eye dominancy is always maintained and not disturbed.

Strong stable ocular dominancy is also important to a feeling of right and left as can be observed while reading. In normal eye teaming the dominant eye orchestrates the tracking of both eyes. The right eye naturally tracks from left to right while the left eye naturally tracks from right to left. People with left eye dominancy will initially want to look at the right side of the page first and then to move to the left, thus causing difficulties in reading languages that move from left to right like English.

There are clinical situations where the demonstration of a preferred eye is a necessary precursor to any proposed ophthalmic therapy or treatment. These occasions include the prescribing of symptom-relieving optical prism as a supplement in corrective spectacle lenses, where all or the greater part of the prescribed prism is located before the non-dominant eye.

It is important to consider dominant eye while taking a decision for under-correcting an eye. In some cases, under-correction in dominant eye can cause the non-dominant eye to work harder to compensate for the lack of visual clarity in the dominant eye, which can result in temporary changes to ocular dominance and may create conflict in the brain while vision processing.

It is considered that the image of the dominant eye will be less easily suppressed by brain as against relative blurred image in the non-dominant eye. Some patients are uncomfortable if their dominant eye is fractionally blurred, for example over-plus by 0.25 D relative to the other eye. On the other hand, a small under-correction in non-dominant eye may not give any discomfort to the patient.

The knowledge of an individual's ocular dominancy is useful also while considering the 'monovision' approach to temporary or long-term unilateral refractive correction with contact lenses or surgery. The monovision technique was initially devised for the convenience of presbyopic contact lens wearers, but ocular surgery has embraced this approach in conjunction with intraocular lens implantation and refractive procedures with a high rate of success and high degree of patient satisfaction. In monovision the dominant eye is usually corrected for distance viewing and the other eye is corrected for near viewing **(Fig. 2.4)**.

Multifocal contact lenses are designed to provide clear vision at different distances. The selection of lens power is typically optimized for each eye individually depending on the individual's ocular dominance. The overall coordination of both eyes is less critical for the fitting of multifocal contact lenses. Therefore, sensory dominance seems to be more important than sighting dominance. If the lens power is not aligned appropriately with the dominant eye, the individual may experience visual discomfort, reduced visual acuity, or difficulty adapting to the lenses. This is because the dominant eye leads in processing vision in the brain. Even though sighting dominance may not be very important for fitting multifocal lenses, it is useful to determine the dominant eye using both concepts while fitting multifocal contact lenses. In a study, Shor et al. found no relationship between sighting dominance and the ability to suppress blur. Robboy et al. (1990) suggested that sighting dominance alone may not be an adequate measure of ocular dominance. They suggest sensory dominance may play an important role. Therefore, assessing

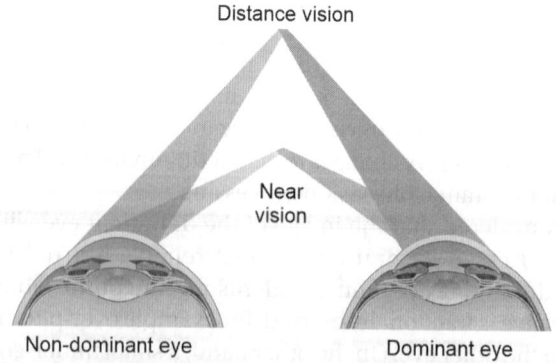

Fig. 2.4: Schematic representation of monovision.

Chapter 2: Vision and Visual Function

both sighting and sensory dominance may be the best approach. When both types of dominance occurred in the same eye, it was easier to suppress blur. This assertion is supported by Collins and Goode (1994) and more recently by Handa et al. (2005) who found binocular summation was influenced by the strength of ocular dominance.

It is also possible to have a situation where the dominancy of eye is not well established. In such case the decision to fit multifocal contact lenses depends on individual's situation and practitioner's recommendations.

There are visually demanding occupations like sports such as archery, shooting, or golf that require precise aiming or alignment. Knowing which eye is dominant can help athletes improve their accuracy and performance in these activities. Research has established that eye dominance is a predisposing factor in sporting ability and contributes in one or more ways to visual performance during sporting activities. One of the objectives of vision correction in sports vision optometry is to restore natural eye dominance.

It seems that eye dominance appears to have a role to play in binocular vision. It is, therefore, important that natural eye dominancy is always maintained and not disturbed.

Tests for Ocular Dominancy

There are different tests that can be used to determine the dominant eye, the common among them are shown in the **Flowchart 2.7**.

The Miles Test

* Extend both arms in front of your body as shown in **Figure 2.5.**
* Place one hand over another, so as to make a small triangular opening.
* With both eyes open, look straight ahead through the opening and focus on a small target. The target may be a doorknob or electric switch.

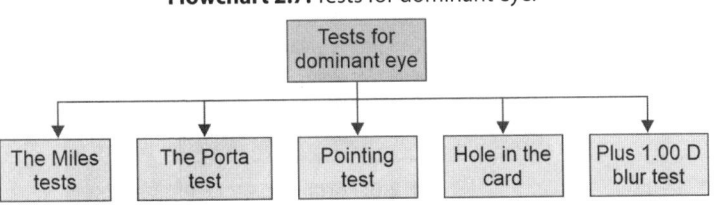

Flowchart 2.7: Tests for dominant eye.

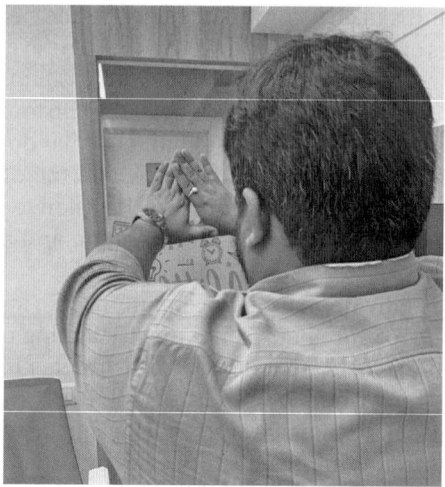

Fig. 2.5: Miles test.

- Close the left eye, if the object remains in view, you are looking with your dominant eye.

The Porta Test

The Porta test **(Fig. 2.6)** is very similar to the Miles test. The only difference is that you ask the patient to bring the opening if the hand closer to his eyes as shown in the figure and you will notice that the opening invariably lines up with the dominant eye of the patient.

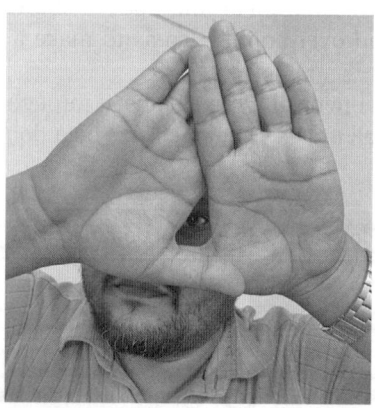

Fig. 2.6: Porta test.

Chapter 2: Vision and Visual Function

Pointing Test (Fig. 2.7)
- Ask the patient to keep both eyes open.
- Identify a target with a vertical line, such as the joining of two walls or a drawn line on a piece of paper hung against a wall.
- Instruct the patient to hold a pencil in their dominant hand.
- Extend the arm with the pencil in front of them, aligning the tip of the pencil with the vertical line.
- Cover their left eye (for example).
- Observe whether the alignment between the pencil tip and the vertical line is maintained.
- If the alignment is still maintained with the left eye covered, the patient is likely looking through his dominant eye.
- If there is a shift in alignment, the dominant eye is the one that was covered.

Hole in the Card

The dominant eye may also be determined using 'Hole in the Card Test' **(Fig. 2.8)**.

Ask the patient to hold a card that has a small hole of 25 mm at its center.

Ask him to extend his hands as shown in the figure and fixate at an object with both eyes open.

The examiner stands right in front of the patient and observes his eyes through the hole.

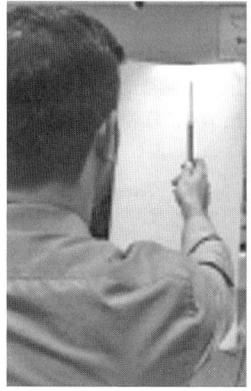
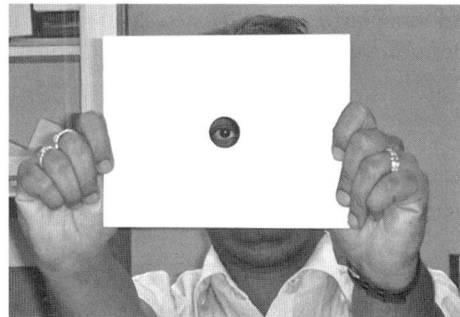

Fig. 2.7: Pointing test.   **Fig. 2.8:** Hole in the card test.

He would be able to observe one eye only which is the dominant eye of the patient.

Plus 1.00 D Blur Test

- Place a +1.00D lens in front of each eye alternately under binocular conditions. This means the patient keeps both eyes open during the test.
- Ask the patient to report if he experiences blurred vision when the +1.00 D lens is in front of each eye.
- The eye that reports greater disturbance is considered the dominant eye.
- Place +1.00 D lens in front of each eye alternately under binocular condition.
- Ask the patient to report if he experiences blur vision.
- The eye with which the patient reports greater disturbances in vision is the dominant eye.

An important caveat is that both eyes must be optimally corrected for distance vision before administering this test.

This test utilizes the blur response to a +1.00D lens and relies on the patient's subjective experience to identify the dominant eye. It is crucial to have proper correction in place to ensure accurate results.

VISUAL FIELD

Visual field of an individual refers to the whole area that is seen while looking straight ahead when the eyes, head and body are still. The peripheral visual field is the outer edge of the field. The monocular visual field is the area in space visible to one eye. The nose prevents the field of the right eye from covering 180% in the horizontal plane. Normal monocular visual field extends up to 60% nasally, 60% superiorly, 70% inferiorly and 100% temporarily as shown in **Figure 2.9**.

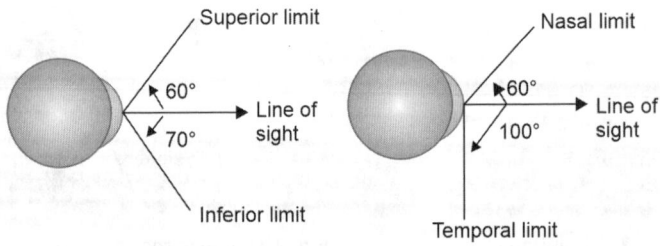

Fig. 2.9: Monocular visual field of an individual.

Blind spot, the physiological scotoma exists at 15° degree temporally where the optic nerve leaves the eye. The monocular visual field of the right and left eye overlap to form the binocular visual field. Objects within the binocular visual field are visible to each eye, albeit from different angles. The binocular visual field is the superimposition of the two monocular fields as shown in **Figure 2.10.**

There are regional differences in color sensation, visual acuity and low-illumination sensitivity within the visual field.

The central visual field is located in a small area of the retina called the macula. The macula contains a large number of cones cells which specialize in seeing detail in color and in relatively bright light. The primary measure of central vision is the visual acuity as determined by reading a Snellen chart. It operates best under high illumination and has the greatest visual acuity and color sensitivity. It represents the operation of the photopic, i.e., light-adapted condition.

The peripheral visual field is more sensitive to dim light and operates under low illumination. It has little color sensitivity and poor spatial acuity and it represents the operation of the scotopic, i.e., dark-adapted condition. The peripheral retina contains rod cells which are more sensitive to low light and, as a group, are very sensitive to movement. It is the primary job of the peripheral vision to make us aware of the location of objects in our visual space and to direct our central vision toward a particular object, if desired. The peripheral retina is not sensitive enough to see much detail on a Snellen's chart.

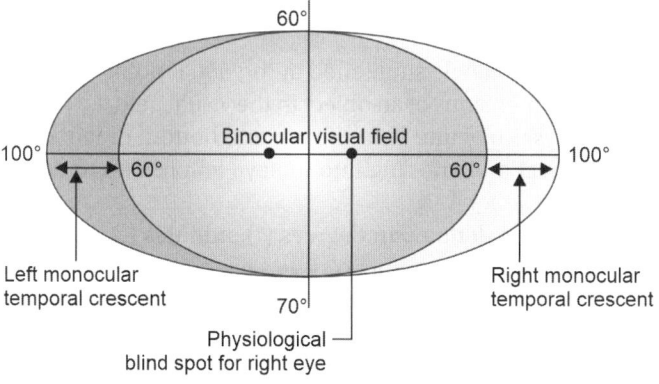

Fig. 2.10: Binocular visual field of an individual.

The image formed by eye is:
- ❖ Smaller than the object viewed
- ❖ Inverted and reversed

Since the image is inverted by the lens system, the superior half of each eye's visual field is projected onto the inferior half of each eye's retina and vice versa. And as because the lens produces a reversed image, the temporal half of each visual field is projected onto the nasal half of each eye's retina which implies:
- ❖ The temporal or left hemifield of the left eye is projected onto the nasal or right half of the left eye's retina.
- ❖ The nasal or left hemifield of right eye is projected onto temporal or right half of the right eye's retina.

Consequently, the left hemifields of both eyes are projected onto the corresponding right halves of the two retinas. It is critical that you understand the relationship between the visual field and the retinal areas and realize that corresponding halves of the two monocular visual fields are imaged on corresponding halves of the two retinas. These relationships form the neurological basis for understanding the visual field defects.

In addition to retina, anatomical structures that connect the retina to visual cortex of the brain make up the complete visual pathway. Any damage to a particular anatomical structure along the visual pathway may produce the characteristic changes in sensitivity of visual field of an individual. The main aim of the visual field testing is to measure the extent of our visual space by determining retinal sensitivity of the selected points at any given point of time.

VISUAL ANGLE

Visual angle is the angle subtended at the nodal point of the eye by the physical dimensions of an object in the visual field, i.e., the angle formed by rays projecting from the top and bottom or left and right end of an object and entering into the eye to focus on to the retina **(Fig. 2.11)**.

Visual angle is denoted in degrees (°), minutes ('), and seconds (") of arc. Two adjacent points can be seen clearly only when they produce a visual angle of 1 minute of arc, which in turn is influenced by two factors:
1. The size of the object
2. The distance of the object from the eye

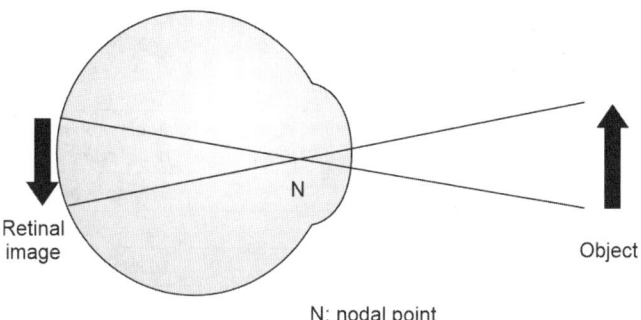

Retinal image

Object

N: nodal point

Fig. 2.11: Visual angle formed at point N.

The bigger objects cast larger images on the retina than smaller objects. Thus, the larger the object is, the larger its visual angle will be. Closer objects cast larger images on the retina than smaller objects. Thus, the closer the object is to the eye, the larger its visual angle will be.

Telescopes are used to alter the angular size of a remote object. The understanding is in order to see an object clearly either the object should be large enough or it should be placed at an appropriate distance. Thus, visual angle is an angular measurement of the size of an object as seen at a given distance. It is a useful and convenient way of specifying the size of the retinal image of the object and the spatial extent of objects.

In terms of the size of the retinal image, it has been studied that two points can be seen clearly when their image size is 4.5 micron. This is so, because the diameter of the cone cell stimulated by the image is 1.5 micron and two cone cells must be stimulated with a gap of one cone cell. If all three cones were equally stimulated, the discrimination would be lacking between two extremes. The computation of spatial relationship of these cones is such as to equal to 1' of arc. Therefore, a good eye can distinguish two points as separate when they subtend an angle of 1' of arc.

The concept of visual angle has been effectively used by Dr Herman Snellen, a Dutch ophthalmologist, while proposing his optotypes for his visual acuity measurement test chart. Snellen's letters were so constructed that their constituent parts, i.e., the limbs and spaces between them, each subtends an angle of 1 minute of arc at a specified distance. The linear size of the Snellen's 6/6 letters is given by the following notation:

Chapter 2: Vision and Visual Function

Table 2.3: Visual angle with corresponding linear size of letters used in Snellen's test chart.

Line	Distance in meters	Linear size of letter	Angle subtended at nodal point
6/6	6	8.75 mm	5 minutes of arc
6/9	6	13.14 mm	7.5 minutes of arc
6/12	6	17.52 mm	10 minutes of arc
6/24	6	35.04 mm	20 minutes of arc
6/36	6	52.50 mm	30 minutes of arc
6/60	6	87.50 mm	50 minutes of arc

1 minute of arc=h/6000 mm (*where* "h" is the size or height of the letter)
Taking the value from log table
0.000292 = h/6000 mm
Or, 0.000292 × 6000 = h
Or, h = 1.75 mm
Therefore, 5 minutes of arc 5 × 1.75 = 8.75 mm

In the clinical environment at a distance each line subtends an angle at nodal point as given in **Table 2.3**.

DEPTH OF FIELD AND DEPTH OF FOCUS

The depth of field and the depth of focus are two different concepts that often create confusion. To simplify the concept depth of field is concerned with image quality of an object as the object is repositioned in its space, whereas depth of focus is concerned with the image quality in the image space for a stationary object.

When an object is accurately focused, it can also be seen clearly if it is placed closer to and farther from the best focus point without changing the accommodation, the range of distance so covered is called the depth of field. Depth of field reduces the precise need for accommodation. However, the concept of depth of field only makes sense when it is defined with a given resolution and contrast.

Depth of focus is the image space complement of depth of field and is related to the range on the retina in which an optical image may move without impairment of clarity while the object remains at the same position. The depth of focus in image space can be regarded as conjugate with depth of field in object space.

The depth of field is influenced by several factors, including the pupil size, focal length, and distance of the subject from the eyes. A larger aperture and a shorter focal length generally result in a shallower depth of field, with only a narrow range of distances in focus. Depth of focus refers to the range of distances over which the optical system can produce a clear, in-focus image. The depth of focus is determined by the size of the pupil, the focal length of the lens, and the distance of the subject from the lens. A larger aperture and a shorter focal length generally result in a greater depth of focus.

Depth of field should not be mistaken for accommodation. The apparent range of accommodation also includes depth of field and tolerance of blur, i.e., depth of focus. However, after the age of 60 years when the accommodating ability is completely declined, the small range of vision that remains is apparently depth of field and not the true accommodation.

In summary, depth of focus refers to the ability of the eyes to produce a clear image, while depth of field refers to the range of distances over which objects in a scene are in focus.

MULTIPLE CHOICE QUESTIONS

1. **Which one of the following is the symptom of visual stress?**
   a. Discomfort while reading
   b. Continually losing the place on the page or skipping lines
   c. Sensations of text moving on the page or screen
   d. All of the above
2. **The ability to judge the distance and speed of approach of a moving object requires:**
   a. Active accommodation and good vergence facility
   b. Visual acuity and binocular coordination
   c. Good contrast
   d. All of the above
3. **The visual acuity is not dependent upon:**
   a. Pupil size
   b. Spherical aberration
   c. Chromatic aberration
   d. Corneal refractive index
4. **Which of the following is not true regarding dominant eye?**
   a. Dominant eye is the fixating eye in the binocular vision.
   b. Dominant eye aims at the object.
   c. Dominant eye leads in receiving the visual inputs.
   d. Dominant eye is the eye with better visual acuity.

Chapter 2: Vision and Visual Function

5. **Which of the following is the progenitor of depth judgment?**
   a. Fusion
   b. Fixation
   c. Suppression
   d. Vergence
6. **Which of the following is associated with close viewing distance?**
   a. The ciliary muscles contract and in effect, reduce the tension that zonule exerts on the lens.
   b. The lens becomes more spherical and has greater refractive power.
   c. Pupil constricts.
   d. All of the above.
7. **Which of the following is not true about normal monocular visual field of human being?**
   a. It extends up to 60% nasally.
   b. It extends up to 50% superiorly.
   c. It extends up to 70% inferiorly.
   d. It extends up to 80% temporarily.

ANSWER KEY

| 1. d | 2. b | 3. d | 4. d | 5. a | 6. d | 7. d |

SELF-PRACTICE QUESTION

1. How would you define vision as against visual perception and visual acuity?

3 CHAPTER

Visual Symptoms

CHAPTER OUTLINE

- Causes of Visual Symptoms
- Common Visual Symptoms
- Optical Correction of Visual Symptoms

Symptoms are manifestations of a disease, disorder, disablement or condition that an individual may experience. These manifestations result from a combination of physical, physiological, psychological, and social factors. Symptoms can be subjective experiences or observable signs that suggest the presence of an underlying issue.

Symptoms related to vision encompass a broad spectrum of experiences that individuals may encounter, indicating underlying issues with the eyes, visual apparatus, or potentially systemic connections. A sense of confusion and temporary blurring of vision, accompanied by discomfort, may be experienced. The eyes may become tired, and lids may feel heavy, while a sensation of weariness or drowsiness progressively may arise, rendering continued attention difficult.

CAUSES OF VISUAL SYMPTOMS

The manifestation of visual symptoms partly depends on the use to which the eyes are put to, partly on the efficiency of visual apparatus and partly on the capacity of the individual to withstand sustained effort. **Flowchart 3.1** shows the principal reasons for the manifestation of visual symptoms.

Flowchart 3.1: Reasons for visual symptoms.

```
          Causes of visual
             symptoms
    ┌──────────┬──────────┬──────────┐
    ▼          ▼          ▼          ▼
  Visual    Ocular   Constitutional Environmental
 apparatus  factors     factors       factors
```

Visual Apparatus

Biologically the eyes were adapted for relatively simple purposes—look for enemies and for food and from long custom we accept the conditions in which we live today as normal. This is by no means absolutely true. Today we live in a more complex world where the modern civilization with its newer function needed for near vision imposes extra strain on our visual system. The convergence, a crucial function required for effective near tasks, tends to break down first, leading to various associated symptoms.

Ocular Factors

Ocular factors encompass conditions directly associated with the eyes, contributing to various visual symptoms and significantly influencing the overall health and functionality of the visual system. Refractive errors, including myopia, hyperopia, astigmatism, and presbyopia, may lead to blurry vision and eye strain. Convergence insufficiency, a condition where the eyes struggle to work together for focusing on nearby objects, can result in eye strain, double vision, and challenges with sustained near vision tasks. Coordination issues between both eyes, such as in cases of strabismus and amblyopia, may cause discomfort, headaches, and difficulties in concentration. Dry eye syndrome can manifest as discomfort, redness, and blurred vision, particularly when there is insufficient lubrication of the eyes. Additionally, eye diseases like glaucoma, cataracts, and macular degeneration have the potential to cause vision problems, emphasizing the diverse range of ocular factors influencing visual health.

Constitutional Factors

The physical health of an individual plays a significant role in the manifestation of visual symptoms. For instance, those with frail health are more susceptible to reaching a breaking point, experiencing symptoms more readily than their robust counterparts. Visual symptoms tend to surface in individuals who are debilitated or convalescing from acute illnesses. Additionally, women may experience visual symptoms after childbirth and during lactation, periods when fatigue is more likely to manifest. This highlights how the constitutional factor, reflecting the overall physical condition of the individual, can influence the occurrence and intensity of visual symptoms. Malnutrition, general exhaustion, insufficient sleep, anxiety and emotional strain may bring about a condition of ocular decompensation even in the otherwise healthy individual.

Environmental Factors

Environmental factors significantly contribute to visual symptoms, with illumination being a principal element. The quality, quantity, and distribution of light, along with the nature of visual tasks imposed—such as the size of targets, their movements, and contrast with surroundings—play crucial roles. The size of objects, in terms of the visual angle they subtend, is particularly important. Small objects, even if not physically small, may require close viewing, adding to accommodative-convergence strain and increasing the challenges of perception. Poor definition and lack of contour in objects pose a notable disadvantage, affecting the clarity of vision. Constant movement of objects introduces the need for continuous and rapid ocular adjustments, contributing to visual symptoms. Therefore, understanding and optimizing environmental factors, especially illumination and task characteristics, are essential considerations in addressing and preventing visual symptoms.

The mechanism of the causation of the visual symptoms is interesting. The intriguing causation mechanism behind visual symptoms challenges the notion that visual capacity alone serves as a true guide for assessment. The condition arises primarily from the strenuous effort to compensate for imperfections, and when such compensation becomes unattainable, sustained efforts diminish. Notably, the intensity of symptoms tends to be more pronounced in cases where overall vision remains relatively good. Interestingly, individuals with minor astigmatism and proportionately reduced vision may lead placid and comfortable lives, while those with a more organized disposition may exhibit noticeable symptoms of disability. Clinicians should remain vigilant, as a subject may vehemently assert excellent vision in response to the suggestion that ocular factors contribute to their symptoms. This underscores the complexity of the interplay between visual perception, compensatory mechanisms, and individual adaptability in the manifestation of visual symptoms.

COMMON VISUAL SYMPTOMS

Common visual symptoms encompass a range of experiences that individuals may encounter, indicating potential issues with the eyes or visual system. These symptoms can vary in nature and intensity. Some common visual symptoms are detailed below:

Blur Vision

Blur vision is characterized by a loss of sharpness in eyesight, resulting in objects appearing out of focus and hazy. This loss of sharpness can occur due to a defocused image or a degraded and deshaped image. Spherical correction is employed to bring a defocused image into focus, while cylinder correction, with its axis appropriately placed, corrects degraded and deshaped images. The correction process involves numerous possible combinations of sphere powers, cylinder powers, and cylinder axes. Blurred vision can manifest in different ways, and each one of types may indicate specific underlying eye conditions, for example:

- Blur vision can be permanent or transient.
- Blur vision can be intermittent and fluctuating.
- Blur vision can be episodic or sudden with the condition worsening over time.

Permanent blur vision can be because of defocused, degraded and deshaped image. It can be caused by ocular condition or refractive error or presbyopia.

Transient blur vision can occur due to local and systemic causes. Pressure from a tumor or swelling of lids may involve transient astigmatic changes. Certain eyedrops and medications can also cause blurring of vision.

Intermittent blur vision in near viewing distance may be because of dry eyes. Insufficient tear production or poor-quality tears can cause blurred vision, particularly when reading, using a computer, or watching TV for extended periods.

Intermittent blur vision at distance may be because of accommodative spasm. Intermittent blur vision may simply mean tiredness, eye strain or over-exposure to sunlight.

Fluctuating vision refers to frequent changes in the clarity of vision. A patient may have blurred vision that comes and goes. Fluctuating vision may be a sign of diabetes or hypertension which are chronic conditions that can damage the blood vessels in the retina. Any damage to the retina can cause permanent vision loss, and so a patient with fluctuating vision should seek immediate medical attention.

Episodic visual blurring is an important clinical indicator of vascular insufficiency in the occipital cortex of the brain.

Sudden blur vision can be a medical emergency and includes stroke, steep increase in blood pressure, hyphema, retinal detachment, concussion, infection of the eye and its tissues, migraine, eye injury.

Double Vision

Double vision, medically termed diplopia, can have various origins, ranging from refractive errors to more complex underlying eye conditions. While it can be associated with common vision issues, it is crucial to recognize that double vision may also indicate more serious health concerns, involving factors such as muscle imbalance, cataracts, neurological issues, or trauma.

Refractive errors, such as astigmatism or anisometropia, can contribute to double vision. Double vision can also be a symptom of more profound eye-related issues. Conditions like strabismus, where the eyes are misaligned, or certain types of eye muscle disorders. Neurological issues, cataracts, corneal irregularities or systemic health conditions like diabetes, stroke, vitamin toxicity, etc. may also cause double vision. Trauma and muscular or nerve damage or head injury may also cause double vision.

Distorted Vision

Distorted vision refers to a condition where objects appear misshapen, blurred, or distorted. This visual symptom can be caused by various eye conditions or abnormalities in the visual system. Astigmatism may lead to distorted vision at all distances, keratoconus may cause distorted vision, and macular degeneration can lead to distorted central vision. Retinal detachment, diabetic retinopathy and glaucoma can cause distorted vision. Some individuals may experience visual distortions during a migraine headache. Certain medications may have visual side effects, leading to distorted vision in some cases. Physical trauma to the eye or head can cause changes in the structure of the eye or affect the visual pathways, resulting in distorted vision. Dislocation or displacement of the eye's natural lens can lead to distorted vision.

Glare, Flare and Haloes around the Light

Glare, flare, and halos around lights are visual symptoms that individuals may experience, and they can be associated with various eye conditions. These symptoms are often related to issues with how the eye handles light, and they can impact visual comfort and clarity. Glare refers to excessive brightness or dazzling light that can be discomforting and may interfere with vision. Flare is the scattering of light within the eye, leading to the perception of scattered light or veiling glare. Halos are circular rings of light that surround a light source, often seen at night. Glare may be caused by oncoming headlights while driving at night, sunlight reflecting off surfaces and bright lights in an indoor environment. The presence of bright light sources in the visual field and light scattering in the eye due to certain eye conditions or abnormalities may cause flare. Cataracts and corneal abnormalities or irregularities may cause glare and halos. Uncorrected refractive errors, particularly astigmatism, can contribute to light sensitivity. Wearing sunglasses with UV protection can help reduce the impact of glare or light sensitivity.

Eye Strain

Eye strain is a condition that arises when the ocular muscles experience fatigue from prolonged and intense use. This phenomenon is akin to muscular strains in other parts of the body, where increased pressure, overuse, or improper use can lead to various symptoms. **Flowchart 3.2** shows the different ocular muscles.

Flowchart 3.2: Ocular muscles.

```
                    Eye muscles
                   /          \
         Intraocular         Extraocular
           muscles             muscles
         /    |    \           /      \
   Ciliary Sphincter Dilator  EOM that    Levator
   muscles pupillae  pupillae controls eye palpebrae
                              movement    superioris
```

(EOM: extraocular muscle)

The ciliary muscles play a crucial role in changing focus from one object to another. When engaged in activities that require sustained near vision, such as reading or staring at a screen, these muscles can become fatigued. Prolonged near work causes the ciliary muscles to constrict continuously, leading to strain and discomfort.

Extraocular muscles control the movement of the eyes, allowing them to move up, down, side to side, and rotate. During extended periods of near work, these muscles are actively involved in maintaining focus on a near object, preventing double vision. This continuous effort can contribute to eye strain.

The levator palpebrae superioris muscle raises the upper eyelid and helps maintain its position. Reduced blinking rate during activities like prolonged gaming or driving can result in increased strain on this muscle, contributing to eye discomfort.

The sphincter papillae constrict the pupil, while the dilator papillae dilate it. Excessive illumination, such as prolonged exposure to bright screens, can lead to sustained maximal papillary constriction, causing discomfort and pain.

Eye strain presents as stabbing pain during prolonged use, accompanied by a subjective sensation of tired and sore eyes due to inflammation and swelling. The eyes exhibit a restricted range of motion, particularly when shifting focus from near to far objects. Reduced blinking rate during extended activities further contributes to the discomfort by impacting natural eye lubrication.

Diagnosing eye strain can be difficult as symptoms may not seem directly related to ocular issues. Vision may appear unimpaired by the patient's own standards, and small errors may escape detection. Eye strain is sometimes linked to general fatigue and may be overlooked. Understanding the specific muscles involved and the activities that contribute to eye strain can help in managing and preventing this condition.

Asthenopia

Asthenopia refers to a cluster of symptoms associated with eye discomfort and fatigue, including tiredness, soreness, headaches, and dizziness. It is often used interchangeably with the more common term "eye strain." While "eye strain" is a widely recognized and straightforward expression, "asthenopia" serves as a medical term encapsulating the same array of symptoms linked to visual fatigue and discomfort. Asthenopia can be transient, typically alleviated with rest; however, in certain instances, it might signal an underlying vision issue or other eye-related problems. It is crucial to recognize that asthenopia may be indicative of temporary strain, but persistent or recurrent symptoms could prompt further investigation into potential underlying eye conditions.

Headaches

Headaches can be associated with various visual symptoms and may arise from different causes related to the eyes and visual system. Prolonged use of the eyes for tasks such as reading or screen time can lead to eye strain, contributing to headaches. Nearsightedness, farsightedness, or astigmatism that is not corrected with appropriate lenses can lead to headaches, especially during activities that require clear vision. Age-related difficulty in focusing on close objects, known as presbyopia, can cause eye strain and headaches during near tasks. Conditions like convergence insufficiency, where the eyes have difficulty working together, can lead to headaches, particularly after prolonged reading. Insufficient tear production or poor tear quality causing dry eyes may contribute to eye discomfort and headaches. Prolonged use of digital devices can cause digital eye strain, characterized by symptoms like headaches, eye fatigue, and blurred vision. Sinus congestion or infections can lead to headaches, and these may be accompanied by discomfort around the eyes. Stress and tension can contribute to tension headaches, causing discomfort in the forehead and around the eyes. While headaches can arise from various systemic conditions, a discussion of these is beyond the current scope. It's important to note that headaches accompanied by visual symptoms can indicate underlying conditions. A comprehensive examination by a healthcare professional, including an eye examination, may be necessary for accurate diagnosis and appropriate management.

Ocular Pain

Ocular pain signifies discomfort or pain localized to the eyes and serves as a distinctive visual symptom indicative of various underlying issues related to ocular health. The pain can manifest in diverse ways, including aching, throbbing, stabbing, or a general sense of discomfort within or around the eyes. When associated with eye strain, ocular pain is of muscular origin, stemming from fatigue. There are various ocular conditions that can contribute to pain, such as lid lesions, episcleral/scleral nodules, corneal edema, keratitic precipitates, cell and flare, angle-closure glaucoma, iritis, anisocoria, and others. Additionally, systemic conditions like rheumatoid arthritis, herpes zoster, sinus infection, gout, and lupus may also be linked to ocular pain. Ocular pain can be a component of migraines or tension headaches, adding another layer to its multifaceted nature.

Eye Rubbing

Eye rubbing is a common behavior with potential implications for ocular health. While occasional, gentle eye rubbing may be harmless, persistent or vigorous rubbing can lead to issues. Dry eyes are often associated with eye rubbing, as individuals may rub to alleviate discomfort caused by insufficient tear production or poor tear quality. Itchy eyes due to allergies can prompt reflexive eye rubbing. Eyes may also be rubbed when tired, especially after prolonged periods of reading or screen use. The sensation of a foreign body, such as dust or an eyelash, can lead to rubbing. Furthermore, eye rubbing can exacerbate certain eye conditions or symptoms associated with uncorrected refractive error. While eye rubbing itself is not a direct cause of refractive errors, it may be a response to the discomfort caused by the refractive error.

Increased Blinking

Blinking is a normal and necessary function of the eyes, helping to spread tears evenly over the ocular surface, protect the eyes from foreign objects, and maintain overall eye health. However, an increase in blinking frequency or duration may be associated with certain conditions or factors, the common among them are dry eye syndrome, eye irritation or allergies, corneal abrasions or foreign bodies, conjunctivitis, nervous system disorders, and medication side effects. Uncorrected or under-corrected refractive errors can lead to eye strain, discomfort, and increased blinking. Prolonged periods of intense visual concentration, such as staring at a screen for extended periods and blepharospasm may lead to increased blinking.

Eye Squeezing

Eye squeezing can be a behavior exhibited for various reasons, and it may be associated with different visual symptoms. Squeezing the eyes can be a natural response to shield the eyes from excessive light. Prolonged periods of visual concentration, such as reading or using digital devices, can lead to eye strain and fatigue. Squeezing the eyes may provide a brief relief from strain. Individuals experiencing headaches or migraines may find relief by squeezing their eyes shut, especially if light sensitivity is associated with the headache. Stress or tension can manifest in various ways, including tightness or discomfort around the eyes. Squeezing the eyes may be a response to stress. During intense concentration or focus, individuals may squeeze their eyes shut momentarily. This behavior can be observed in various activities, such as problem-solving or deep thinking. Allergic reactions, especially those affecting the eyes, can cause itching and discomfort. Squeezing the eyes may be an attempt to relieve the itching. Some individuals may habitually squeeze eyes.

Loss of Peripheral Vision

The loss of peripheral vision, also known as peripheral visual field loss or tunnel vision, refers to a reduction or absence of vision in the outer areas of the visual field. This can affect an individual's ability to see objects or movement to the side or around the edges of their visual field. Peripheral vision loss can be associated with various eye conditions or neurological disorders. Some of the common among them are glaucoma, retinitis pigmentosa, optic nerve disorders, stroke or brain injury, retinal detachment, chronic retinal diseases, hypertensive retinopathy.

Flashes of Light

Flashes of light are visual symptoms characterized by the perception of brief, flickering, or flashing lights in the visual field. These flashes can appear as sparks, streaks, or arcs of light and may be described by individuals as seeing "stars" or "lightning." Flashes of light can be associated with various underlying causes that may include retinal detachment, posterior vitreous detachment, and vitreous floaters. A blow to the head or eye can stimulate the retina and cause flashes of light.

OPTICAL CORRECTION OF VISUAL SYMPTOMS

Visual symptoms should not be treated solely through optical correction, as it is crucial to recognize that the individual reports these symptoms, not just his eyes. The treatment of visual symptoms should be viewed as integral parts of the body, sharing with other organs in its constitutional variations and in the effects of ills with which it may be afflicted. The optical correction of visual symptoms should be guided by the clinician's understanding of the underlying organic conditions, the demands placed on the patient, and the clinician's ability to meet those demands. A comprehensive approach requires the clinician to consider the patient's entire life, encompassing activities, habits, diet, environment, workload, personality, and intelligence. While optical correction is often emphasized, it is essential to remember that not every small error necessitates correction.

It is worth noting that gross visual errors typically do not manifest in typical symptoms but rather result in a failure of visual function. In contrast, when errors are small, individuals can often compensate to some extent through their own efforts, unconsciously imposing difficulties upon themselves. Thus, it becomes evident that the error itself may not be the primary issue; rather, it is the continuous effort to correct it that poses a challenge. Therefore, thoughtful consideration is essential when choosing correction, as small errors may persist in a different form if not addressed appropriately.

Thorough examination of refractive error, accommodation and convergence function, muscular balance, binocular vision, and the size relationship of retinal images is crucial in the optical correction of visual symptoms. Rule-of-thumb approaches should be avoided, as correcting small refractive errors unnecessarily may have adverse effects, such as depriving individuals of necessary stimuli or causing issues related to muscular deficiency.

The wholesale correction of small amounts of astigmatism is cautioned against, considering that absolute optical perfection in the eyes is rare. The eyes possess inherent errors, and attempts to correct every minute, symptomless error may misinterpret the complexity of the living organism. Correction should be based on the clinician's assessment of visual requirements and personality, particularly when symptoms are associated with the identified error.

In the treatment of smaller corrections, precision is paramount, given that even minor errors can lead to significant systemic disturbances. Addressing these errors requires punctilious care to prevent perpetuating the issue in another form. Discomfort experienced by patients with marked refractive anomalies upon wearing spectacles may result from slightly inadequate correction, emphasizing the need for accurate adjustments.

It is undisputed that orthoptic exercises, crafted to address the detrimental habits of binocularity, foster the development of fusional reflexes, and through repetitive tutoring, instil skill in an imperfect neuromuscular mechanism. These exercises play a distinct role in the treatment of certain visual symptoms, facilitating the acquisition and seamless execution of binocular habits.

We understand that vision extends beyond the mere creation of a retinal image through the dioptric system of the eyes and its transmission to the cortex via physiological processes. It involves the perceptual appreciation of presented patterns imbued with meaning. The interpretation of such patterns is significantly influenced by memories of past experiences, playing a dominant role in the ease and efficiency of the visual process. Unfortunately, the conventional approach predominantly focuses on lower level events, emphasizing the attainment of appropriate retinal images, often neglecting considerations at the higher level without apparent justification. It is crucial to recognize that difficulties in interpretation at the higher level can be as impactful in causing strain as disturbances at the lower level. Consequently, clinicians should actively consider both aspects. Repetitive exercises play a vital role in facilitating perceptual processes and providing an accumulated reservoir of memories and associations to aid in interpretation, proving immensely beneficial in refining the art of seeing. Undoubtedly, repetitive exercises can dramatically enhance the efficiency of macular perception, especially in cases of amblyopia. Similarly, focused training has demonstrated the potential to increase the efficiency of peripheral vision. With consistent practice, individuals can acquire proficiency in the nuances of color vision tests, resulting in significant improvements in the interpretation of such tests.

Therefore, it is imperative to recognize that providing suitable lenses is not an isolated treatment; the clinician must consider the patient's entire life, encompassing habits, diet, exercise, workload, and individual characteristics.

MULTIPLE CHOICE QUESTIONS

1. **What is the primary consideration when addressing visual symptoms in an individual?**
   a. Isolating the symptom to the eyes alone
   b. Treating the symptom solely with optical correction
   c. Recognizing the individual as the reporter of symptoms, not just the eyes
   d. Emphasizing the correction of even minor errors

Chapter 3: Visual Symptoms

2. **Why is careful consideration essential when opting for the correction of small visual errors?**
    a. Small errors are always indicative of significant underlying issues.
    b. Small errors tend to resolve on their own without intervention.
    c. Small errors may be perpetuated in another form if not addressed appropriately.
    d. Correction of small errors is a routine procedure with no potential consequences.
3. **What is the purpose of orthoptic exercises in the context of visual symptoms?**
    a. To prescribe corrective lenses
    b. To develop fusional reflexes and rectify binocular habits
    c. To induce permanent changes in refractive error
    d. To replace traditional medical treatments
4. **Why is it crucial to consider both lower level and higher level events in the context of visual symptoms?**
    a. Lower level events are always more critical.
    b. Higher level events have no impact on visual comfort.
    c. Strain can arise from difficulties at both lower and higher levels.
    d. Clinicians prefer focusing on one level for simplicity.
5. **How does astigmatism contribute to blurred vision?**
    a. It causes a loss of central vision.
    b. It results in distorted or elongated images.
    c. It leads to color blindness.
    d. It only affects peripheral vision.
6. **Which manifestation is often associated with sudden onset of blurred vision and may indicate a medical emergency?**
    a. Eye fatigue
    b. Presbyopia
    c. Retinal detachment
    d. Dry eyes
7. **Constant blurred vision is an indication of:**
    a. Uncorrected refractive error
    b. General accommodative dysfunction
    c. Poor convergence function
    d. None of the above
8. **Intermittent blurred vision in distance is an indication of:**
    a. Uncorrected refractive error
    b. General accommodative dysfunction

c. Poor convergence function
d. Poor binocular balancing
9. **Glare can be caused because of:**
   a. Light sensitivity
   b. Binocular vision disorder
   c. Light scatter within the eye
   d. All of the above
10. **Intermittent blurred vision at near is an indication of:**
    a. Uncorrected refractive error
    b. Accommodative spasm
    c. Dry eyes
    d. Inadequate near addition

ANSWER KEY

1. c	2. c	3. b	4. c	5. b	6. c	7. a	8. b
9. d	10. c						

SELF-PRACTICE QUESTION

1. Elaborate on the potential causes and consequences of smaller visual errors compared to gross visual errors. Why careful consideration is necessary before opting for the correction of small errors, and how can such errors be perpetuated if not addressed appropriately?

CHAPTER 4

Retinal Image

CHAPTER OUTLINE

- Retinal Image: Foundation of Vision
- Chromatic Aberration
- Monochromatic Aberration
- Rationale for Higher Order Aberration

RETINAL IMAGE: FOUNDATION OF VISION

The rays of light after having passed through the cornea and the lens of the eye are focused on the retina to form an image on the retina. The image formed on retina is labeled as real because it is formed by the converging optical system of the eye and the real images are always inverted. The image so formed on retina forms the foundation of vision.

The retinal image contains important visual information such as the location, size, shape, color, and texture of objects in the visual field that is being transmitted to the brain via optic nerve. The brain then processes and interprets retinal image to form a coherent visual perception of the world around us.

However, it is important to note that vision is not solely based on the retinal image. The brain also plays a critical role in processing and interpreting visual information, using cognitive processes such as perception, attention, memory, and decision-making. Therefore, while the retinal image is an important foundation of vision, it is only one part of the complex process that allows us to see and understand the world around us.

Chapter 4: Retinal Image

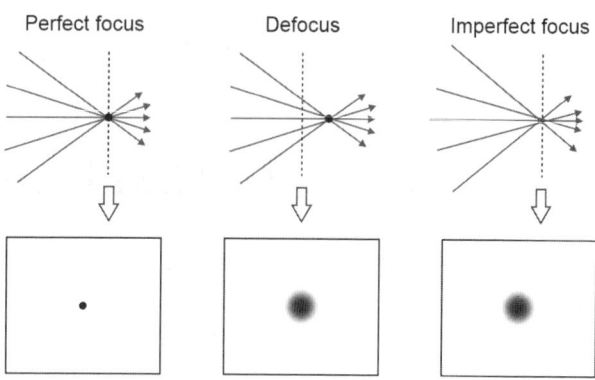

Fig. 4.1: Image quality is the function of how well the light focuses on retina.

The quality of the retinal image is determined by how well the light focuses on the retina which ultimately determines vision clarity and visual acuity. Three types of imagery are possible depending upon the ocular structure, especially the cornea and the lens, axial length of the eye and proper functioning of ocular muscles—perfectly focused image, defocused image and imperfect image as shown in **Figure 4.1**.

A focused image is one in which the light rays from an object being viewed converge precisely onto the retina, the light-sensitive tissue lining the back of the eye. The retina then sends signals to the brain, which interprets these signals as a clear image. This precise focusing is possible when the cornea and lens have normal shapes and refractive indices, and the muscles controlling the lens function correctly. When these conditions are met, the image formed on the retina is sharp and clear.

A defocused image, on the other hand, occurs when the light rays from an object do not converge onto the retina but instead converge either in front of or behind it. This can happen when the shape and the refractive indices of ocular structure, especially the cornea and lens are not normal and the muscles controlling it are functioning correctly. A defocused image will appear blurry or out of focus. Defocus is one of the simplest Zernike modes, expressed in diopters and is reciprocal of focal length in meters. Clinicians have been correcting defocus with spherical correction.

An imperfect image can result from a variety of conditions affecting the eye. For example, astigmatism is a common condition in which

Chapter 4: Retinal Image

the cornea, the clear front surface of the eye is irregularly shaped, causing images to appear degraded and deformed. An imperfect image can also result from various conditions or abnormalities of the eye. Cataracts are common conditions that can cause images to appear blurry or dim. Other conditions such as glaucoma, macular degeneration, and diabetic retinopathy can also affect the clarity of vision. Ocular aberrations are also the reason of imperfect image.

Defocused and imperfect images result in blur images. There are basically three sources of image blur in human eye as shown in **Flowchart 4.1**.

Among the three, scatter is the minor source of image blur in young and normal eyes. Diffraction at the eye's pupil is an important source of image blur with small pupil. However, it becomes less important with increasing pupil size. The image formed on the retina from the light entering through the pupil is not a perfect point but a light disc surrounded by concentric dark and light rings. This is because of the wave nature of the light and is pupil size dependent. No point image is formed, only a diffraction pattern is formed. The diffraction pattern varies directly with the wavelength of the light and the focal length of the optical system and inversely as pupil size (aperture size) through which light rays enter into eyes **(Figure 4.2)**.

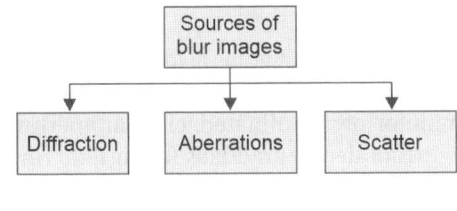

Flowchart 4.1: Three sources of blur image.

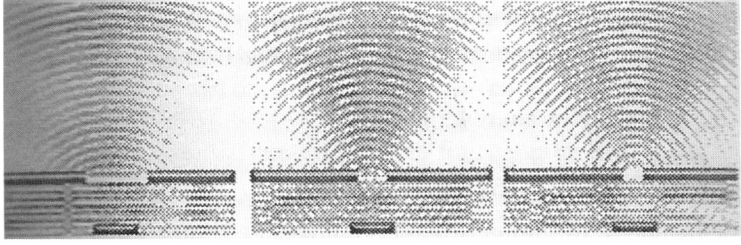

Fig. 4.2: Schematic representation of diffraction of light after passing through an aperture.

Chapter 4: Retinal Image

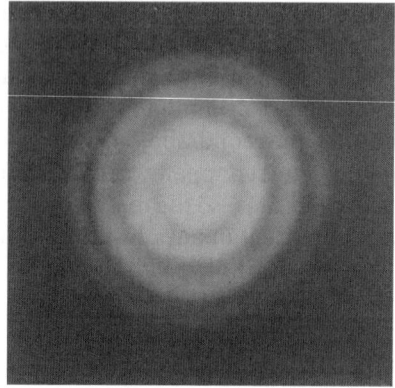

Fig. 4.3: Diagrammatic representation of airy disc.

Flowchart 4.2: Optical aberrations

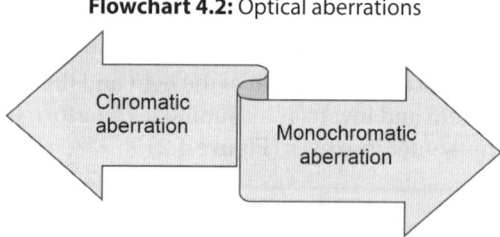

The diffraction pattern of light is also known as Airy disc, named after George Biddell Airy, who showed that the diffraction pattern resulting from uniformly illuminated, circular aperture has a bright central region surrounded by gradually fading light rings as shown in **Figure 4.3**.

This diffraction visibly reduces image sharpness. The edges of an image are never sharp. No matter to what extent the system is optically perfect, the limits of efficiency are determined by the diffraction.

Optical aberrations can be categorized into two subcategories as shown in the **Flowchart 4.2**.

CHROMATIC ABERRATION

Refraction by the human eye is also subject to chromatic aberration. As a result, the focusing power of the eye is different for different

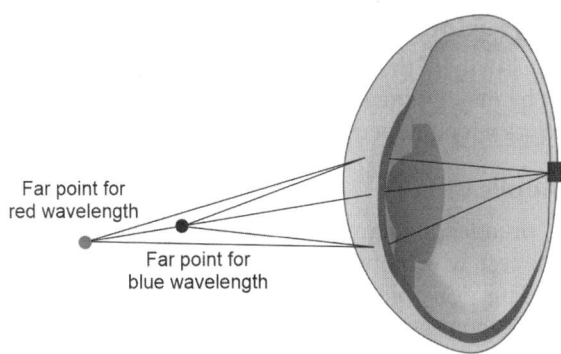

Fig. 4.4: Far point of an individual's focus varies with the wavelength of light.

wavelengths of light in the real world of polychromatic objects. Consequently, there is no place in the visual space where one can place an object and expect it to be well focused on the retina for more than one wavelength of light at a time. Hence blue wavelength focuses before the retina and red beyond the retina, i.e., the far point of an individual's focus varies with the wavelengths of light (**Fig. 4.4**). There are two types of chromatic aberration—longitudinal chromatic aberration and transverse chromatic aberration. Longitudinal chromatic aberration, also known as axial chromatic aberration, is the chromatic difference of focus on the optical axis of the eye. Transverse chromatic aberration, also known as lateral chromatic aberration, on the other hand is because of difference in image sizes and result in colored 'ghost' images. In terms of foveal vision, the dominant chromatic aberration is axial or longitudinal chromatic aberration.

The causes of chromatic aberration are dispersion in the cornea, aqueous, crystalline lens and vitreous humor. Dispersion is simply a variation in the refractive index of the material with various wavelengths of light and causes white light to be dispersed into the various spectral colors, just as prism disperses light into a rainbow. Refractive surgery techniques cannot correct chromatic aberration as this error is inherent to the properties of ocular structures and not to the shape of the ocular components.

Influencing Factors

Spectral sensitivity of the eyes helps reduce the effect of chromatic aberration by making the visual system more sensitive to the green and yellow wavelength focused onto the retina.

Clinical Application

In clinical practice, ocular chromatic aberration is utilized in the duo chrome test, which operates on the principle of axial chromatic aberration. This principle states that green light is refracted more by the eye's optics compared to red light.

MONOCHROMATIC ABERRATIONS

Monochromatic aberrations are surface-related aberrations and can be broadly classified into two categories:
1. Lower order aberrations
2. Higher order aberrations

The most common lower order aberrations are defocus and astigmatism. Defocus is one kind of aberration in which an image is simply out of focus. Defocus is commonly caused by myopia and hypermetropia. Myopia causes positive defocus and hypermetropia causes negative defocus. These are commonly corrected by using spherical lenses, positive defocus is corrected by negative lenses and negative defocus is corrected by positive lenses.

Astigmatism occurs when the cornea or lens of the eye has an irregular shape, causing the light to focus unevenly on the retina. Instead of the light coming to a single point of focus on the retina, it creates two points of focus. This results in imperfect image that degrades and deforms the image quality, making it difficult to see fine details, both at a distance and up close. Astigmatism can occur on its own or in combination with other refractive errors such as myopia or hyperopia. Only astigmatism is corrected with cylinder lenses and astigmatism in combination with defocus is corrected by using spherocylinder lenses.

In the majority of clinical situations, the spherocylinder correction addresses adequately the visual needs of the most patients. However, human eyes also suffer from some higher order aberrations. Higher order aberrations are more complex than lower order aberrations. They cannot be corrected with regular spectacle lenses or contact lenses. These aberrations degrade and deform the image quality

Chapter 4: Retinal Image

Flowchart 4.3: Higher order aberrations.

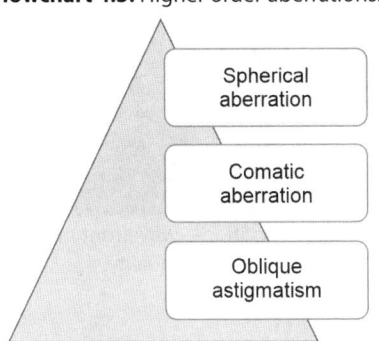

and are also associated with double vision, blurriness, ghosts, halos, starbursts, loss of contrast and poor night vision. Although there are several higher order aberrations, the three most commonly heard among them are given by **Flowchart 4.3**.

Spherical Aberration

The refractive power of ocular structure is greater for peripheral rays than paraxial rays which means the peripheral rays of light bend more quickly than the paraxial rays as shown in **Figure 4.5**. The effect of spherical aberration on retinal image is a symmetrical blur like defocus which is reduced by the size of pupil (**Fig. 4.6**). In human eye spherical aberration is the result of positive spherical aberration of the cornea and the negative spherical aberration of the crystalline lens. It is because of this spherical aberration is low in young eyes as compared to aging eyes.

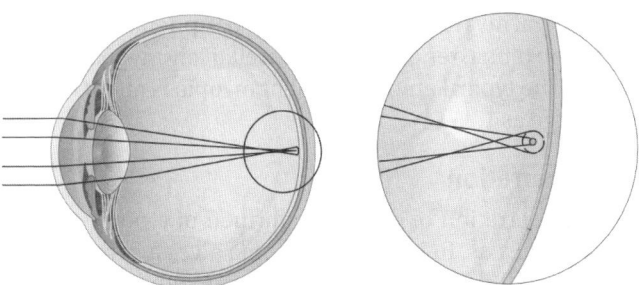

Fig. 4.5: Spherical aberration.

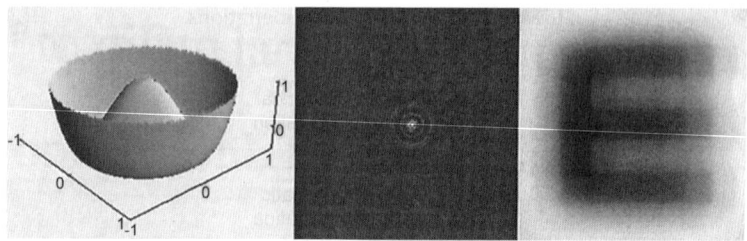

Fig. 4.6: Spherical aberration—wavefront map, retinal image and visual quality.

Influencing Factors

The effect of spherical aberration in the human eyes is reduced by several factors:

❖ The anterior corneal surface is flatter at the periphery than at its center, and therefore acts as an aplanatic surface.
❖ The iris acts as a stop to reduce spherical aberration. The impairment of visual acuity that occurs when pupil is dilated is almost entirely due to spherical aberration.
❖ The nucleus of the lens of the eye has a higher refractive index than the lens cortex. Hence, the axial zone of the lens has greater refractive power than the periphery.
❖ The retinal cones are more sensitive to light which enters the eye paraxially than the light which enters obliquely through peripheral cornea. This directional sensitivity of the cone receptors limits the visual effects of the residual spherical aberration in the eye.

Clinical Application

Spherical aberration accounts for much of the phenomenon known as "Night Myopia". At low light levels, the pupil enlarges and allows more peripheral rays to enter the eye. The peripheral rays are focused anterior to the retina, rendering the eye relatively myopic in the lower light levels. The typical amount of night myopia is about 0.5 D, but it can be as large as 1.25 D.

Comatic Aberration

Coma is an aberration of the image formed of a point object lying off the principal axis. In human eyes coma gives a comet-like image because of small decentration of the cornea and the lens, which

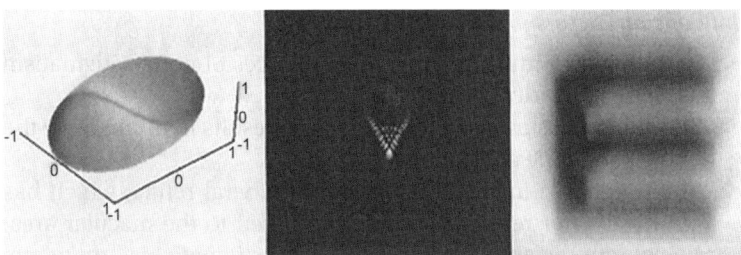

Fig. 4.7: Coma—Wavefront map, retinal image and visual quality.

results in different magnifications in the different parts of the pupil (**Fig. 4.7**). Coma degrades and deforms the image, i.e., the center of the image is clear but it becomes increasingly blur towards the edges. Coma is a wide beam aberration. Since most of the daytime undilated pupil is around 2–3 mm in size, the ocular cometic aberration does not carry much of practical importance.

Oblique Astigmatism

If the point object is in the peripheral field of vision, the light rays from it will focus in such a way so as to produce comatic aberration. Imagine that coma is eliminated; human eye may still suffer from another aberration known as oblique astigmatism. The oblique incident rays emerging from the object create oblique astigmatism after refraction in the human eye. The more oblique is the object, the worse is the resulting astigmatism. Oblique astigmatism is a narrow beam aberration, and the visual effect is not more than reduction of contrast (**Fig. 4.8**).

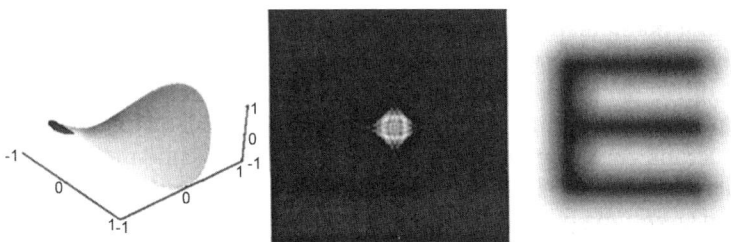

Fig. 4.8: Oblique astigmatism—wavefront map, retinal image and visual quality.

Chapter 4: Retinal Image

Influencing Factors
- Aplanatic curvature of the cornea reduces oblique astigmatism as well as spherical aberration.
- The spherical surface of the retina also results in minimizing the effect of oblique aberration.
- The astigmatic image falls on the peripheral retina, which has relatively poor resolving power compared to the macular area. Visual appreciation of the oblique astigmatic is, therefore, limited.

Clinical Application
Oblique astigmatism aberration can also be a problem when objective measure of the refractive error of an eye is attempted. This is especially important when retinoscopy is performed on a patient who does not maintain fixation, as commonly seen in small children.

RATIONALE FOR HIGHER ORDER ABERRATION

Aberrations exist throughout the ocular system, in the cornea and the crystalline lens. There have been a number of methods developed to quantify these aberrations. Most popular among them is the Hartmann-Shack principle that provides a rapid and objective measure of the wave aberrations at large number of points across the pupil. The three-dimensional picture of wave aberration so captured can be described as the sum of the various components of lower order and higher order aberrations which can be decomposed into component aberrations like defocus, astigmatism, coma, spherical aberration and other higher order aberrations trefoil, tetrafoil, quadrafoil and many more. Frits Zernike, a physicist, developed a set of mathematical functions to describe the wavefront aberration for circular pupils that incorporates as many as 65 individual Zernike modes. Each Zernike mode represents a particular aberration and has a value that indicates its magnitude, usually expressed in microns, corresponding to its root mean square or standard deviation across the pupil. Defocus is the lower order aberration which has the largest magnitude, followed by two Zernike modes representing astigmatism. Higher order aberration corresponds to those beyond the first three.

A conventional refraction that detects spherical, cylinder and axis typically corrects only low order aberration—defocus and two astigmatic modes.

Wavefront data provides the basis for several other functions that can be used to define the image quality on retina using modulation transfer function and point spread function. The advantage of these functions is that we can compute from aberrations which are captured at eye's pupil, the impact they will have on the quality of the image formed on the retina. This computational link between pupil and retina is very valuable as we can deduce the relative importance of different aberrations on image quality before taking decision for correction.

The point to be remembered is that the higher order aberrations are not static and can be altered by several factors in the optical system of the eye. Larger the pupil size, greater is the amount of aberrations which means visual performance will automatically be affected in scotopic condition. In smaller pupils, diffraction dominates and the higher order aberrations are relatively unimportant.

The effect of higher order aberration also grows with age. As the patient grows in age, the lens properties change which results in an increase in the amount of aberration.

Accommodation is also said to have the effect on these aberrations as the amount and characteristics of these aberrations change significantly when the eye accommodates.

Probably, it is because of these reasons there is considerable amount of debate concerning the visual benefits of correcting these higher order aberrations of the eye. There are some prevailing opinions for correcting these higher order aberrations as there is a possibility of improving contrast sensitivity. But there is more to vision than just high contrast resolution. Visual need depends upon a person's age, vocations and activities. A 42-year-old person may be happier sacrificing 20/20 line for 20/30 for his distances vision so that he can read without using his reading glasses. In contrast, a 20-year-old athlete may have the need for highest possible resolution to see the fast approaching object. So the more important question is not whether to correct these higher order aberrations but to see how many people will benefit and whether or not they really need.

Chapter 4: Retinal Image

MULTIPLE CHOICE QUESTIONS

1. Which of the following describes a retinal image that is not properly focused?
   a. Distorted image
   b. Deformed image
   c. Defocused image
   d. Degrade image
2. Which of the following refractive errors is most likely to result in a degraded retinal image for both near and distant objects?
   a. Hyperopia
   b. Myopia
   c. Astigmatism
   d. Presbyopia
3. What impact does a defocused retinal image have on visual acuity?
   a. Enhanced acuity
   b. No impact on acuity
   c. Reduced acuity
   d. Improved color discrimination
4. What does astigmatism in the eyes primarily affect in the formation of the retinal image?
   a. Central vision
   b. Color perception
   c. Peripheral vision
   d. Image clarity
5. Which part of the eye is responsible for focusing light onto the retina?
   a. Lens
   b. Cornea
   c. Retina
   d. Optic nerve

ANSWER KEY

1. c	2. c	3. c	4. d	5. b			

SELF-PRACTICE QUESTIONS

1. Retinal image serves as the foundation of vision—Explain.
2. While correcting higher order aberrations can be beneficial in specific cases, especially for individuals with specific visual complaints, the overall impact on visual acuity and daily visual tasks may not be impacted significantly. Explain the rationale behind correcting higher order aberration in light of its impact in daily life.

5 CHAPTER

Refractive Error

CHAPTER OUTLINE

- Myopia
- Hypermetropia
- Regular Astigmatism
- Pathological Hypermetropia
- Pathological Myopia
- Irregular Astigmatism

Refractive errors are visual disorders that affect the ability of the eye to refract or bend the light. The rays of light are not correctly focused on retina and therefore blur image is created, troubling the subject to see the world clearly. The condition may develop because of the axial length of the eye, abnormalities in the shape of cornea or changes in the refractive power of the optical elements of the eye with respect to the location of the retina. The vast majority of refractive errors are simple that present no medical problem and are not meant to be worried about. From the clinical point of view, they may be said to be simple refractive errors. These types of refractive errors are primarily hereditary or of chance incident. They are not progressive beyond the amount included within normal development and are associated with good vision. They do not require any treatment other than their optical correction. Some refractive errors are pathological in nature. Pathological refractive error is because of the presence of refractive anomalies in the optical system of the eye which is outside the limits of the normal biological variations.

Simple refractive errors are broadly classified into three categories:
1. Myopia
2. Hypermetropia
3. Regular astigmatism

MYOPIA

Myopia is the form of refractive error in which parallel rays of light are brought to focus in front of the sentient layer of retina, when the eye is at rest as shown in **Figure 5.1**. The image on retina is made of circle of diffusion formed by the diverging beam. The effect of which is seen as blurred distance vision. In order to see the object clearly, it must be brought closer to the eye so that rays of light coming from it are pushed onto the retina. That is why myopia is often termed as shortsightedness or nearsightedness. The far point in myopia is a finite distance away. It is between infinity and the eye, in front of the eye. Higher the myopia, shorter is the far point.

Symptoms

Myopia is a one-symptom refraction problem, i.e., blurring of distance vision. Patients may adopt a habitual squint to simulate the effect produced by a pinhole pupil and a 'furrowed brow', both of which are classic manifestation of uncorrected myopia. In smaller degree of error, eye strain may become evident, although not so obvious as in the case of hypermetropia. The constant screwing of lids in an attempt to clear vision may induce headache.

The myope often fails to recognize his visual limitations when he begins to look upon the world, especially when his close work is not affected. He accepts his distance blurring as normal and neglects

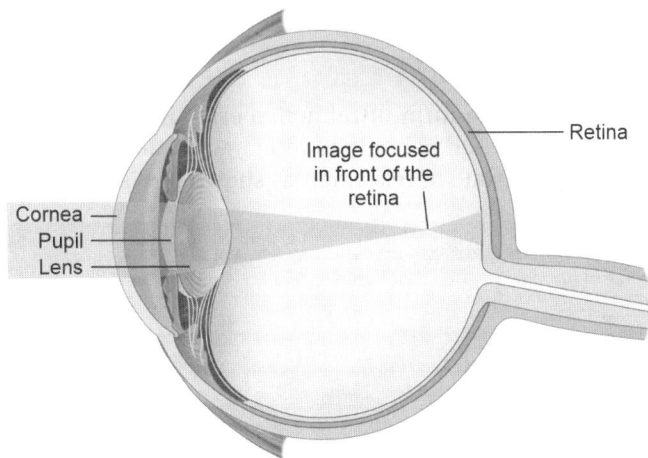

Fig. 5.1: Myopic eye.

until it affects his visual performance. In middle age, when the accommodation fails, he has an additional advantage as he does not require additional correction for near vision. In old age his contracting pupil cuts down diffusion circles and as the senile changes in his lens bring on a relative hypermetropia, he is in happy position of finding his vision gradually improving.

The blur in reading results when the patient holds the print at a reading distance which is farther than his far point. Reading while uncorrected at near point may lead to asthenopia. This may be because of the greater proximity of the target that calls for increased convergence. Sometimes patient moves the object closer than the far point in an attempt to relieve.

Visual Acuity in Myopia

Visual acuity beyond the far point is seriously affected in uncorrected myopia, being reduced by almost the same ratio as occurs in absolute hypermetropia. Although it is difficult to predict what would be the loss of visual acuity in different degrees of myopia, it has been found to be closely related to what is given in **Table 5.1** in most cases.

The corrected visual acuity, in the absence of degenerative changes, in contradistinction to the vision in hypermetropia is usually good. However, it is to be remembered that individuals who use spectacles habitually see less without the spectacle as compared to those who wear spectacle intermittently or not at all. This is because of perceptual reasons and not because of any physical reasons.

HYPERMETROPIA

Hypermetropia is the form of refractive error in which parallel rays of light are focused behind the retina, while accommodation is maintained in a state of relaxation as shown in **Figure 5.2**. In a

Table 5.1: Visual acuity in different degree of myopia.

Degree of myopia	V/A based on feet	V/A based on meter
−0.50 D	20/25	6/7.5
−1.0 D	20/40	6/12
−1.50 D	20/80	6/24
−2.00 D	20/160	6/48
−3.00 D	20/250	6/75
−4.00 D	20/400	6/120

Chapter 5: Refractive Error

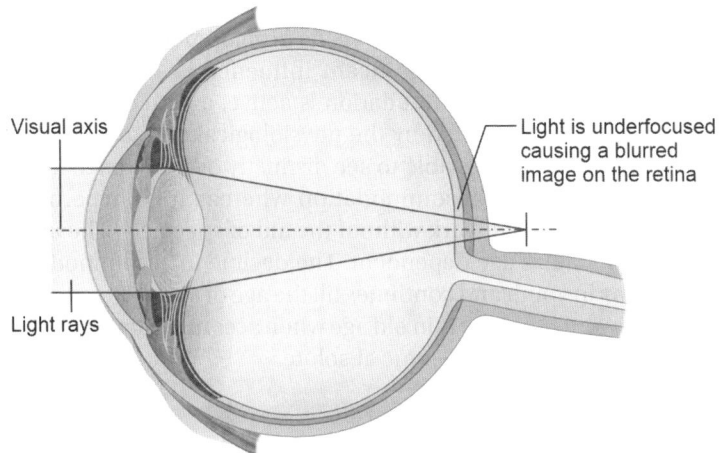

Fig. 5.2: Hypermetropic eye.

hypermetropic eye the focal point is located behind the retina and therefore the image formed on retina is made up of circles of diffusion and is consequently blurred. The patient can manage to see the distant objects clearly by exerting accommodation. But they have difficulty in focusing on close objects. That is why hypermetropia is often termed as farsightedness. However, more severe farsightedness would also cause problems with seeing objects in the distance clearly.

The following variations in the optical components of eye are most commonly responsible in simple hypermetropia:
- Flattening of cornea or the lens
- A deep anterior chamber
- A low refractivity of the lens
- A small axial length of the eye

Children are typically born with a certain degree of hypermetropia. In infancy, a range of +2.00 D to +3.00 D of hypermetropia is commonly observed. This hypermetropia tends to increase initially, reaching its peak around 6 months of age, and then gradually decreases through a process known as emmetropization. By the age of 6 years, the visual system typically stabilizes around emmetropia, with a deviation of approximately ± 0.75 D. Any residual hypermetropia that persists at this stage tends to remain relatively stable until mid-life. However, due to changes in the crystalline lens, there is a tendency for hypermetropia to increase again in the later stages of life. This natural progression highlights the dynamic nature of refractive errors throughout the different stages of visual development and aging.

Accommodation has significant influence in hypermetropic patients. As long as accommodation is active, a certain amount of refractive error is corrected by the physiological tone of the ciliary muscle. Low hyperope is able to see distinctly over all range like an emmetrope by using accommodation whereas high hyperope is incapacitated for near work without the aid of spectacle. The ability to accommodate is age dependent. The decline in accommodation ability starts in youth and continues till the age of about 60 years. The straightforward meaning is in old age when accommodation fails; all hypermetropia tends to become absolute.

Type of Hypermetropia

Flowchart 5.1 shows the different types of hypermetropia.

Absolute Hypermetropia

Absolute hypermetropia is a type of hypermetropia which cannot be corrected by accommodative efforts. It is given by the weakest convex lens with which maximum visual acuity can be achieved. Absolute hypermetropia affects distance visual acuity much in the same proportion as myopia.

Facultative Hypermetropia

Facultative hypermetropia is the type of hypermetropia which can be overcome by accommodative efforts. It is given by the difference

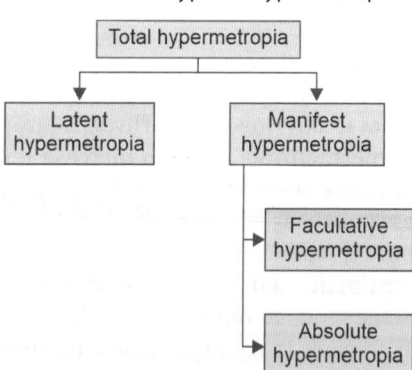

Flowchart 5.1: Types of hypermetropia.

between strongest and weakest convex lens with which maximal visual acuity can be achieved. Importantly, the presence of facultative hypermetropia, in and of itself, does not lead to a decrease in visual acuity. The ability to overcome this hypermetropia through accommodation contributes to maintaining clear vision without a significant impact on visual acuity.

Manifest Hypermetropia

Manifest hypermetropia is the total of facultative and absolute hypermetropia. The strongest convex lens with which the maximum visual acuity can be obtained, is the measure of manifest hypermetropia.

Latent Hypermetropia

Latent hyperopia is a term used to describe the amount of farsightedness that is 'masked' when the accommodative muscles are used to increase the eye's focusing power. Since children under 10 years of age have tremendous focusing ability, they can partially correct their farsightedness by accommodation. It is totally by eye's own accommodative ability and can be detected only by cycloplegia.

Total Hypermetropia

Total hypermetropia is the sum total of latent and manifest hypermetropia. It is given by the strongest lens with which maximum visual acuity can be obtained under complete cycloplegia.

Visual Acuity in Hypermetropia

The uncorrected visual acuity in hypermetropia is refractive error dependent and the proportion which cannot be overcome by accommodation. Therefore, visual acuity is poor in high degree of refractive error but for lower degree as usually seen in youth when the accommodation is active, there may not be any visual symptoms. Facultative hypermetropia does not by itself involve any decrease in visual acuity, but absolute hypermetropia which cannot be overcome by accommodation affects the visual acuity in the same proportion as myopia.

The corrected visual acuity often does not come up to standard especially in higher degree of hypermetropia. This is mostly because of perceptual factor. It may also be due to lack of retinal development in some cases. However, in smaller degrees of hypermetropia poor visual acuity is found to be rare.

Symptoms

The clinical symptoms in hypermetropia significantly vary in lower degree than that of higher degree of hypermetropia. In lower degree of hypermetropia, particularly in young patients, whom accommodation is active, both visual and clinical symptoms are usually entirely absent. However, if accommodation falls short of the task as it may be seen in advancing age or may come on in states of physical and nervous debility, visual troubles occur after long-continued application to close work when the vision becomes temporarily blurred and only recovers when the patient rests his ciliary muscles for some time. Symptoms of eye strain are frequent in these conditions which the patient expresses as:

- Headache and asthenopia are common problems of uncorrected hypermetropia.
- General physical disturbances
- Mental unhappiness
- Dislike of work
- Early tiring
- Rubbing of the eyes, this may be because reflex response to discomfort due to prolonged near work
- Itching
- Twitching of the lids

In higher degree of hypermetropia both visual and clinical symptoms are marked. The patient may complain of:

- Nothing is seen clearly unless with significant effort is made.
- Nearby objects are completely blurry.
- The object is held farther away.

REGULAR ASTIGMATISM

Astigmatism is an imperfection in the curvature of cornea or lens, in which no point focus is formed because of the unequal refraction of incident light by the optical system of the eye in different meridians as shown in **Figure 5.3**. The astigmatic eye is unique in the sense that it has two far point planes, one for each of the two principal meridians of the refractive error. In simple myopic astigmatism, one plane is located at infinity and the other is at a finite distance in front of

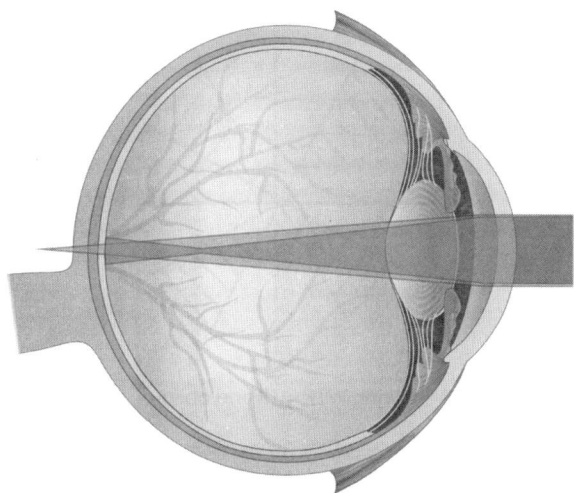

Fig. 5.3: Astigmatic eye.

the eye. In compound myopic astigmatism, the two far point planes are located at different distances in front of the eye. Similarly, in simple hyperopic astigmatism, one plane is located at infinity, and the other is located behind the eye, whereas in compound hyperopic astigmatism, both planes are located at different distances behind the eye. In mixed astigmatism, one far point plane is located in front of the eye, and the other is located behind the eye.

Patients with astigmatism cannot achieve perfect retinal clarity by holding an object at a single position, unlike myopic individuals. Additionally, accommodative effort does not help astigmatic patients achieve proper focus, unlike pre-presbyopic hyperopic patients. For astigmatic individuals, optical correction is the only option for creating sharp retinal imagery.

Classification of Astigmatism

Astigmatism may be with the rule, against the rule and oblique as shown in **Figure 5.4**.

In with-the-rule astigmatism, the focusing elements of the eye require more convergent power in the 180° meridian, which is corrected by plus cylinder at axis 90° or minus cylinder at axis 180°. In against-the-rule astigmatism, the focusing elements of the eye require more convergent power in the 90° meridian, which is

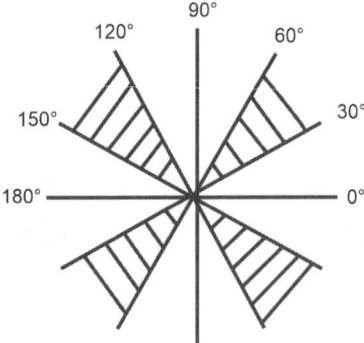

Fig. 5.4: Axes showing WTR, ATR and oblique astigmatism.

corrected by plus cylinder axis 180° or minus cylinder axis 90°. It is believed that newborn babies have a high prevalence of against-the-rule astigmatism, which decreases over the first few years of life. After 5 years of age, with-the-rule astigmatism gains the prevalence, the etiology of which is still not very clear. One common hypothesis is for such shift is the pressure exerted by the eyelids which steepens the vertical corneal meridian and causes with-the-rule astigmatism. Oblique astigmatism is characterized by the axes lying somewhere in between the axes defining either WTR or ATR astigmatism, between 120 and 150° and 30 and 60°.

Astigmatism may be corneal or lenticular in origin. Corneal astigmatism occurs when the curvature of anterior surface of cornea is different and is responsible for the majority of cases of astigmatism. The average difference between refractive power of two corneal meridians lies between 0.50 D to 0.75 D. When the astigmatism is because of difference in the refractive power of the two meridians of the crystalline lenses, it is called lenticular astigmatism. Lenticular astigmatism may also be because of tilted or decentered lenses.

Visual Acuity in Astigmatism

The vision in astigmatism is typically characteristic, affected by three factors—amount of astigmatism, type of astigmatism and the axis direction. Given the other factors remaining same, the dimensions of the focal line and the circle of least confusion of astigmatic pencil are directly proportional to the amount of astigmatism in Diopter.

Given the pupil size, the retinal blur depends on which the cross-section of the astigmatic pencil lies on the retina and whether any improvement can be brought about by accommodation. In simple and compound myopic astigmatism, the distance vision cannot be improved by accommodation. In such cases the vision would be expected to be approximately the same as in spherical ametropia equal to the spherical equivalent. In simple and compound hypermetropic astigmatism, the subject can place the most favorable cross-section of the astigmatic pencil on the retina, provided the sufficient accommodation is available. In case of mixed astigmatism, only one focal line is behind the retina which means more limitation is imposed on the scope of improvement in vision by accommodation. However, it depends more on the position of circle of least confusion, which one is in front of the retina or behind the retina.

Since vertical and horizontal lines predominate in test letters as well as in most objects in our environment, vision is poorest when the astigmatism is at oblique axis, all other factors remaining the same. Another important factor is that in printed matter there is usually less space between the letters on a line than between the lines themselves. Consequently, if the horizontal focal lines or ellipse are being formed on the retina, the letters will appear to 'run together' and become indistinct.

The corrected visual acuity in the low degree of astigmatism can be brought back to normal standards or above, but in higher degree this is not always possible, particularly if the correction is not made in early life and also if the astigmatism is oblique.

Symptoms

Astigmatic patient usually does not complain of visual difficulties excluding significantly larger astigmatism. However, constant effort to see clearly in hypermetropic and mixed astigmatism may cause symptoms of eye strain. In the majority of cases small error does not give rise to discomfort, they may be accepted as physiological and may not require correction. In some cases, all symptoms of eye strain including headache, dizziness, fatigue, irritability may be observed.

PATHOLOGICAL HYPERMETROPIA

Pathological hypermetropia is seldom found. The major reasons that have been cited for pathological hypermetropia are either shortening of anteroposterior axis of the eye and abnormal small curvature of the cornea. A developmental flattening of corneal curvature is seen that may result in hypermetropia. Acquired flattening of cornea may result from injury or disease with contraction of wounds or corneal ulcers with irregular astigmatic changes as most common. Flattening of cornea has also been seen in some cases of glaucoma with increased intraocular pressure.

PATHOLOGICAL MYOPIA

Pathological myopia, also known as degenerative myopia, is a severe form of myopia that can lead to vision loss and other eye problems. It is characterized by a refractive error of at least −6.00 diopter or more, along with changes in the retina and other parts of the eye. In pathological myopia, the eyeball grows longer than normal, causing the retina to stretch and thin which can increase the risk of other eye conditions, such as retinal detachment, cataracts, glaucoma, and myopic macular degeneration. There are several potential causes of pathological myopia, including genetics, environmental factors, and certain medical conditions. The gross appearance of the highly myopic eye is characteristic both in shape and size. Pathological changes in the posterior segment of the globe are more than the anterior segment of the globe. The clinical features of pathological myopia are:

- ❖ The pupil is usually dilated and somewhat sluggish in reaction.
- ❖ Myopic crescent becomes evident as it appears as white sharply defined area lying on the temporal side of the optic disc.
- ❖ Choroidal atrophy, changes in optic disc, changes in retina, sclera ectasias and degenerative changes in vitreous, detachments and formation of hyaloids holes are also common.

IRREGULAR ASTIGMATISM

Irregular astigmatism can be caused by a number of factors, including corneal scarring, keratoconus, trauma to the eye, or previous eye surgery. The condition is characterized by refraction in different meridians conforms to no geometrical plan and refracted rays have no planes of symmetry.

PRESBYOPIA

Presbyopia is an age-related loss of ability to focus on things up close **(Fig. 5.5)**. It affects almost everyone around the age of 40 years. It is the failure of accommodation to provide a clear image of the near object at a normal reading distance. Failure of accommodation may be because of two factors:

- Physical changes in crystalline lens rendering its deformation difficult.
- Functional incapacity of the ciliary muscles to bring changes in crystalline lens.

If the lens scleroses and becomes hard as it does with advancing age or in cataract, it is no longer sufficiently elastic to allow its deformation. Thereby accommodation cannot be affected by the contraction of the ciliary muscle. On the other hand, weak ciliary muscle will not be able to induce changes in a normally elastic lens. These two elements are fundamentally distinct and are often termed as physical and physiological accommodation. Physical accommodation fails in presbyopia such that accommodation becomes difficult, on the other hand the ability of ciliary muscles may decrease in situation of debility at any age, diminishing or abolishing the accommodation. The changes in crystalline lens are gradual and it advances with age throughout whole life without any sudden alteration. At first no difficulty is experienced, but eventually the near point recedes beyond the usual distance at which the subject is used to reading and then it becomes difficult, the stage so reached is called presbyopia.

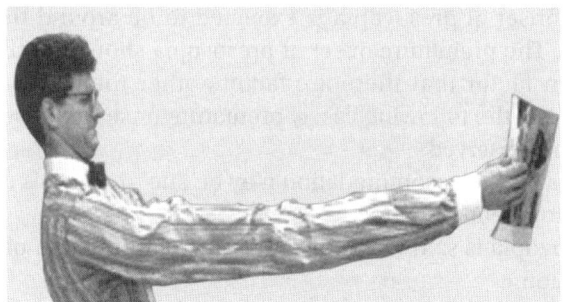

Fig. 5.5: Presbyopic patient.

Symptoms

The common symptoms that the patient reports in presbyopia are:
- Blurring of vision at near vision distance is most common. Small print becomes indistinct especially in reduced illumination.
- The eyes tire quickly so that the print becomes indistinct after reading for a few minutes.
- The lines run together and overlap and sometimes double.
- Gradually symptoms of eye strain start. The ciliary muscle working near its limit tire and accommodative effort strained to its limit and acting in excess of convergence, gives rise to distress—the eyes feel tired and ache, headache comes on.
- Some patients complain of glare while reading books.

The patient may complain in different ways. Some of the examples that are commonly seen in practice are:
- I have to stretch my hands to read as shown in **Figure 5.5**.
- I have difficulties in threading a needle.
- Myopes report removing of their spectacles for near vision task.

A hyperope starts life with his near point considerably farther away, the decline in accommodative power is noted sooner. The opposite holds true in case of myopes. In case of low myopia, presbyopia will be delayed. Emmetrope in most situation, behaves in the same way as hyperopes behave. Thus, presbyopia is a relative term. It varies with the individual and also with his habit. A person with a habit of reading complains of discomfort sooner than a person who does not have a reading habit.

Premature Onset of Presbyopia

Usually onset of presbyopia is expected to be around the age of 40 years. The premature onset of presbyopia should always excite suspicion factor that there are factors other than physiological involved. In the following cases, premature onset of presbyopia is commonly observed:
- The failure of accommodation may be due to sclerosis of lens or development of cataract.
- Presbyopia is said to appear early after suppression of ovarian function.
- Glaucoma is said to be the reason for early presbyopia.
- The general health is also frequently associated with ciliary weaknesses. It has been noted that conditions like anemia,

Chapter 5: Refractive Error

diabetes, lactation, tuberculosis are all associated with early presbyopia.

MULTIPLE CHOICE QUESTIONS

1. **What is refractive error?**
   a. Refractive error means that the rays of light are not focused properly on retina, resulting in a blurred image.
   b. Reduction in visual field
   c. Recent onset may be disease in eye
   d. All of the above
2. **What is myopia?**
   a. Myopia is a vision defect in which case rays of light coming from infinity focus before retina.
   b. Myopia is a disease in which case rays of light coming from infinity focus before retina.
   c. Myopia is a condition in which case rays of light focus on retina.
   d. Myopia is a vision defect in which case rays of light coming from infinity focus after retina.
3. **What is hypermetropia?**
   a. Hypermetropia is a vision defect in which case rays of light coming from infinity focus before retina.
   b. Hypermetropia is a disease in which case rays of light coming from infinity focus before retina.
   c. Hypermetropia is a condition in which case rays of light focus on retina.
   d. Hypermetropia is a vision defect in which case rays of light coming from infinity focus after retina.
4. **What is astigmatism?**
   a. Astigmatism is a condition where rays of light that propagate in two perpendicular planes have different foci.
   b. Astigmatism is a condition where rays of light that propagate in two perpendicular planes focus before retina.
   c. Astigmatism is a condition where rays of light that propagate in two perpendicular planes focus at one point.
   d. All of the above
5. **Presbyopia commonly occurs due to:**
   a. Elongation of the eyeball
   b. Shortening of the eyeball
   c. Loss of flexibility in the lens
   d. Irregular corneal curvature

Chapter 5: Refractive Error

ANSWER KEY

1. a   2. a   3. d   4. a   5. c

SELF-PRACTICE QUESTIONS

1. Explain the impact of astigmatism on visual perception. Discuss how uneven corneal curvature or lens shape contributes to astigmatism.
2. Elaborate on the symptoms of astigmatic patient.

CHAPTER 6

Fundamentals of Clinical Refraction

CHAPTER OUTLINE

- Laws of Clinical Refraction
- Goal of Clinical Refraction
- Cardinal Principles of Clinical Refraction
- Clinical Refraction: An Intellectual Procedure
- Methods of Clinical Refraction
- Correction of Refractive Error
- Trial Framing

Clinical refraction refers to a set of clinical procedures applied to measure refractive error or determine the refractive state of the eye and arrive at a clinical decision as to the prescription for corrective lenses. The procedure is the part of the total eye care examination that provides an intimate opportunity for the examiner to know the patient and his visual system—how exactly his visual system is behaving. The methods adopted to measure the refractive error are numerous. The practitioners often have their preferences for specific techniques. The diversity in methods reflects the evolving nature of clinical refraction, allowing for a personalized approach tailored to individual patient needs. It is important to note that what is measured during clinical refraction may not always align precisely with what is ultimately prescribed. This variation underscores the nuanced nature of determining the most suitable corrective lenses for an individual, considering factors beyond just numerical measurements.

Clinical refraction is best approached as a problem-solving procedure. Finding a suitable solution for the problem can be accomplished by following the basic rules of the problem-solving approach, which includes diagnosing and determining the presence of the problem, evaluating the implications of what has been diagnosed and determined, and finally implementing and following up on the solution. In light of the above, clinical refraction can be defined as an art and science that includes:

- Assessing the refractive state of the eye and measuring the refractive error
- Prescribing the appropriate refractive corrections
- Counseling the patient as to the use of refractive correction

A good refraction requires patience and a good connection with the patient. The lenses that are prescribed must address the patient's problem, and at the end, it is the patient's satisfaction, not the precise prescription for refractive correction, which is of paramount significance.

The examiner must apply his knowledge of optics, ocular structure, their functioning, and techniques of measurement together with a combination of other skills and intellectual processes to examine the eyes and visual system of an individual with the objective of prescribing a suitable correction so that he is able to perform his visual task comfortably. Practice and experience add to the skills of the examiner.

Additionally, the examiner must be congenial and a little talkative to understand the patient in terms of his profession, work, hobbies, and special interests, be able to elicit the visual needs, understand his concern, and thereafter apply his clinical judgmental ability to prescribe the appropriate correction to meet the objective. Finally, an explanation and binocular demonstration of what he prescribes always help to win patient's confidence.

Refraction is done in a clinical setting with the help of a set of trial lenses, a visual acuity test chart, and other equipment. Room illumination and test distance are two critical elements that are specific to the test employed. The patient needs to be relaxed; sitting on a chair throughout the procedure, and the clinician may either stand beside the patient or sit right in front of him, depending on his own comfort.

▌LAWS OF CLINICAL REFRACTION (TABLE 6.1)

There are innumerable tests and techniques used in the examination of the eye for the determination of the refractive error. These procedures include tests for assessing various visual functions like

Chapter 6: Fundamentals of Clinical Refraction

Table 6.1: Laws of clinical refraction.	
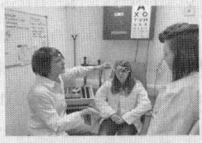	All tests and techniques applied for the purpose of assessment of refractive state of the eye can be categorized in three broad categories for the purpose of understanding their implications.
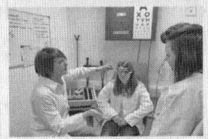	All patients that we see in the clinical practice for the purpose of assessment of refractive state of the eye can also be classified in three broad groups for the purpose of driving the objective driven clinical procedure.
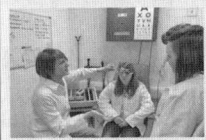	A routine procedure comprising a set of tests and techniques may be devised for an individual practice that may be applied in each case as a part of basic routine procedure.
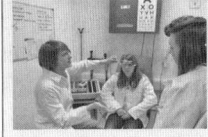	Additional tests or techniques may be adopted on case-to-case basis.

visual acuity, tests for accommodative function, detection and refinement of spherical and cylindrical correction, a near vision test, the binocular coordination of the eye, and others as needed. Each function can be examined by a number of tests, and for each test there are specific equipment, tools, and charts that are used. It is not possible to apply all tests to each patient, nor is it possible for a clinician to possess equal competence in all tests. Most clinicians therefore select their own preferred tests and techniques for their day-to-day practice and apply them to their patients. The refractive state of the eye can be determined objectively by a retinoscope or an auto-refractometer, and then it is verified subjectively by trial lenses using a trial frame or phoropter together with Snellen's test charts. Subjective method may be manifest monocular subjective refraction, fogging method of refraction, or other. When the results of the refraction are attained, the measured correction is normally refined using refinement tests.

There are different types of patients that are seen in clinical practice, differing because of age, gender, occupation, and intellectual level. The specific vision requirements of each individual patient may vary because of these factors. Moreover, different patients present with different types of symptoms. Blurring of vision is the most common symptom. Blurring may be at distance vision or it may be at near. Blurring may be intermittent, or it may be transient. The ciliary muscle may give up any attempt to focus or go into spasm, and the image may become indistinct. Also, the external muscles may also fail to work together, and the transient diplopia may result or the convergence function may fail, and therefore the letters may seem to run together. Pain is another common symptom. Ocular pain, not related to inflammation, is almost always muscular in origin and is due to fatigue. The reflective symptoms may arise from eye strain and may include headache, mild vertigo, and a host of other manifestations. In most cases, the vision may be affected, which may add to the difficulties.

Several factors affect the refractive correction of the eye. Ocular disease, systemic disease, medications, psychological state, physical health, occupational need—all of these factors must be considered before prescribing the correction. Visual fatigue has a profound effect on the visual system, especially when the visual demand exceeds the visual skills. Therefore, nothing is more detrimental than the routine correction of optical defects by rule-of-thumb methods. Not only is the eye to be treated as an optical system, but it ought to be considered an integral part of the body, sharing with other organs in its constitutional variations.

The above explanation clearly states that vision is affected by multiple factors, and when things go wrong with the visual system, it can have a profound effect on everything that we do. Therefore, the objective of clinical refraction is not to treat the eyes but to treat the patient as a whole. It is important to analyze previous corrections and the current visual status of the visual system and understand the visual needs of the patient before prescribing the new correction, and the decision to change the correction should be considered based upon the patient's lifestyle, profession, working environment, and other related factors. It is prudent to avoid large changes in prescription. In the event that it becomes necessary, it is crucial to conclude with a thorough explanation to the patient. This should include detailed information about the potential for initial difficulties and the expectation of a brief adaptation period.

Occasionally, there are temporary and sudden changes in the refraction due to local or systematic reasons, as has been observed

Chapter 6: Fundamentals of Clinical Refraction

in cases of accommodative paralysis, accommodative spasm, uveitis, changes in crystalline lenses, diabetes, and other ocular and systemic conditions. The examiner must adopt a different approach in such cases to address the symptoms resulting from such conditions. The prescription for the lenses should always be regulated by the physician's grasp of the organic condition underlying the symptom.

Hence, the prescription of refractive correction necessitates a thoughtful intellectual process that considers various aspects of the patient's life, activities, occupational demands, and individual traits such as personality and intelligence. This holistic approach is crucial in tailoring the refractive correction to align with the patient's specific needs and lifestyle. Building upon this understanding, fundamental laws of clinical refraction can be formulated, as presented in **Table 6.1**. These laws serve as a foundation upon which an effective clinical assessment methodology can be devised for each individual patient. This methodology takes into account not only the numerical measurements of refractive error but also the broader context of the patient's daily life, work commitments, and personal characteristics. The goal is to provide a comprehensive and personalized prescription that optimally addresses the visual requirements and preferences of the specific patient.

> *All tests and techniques applied for the purpose of assessment of refractive state of the eye can be categorized in three broad categories for the purpose of understanding their implications.*

The clinical refraction starts with an extensive history of the individual and ends with an individualized prescription and appropriate management provided to the patient. A quick and efficient refraction involves a number of procedures that, if done in a logical order, really provide the most predictable results. In order to develop one's own strategy, the clinician may categorize all tests into three broad categories, as shown in **Flowchart 6.1**.

Entrance tests are the first procedure performed to initiate the whole process of clinical refraction. They are relatively simple

Flowchart 6.1: Classification of tests used for the purpose of clinical refraction.

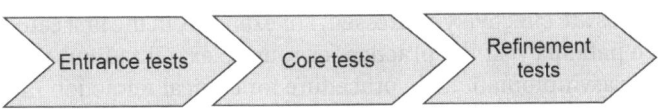

procedures and help assimilate preliminary data and set up the goal of clinical refraction. Core tests are routine procedures that are applied almost in every case for the purpose of refractive error assessment after the completion of entrance tests. They can be viewed as the tests that verify and establish the error detected at the entrance test level. The clinician's practice philosophy and demographic characteristics of patients influence what tests will be included in the core tests. It is, therefore, possible to see the overlapping of different tests between the two categories in different practices. The end point of the whole process aims to refine the results as derived and verified from the aforementioned two sets of test procedures. This seems to be a meaningful categorization as it entails spontaneously strong concentration and attention towards each test.

> *All patients that we see in the clinical practice for the purpose of assessment of refractive state of the eye can also be classified in three broad groups for the purpose of driving the objective-driven clinical procedure.*

The hypothesis is that all the patients who visit the practitioner for the purpose of assessment of refractive error, irrespective of age, gender, and occupation, may be divided into three broad categories, and therefore, specific goals and objectives for each category may be set to achieve out of the whole process of clinical refraction. The objective is to apply the relevant tests, which may be termed minimum tests needed, to achieve the desired objectives. In this age of managed health care, there is no scope to perform all the tests on every patient simply to collect data. It is important that the problem is detected efficiently within minimum possible time, allowing probing each problem with more specific tests. It is important to keep in mind that both patients and practitioners want a positive interaction to ensure the best possible health outcome, as time spent in consultations is valuable for both parties. The author's opinion as to such a classification is given in **Flowchart 6.2**.

This categorization proves advantageous as it allows for a targeted approach in guiding the clinical assessment of the refractive state of the eye within each category, ensuring that the specific objectives for routine examinations, symptomatic cases, and non-adaptation instances are effectively addressed. For example, in the first category, where patients visit the practice for routine examinations, they are usually asymptomatic. The procedure for clinical refraction may be

Chapter 6: Fundamentals of Clinical Refraction

Flowchart 6.2: Categorization of patients.

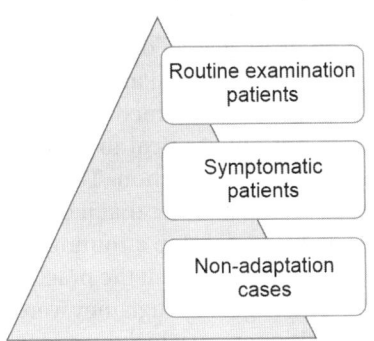

carried out with a simple routine set of tests to determine the state of the refractive error of the eye and to detect the early symptoms of any abnormality. In the second category, the primary objective is to diagnose the cause of the symptoms. The clinician's primary obligation is to understand the symptoms and apply relevant tests so that he can treat the patient's symptoms. However, for the third category of patients, the clinician must think beyond the paradigm of the routine process and drive all the tests and procedures to alleviate the patient's complaints and restore his lost confidence. The straight-forward understanding is that a set of different mechanics of refraction is warranted in each of these categories to achieve the desired objectives.

> *A routine procedure comprising of a set of tests and techniques may be devised for an individual practice that may be applied in each case as a part of basic routine procedure.*

The assumption here is that there are multiple tests for the assessment of each element of visual skill. A clinician may be more comfortable with one particular test than another. Patients also walk into the clinic with a set of beliefs and expectations affected by their personality, perceptions, and their own knowledge about the test procedures. They may also have had negative experiences and previous disappointments within the healthcare system that may be challenging to overcome and may generate some mistrust. They may feel that the clinician has not applied all the relevant tests before arriving at the conclusion or has not given him sufficient time to hear his complaints. Such circumstances can, understandably, make a patient feel anxious, worried, hopeless, and uncertain about their health, which can be displayed as disappointments and negative reactions towards the practitioner. Patients seek professional help because they are in pain or are concerned. The clinician must consider such factors that are not only critical to establishing the practice but also critical for patient satisfaction. Therefore, he must set up his practice model in such a manner that it delivers comprehensive care. All that is needed is to develop a routine set of tests that must be applied to all the patients who visit the practice. Thoroughness is the key, i.e., doing little things as though they were the greatest things in the world. The practitioner must feel the patient's pain, and at the same time, never forget that he is in the professional practice.

> *Additional tests and techniques may be adopted on case-to-case basis.*

There may be situations when the patient needs a problem-specific test that is equally important as the main procedure. When indicated, the clinician should be prepared to take a 'side trip', i.e., he must perform tests that are supplemental to the main tests. When the clinician follows the sequential flow of the procedure, he will be easily able to understand when the additional tests are indicated. Once the additional tests are completed, he should return to his main route and complete the examination. Sometimes, for the sake of efficient delivery of a specific test, the clinician may need to refer the case to an appropriate professional. There should not be any hesitation. The entire practice must be built around three factors: care, concern, and conviction.

▌GOAL OF CLINICAL REFRACTION

The laws of clinical refraction clearly state that setting up a precise goal for a patient is very critical for the effective application of a refraction procedure. The theoretical goal of the clinical application of a refraction procedure may be to prescribe a pair of lenses that ensure the retina is in conjugate with optical infinity. However, while correcting the refractive error, the practitioner should always remember that the patient will use the correction in real life to navigate through his occupational and visual needs. So, the importance of the real-life objective should be more important than the theoretical objective. In real life, during day-to-day activities, the process of vision has to be a subconscious function. The patient's visual satisfaction manifests only when he is able to cope with his occupational needs unconsciously and develops a positive feeling with his correction. If that happens, he continues with it comfortably for a prolonged period of time. Therefore, the true objective must be set for each patient individually before embarking on the procedure for assessing the refractive state of the eye. In general, the true objective of clinical refraction is always to prescribe correction that provides the patient with clear and comfortable vision to which he adapts quickly and also allows him to work for a longer period of time without any symptoms.

The law also states that there are three different categories of patients, and they must be treated to achieve specific objectives, which means goals may also vary accordingly. The objective behind setting up the objectives is to apply the mechanics of refraction that not only aim to enhance the vision but also focus on minimizing the disadvantage, if any. 6/6 or 20/20 is the end point of the procedure, which is usually achieved in most cases but not all.

CARDINAL PRINCIPLE OF CLINICAL REFRACTION

At the most fundamental the principle of clinical refraction states that the clinician should always keep in mind during clinical refraction that he should follow the principle of keeping the sleeping dog lie, i.e., he should avoid interfering with the lens prescription that is currently causing no difficulties but may cause difficulties if altered for no reason. This makes clinical refraction an art, a skill, and a science. It should also be understood that vision is a complex phenomenon. Achieving single, clear, and comfortable binocular vision is a task that is too demanding. Although the new sophisticated, technologically driven equipment have changed the way the refraction was done before and is done now, they could not yet replace clinical judgment of the clinician which is intellectually driven process.

Clinical judgment plays a critical role in clinical refraction, as it involves the clinician's subjective assessment and interpretation of the patient's visual needs, visual environment, responses and habitual correction. Clinical judgment also allows the clinician to tailor the refraction process to each patient's individual needs and provide the best possible visual correction. The cardinal principles of clinical refraction involve a series of steps that the clinician follows to determine a patient's refractive error and prescribe the appropriate corrective lenses. The following explanation sets out the key principles:

Principle 1: Pretest the Patient

Before beginning the measurement of refractive error, it is important to assess the patient's visual acuity, eye health, and current refractive status; take a complete case history; measure the patient's habitual glasses or contact lens prescription; and measure uncorrected visual acuity. This is important to gather initial data and rule out any ocular pathology before getting into process clinical refraction. It is also important that the clinician makes full attempt to build rapport with the patient during initial stage of interaction.

Principle 2: Proceed with a Purpose

Use a systematic and methodical approach to measure the refractive error. Every action and decision must be in line with the goal of clinical refraction. Avoid changing more trial lenses. A lengthy procedure creates boredom and fatigue, which can result in poor subjective responses. Do not offer more choices than are necessary to establish the endpoint. Remember that the differentiating gets harder as we get closer to the end point.

Principle 3: Measure Refractive Error Using Appropriate Tests

Use the appropriate tools, equipment and techniques to obtain accurate and reliable measurements. This includes using trial frame or a phoropter, with appropriate testing charts in appropriate environment for the respective test including test distance and room illumination.

Principle 4: Verify and Confirm What is Measured

Use a systematic and methodical approach to measure the refractive error of the patient and keep verifying the results at every stage. For example, the results of the objective refraction must be verified subjectively, and the results of the subjective refraction must be refined before prescribing using both techniques of refinement: monocular and binocular.

Principle 5: Prescribe to Treat Symptoms

Measuring refractive error and prescribing refractive correction are best approached as problem-solving procedures. It is, therefore, not necessary that what is measured is prescribed always. All decisions taken to prescribe refractive correction and counsel patient should be taken and executed in light of treating the patient's symptoms. If needed, for the sake of efficient management of specific symptoms, the clinician may need to refer the patient to an appropriate professional. Not only is the eye treated as an optical instrument, but it should always be considered as an integral part of the body, sharing with other organs in its constitutional variations and in the effects of the ills with which it may be afflicted.

Principle 6: Be Proactive as well as Reactive

As an optometrist, it is important to be both proactive and reactive in order to provide the best care to the patients. As a part of a proactive approach, he should educate patients on the importance of eye health, regular eye checkups, advice on the right solution, and the importance of preventive treatment. Being reactive means responding to patients' needs when they are experiencing eye problems or conditions.

This can include diagnosing and treating eye conditions as well as prescribing glasses or contact lenses to correct vision problems. By combining both proactive and reactive approaches seamlessly, the optometrist can help their patients maintain good eye health throughout their lives, and also provide effective treatments and support when issues do arise.

Principle 7: Avoid Making Large Changes

Making larger changes in the refractive correction may lead to non-adaptation and may also cause discomfort and even confusion in the patient. It is, therefore, prudent to follow a logical guideline for making changes in the spherical, cylindrical, and cylinder axes. Changes in near addition must be based on considering the changes made in distance correction so that the resultant change is within acceptable limits.

Principle 8: Be Empathetic to the Patient

Empathy involves understanding and sharing the patient's feelings, thoughts, and experiences, and being sensitive to their needs and concerns. During a clinical refraction, the patient may feel anxious or uncertain about the process or their visual health. It is important to create a safe and welcoming environment and to listen carefully to the patient's concerns. Communicate clearly and effectively with the patient throughout the refraction process. Keep explaining each step and the rationale behind it. It is important to note that the clinician should also take into account the patient's comfort level and any signs of eye fatigue or strain during the refraction. This will help to build trust and confidence in the patient and ensure that they are satisfied with their final prescription.

Principle 9: Allow Time for the Patient to Respond

Rushing to complete the procedure is never advisable. When changing a trial lens, it is important to wait for the patient to adjust to the new lens and give feedback on how the lens is affecting their vision. The patient may take some time. The process of changing a trial lens should be swift and deliberate, with ample time given to the patient to observe and evaluate the effect of the new lens. The clinician should also inform the patients when they have responded incorrectly on the Snellen's Visual Acuity Test chart in the most supportive and encouraging manner. By doing so, the clinician can help the patient understand the importance of providing accurate responses.

Principle 10: Record Everything that you Measure and Prescribe

Document all measurements and prescriptions accurately and legibly in a standard manner and include any relevant notes or observations. This will ensure that the information is available for future reference and can be used to monitor changes in the patient's visual status over time.

Principle 11: Counsel and Follow-up with the Patient

While prescribing the appropriate correction, the optometrist must counsel the patient to explain the prescription and the appropriate solution. Also, advise them on a follow-up program to ensure that the lenses are providing the intended visual correction. If necessary, make adjustments to the prescription or recommend further testing to address any unresolved visual issues.

The end point of clinical refraction is the clinical judgment of the clinician. It is important to keep in mind that the endpoint of clinical refraction is subjective and can vary between patients. It is essential to work with the patient to ensure that the final prescription provides

clear and comfortable vision in all viewing conditions. There are several signs that may indicate that the refraction is complete and that you are at or near the end point. These signs are listed below:
* The patient achieves the best-corrected visual acuity.
* The patient is happy with the correction.
* The further change in the correction does not improve visual acuity.
* The optometrist has exhausted all testing methods.
* The results are stable and consistent.

CLINICAL REFRACTION: AN INTELLECTUAL PROCESS

The law of clinical refraction is very intuitive. It makes the clinical refraction extremely perceptive and sensitive, making the entire procedure a powerful force of the mind that can help the clinician make better decisions. It applies to every element of clinical refraction at every stage.

The correction of visual defects involves examination of the refractive state of the eye, accommodation and convergence function, their mutual relationship, the muscular balance, the degree of binocular vision disorder and finally if possible and indicated, the size relationship of the retinal images of the two eyes.

It must be remembered that the eye is neither an accurately centered nor corrected optical system. It is characterized by inaccessible errors of spherical, chromatic, diffractive and astigmatic aberration, so that in no case an optically perfect image is formed.

The patient also presents myriad of symptoms which can be classified as visual, ocular, referred and functional. Prescribing of correction, therefore, should never degenerate into a routine correction of refractive error by rule of thumb method. It should also include a survey of patient's lifestyle, nature of work, amount of work, visual environment, physical abilities, his psychological reaction to life, established visual habits, changing visual demands and his habitual correction.

Clinical refraction is a patient centric and collaborative process to problem solving that helps patient get rid of their visual symptoms and navigate smoothly through the occupational and visual needs of daily life. The patient is at the center of everything that the examiner does. A good approach is all about empathy, so the examiner starts by understanding the patient and patient's visual needs. The initial phase consists of baseline data assimilation so he starts with extensive history taking to gather key information about his symptoms, his lifestyle and his visual needs and also tries to link to possible causes as a part of data analysis and data synthesis. This is when the examiner distils all information into critical thinking and discovers valuable insights about patient's ocular and visual condition. The process does not end there. The examiner goes beyond and implements several tests to measure the refractive error and then sits with the patient to optimize the results before prescribing. In this way the clinical refraction is a highly intellectual process as it involves mental exercise, intuition, thinking, ability to analyze and make judgment and other similar skills. It is absolutely not a trial-and-error method. While trial-and-error is a good way to test and experiment what works and what does not, it is often time-consuming, expensive, and ultimately ineffective. Clinical refraction requires setting objectives, making premises, looking at alternatives and finally prescribing the best one. All these require a lot of thinking process at every stage of the procedure. The entire procedure of clinical refraction can be articulated in six steps or phases as shown in **Flowchart 6.3**.

Data Assimilation

There are multiple ways that an examiner can adopt to collect objective and subjective data during the clinical refraction. Observation, communication, investigation and measurement are commonly used techniques. Applying them systematically and logically with purpose yields sufficient information that can be used effectively to achieve desired objectives. It requires application of wits and intelligence and knowledge of eye, visual system, patient's psychology, knowledge of relevant tests and procedures.

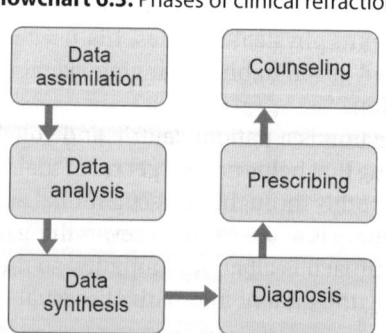

Flowchart 6.3: Phases of clinical refraction.

Chapter 6: Fundamentals of Clinical Refraction

Observations of visual behaviors of the patient can provide lot of clues regarding the condition of the patient's eye. It provides insights and these insights enable the examiner to implement appropriate tests and techniques. Observation has to be done empathetically and in a very discreet manner so that the patient does not understand. Using these observations, the examiner can design relevant questioning for history taking and implement the relevant tests and procedure. Some of the visual observations that help are downward head tilt, head tilts to one side, frequent head and eye movement, unusual head posture, squinting of eyes, erratic eye movement, eye poking, disheveled and fatigued appearance.

Communication is the key to the entire process as the examiner and the patient needs to interact continuously throughout the procedure. The optometrist must communicate effectively with the patient in order to gather information, provide instructions, educate and explain the diagnosis and treatment plan. During the process he also discusses specific needs, if any. In addition, he interprets the patient's feedback to guide the refraction process. During the process he invariably uses some phrases, the common among them are given below:

- ❖ "I am going to have you look through two different lenses. Although neither lens may be perfect, I want you to tell me which one looks clearer".
- ❖ When the patient becomes indecisive, he adds - "Do they look the same?"
- ❖ "Which is better, number one or number two?"
- ❖ "Does letter appear darker and smaller?"

He also explains how he expects the patient to answer his question.

Investigation starts with history taking and is followed by use of appropriate equipment to examine the eyes from outside to inside to assess the ocular health to diagnose the condition and application of objective method of refraction. Throughout the investigation process the examiner uses his knowledge, experience, observation and communication skills, attention to detail to integrate the information.

The measurement of refractive error involves several distinct steps. The first phase of testing is the collection of initial data. It starts with history taking and then goes into measuring UCVA, vision with habitual correction, habitual correction, and objective measurement of refraction. These data are needed to set the goal for the end result. Once the goal is set, subjective refraction is carried out to measure the refractive error in terms of spherical, cylinder, axis and near addition. In fact, subjective refraction may also be considered as verification of what is measured objectively. Phoropter or trial lenses are used that simulate the effect of potential eyeglasses that the patient will use eventually in his day to day life. Trial lenses are interchangeably placed in the trial frame and the patient is asked to read out the letters on the test chart.

Data Analysis

Data analysis is the process of organizing and classifying data that have been collected, comparing the results with other appropriate information and presenting the results in an appropriate manner. During the entire procedure of clinical refraction the examiner gathers several objective data as measured by different tests. These data are important individually as well as collectively. A good examiner keeps analyzing them throughout the process as he proceeds from one test to another and finally to the lens prescription for each eye. The examiner also analyzes the gathered data at every milestone, for example after completing all entrance tests as well as all core tests and also after refinement tests and before prescribing. All data are analyzed against their expected values which can indicate the current stage of development of vision problem and subtle changes can be detected early. If the data collected does not yield conclusive information to address patient's symptoms, additional tests may be considered to execute on case-to-case basis.

Data Synthesis

Data synthesis means combining the main points of each source of data including objective and subjective measurements together with examiner's opinion as developed through his knowledge and experience to see the overall pattern, how things come together. Data synthesis is perhaps the most important element of the refraction procedure. It enables the examiner to look at the entire data in a holistic manner. In real practice, patients do not come with only vision-related problems. They do present the symptoms of eye strain and ocular symptoms. The manifestation of eye strain is not just because of the visual system. It is multifactorial and a very complex phenomenon. As a general rule, gross visual errors do not give rise to the typical symptoms of eye strain. It is the failure of the visual function because of a small error that causes eye strain in most cases.

The patient often can correct a small error to a greater or lesser extent by muscular effort. The constant effort unconsciously imposes upon him the symptoms of eye strain. This implies that it is not the error itself that causes so much trouble but the continuous effort to correct it. Moreover, different patients respond to difficulties differently. While a feeble individual may reach the breaking point more readily, a robust may even live peacefully and comfortably with a small degree of difficulty. A good optometrist synthesizes the entire set of data to decide the treatment plan, considering the eye not just as an optical instrument but also as an integral part of the body, sharing with the other organs in its constitutional variation.

Diagnosis

Diagnosis is the process of identifying and determining the nature and cause of a health condition. It involves analyzing a patient's symptoms in relation to clinical signs together with medical history, and clinical procedures to identify the underlying disorder and ruling out other possibilities. Diagnosis requires a combination of analytical and critical thinking skills, as well as the ability to integrate information from various sources to arrive at an accurate conclusion. The clinical refraction involves diagnosis of a variety of refractive errors such as myopia, hyperopia, astigmatism, and presbyopia. It also involves the diagnosis of eye conditions such as cataracts, glaucoma, macular degeneration, or diabetic retinopathy that may be impacting the patient's vision. The clinician performs a series of tests including visual acuity, refraction, binocular vision, and ocular health assessments. These tests are designed to help the clinician identify any issues with the patient's vision or the health of their eyes. Based on the results of these tests, the clinician can make a diagnosis and determine the appropriate treatment plan, which may involve prescription eyeglasses or contact lenses, vision therapy, or referral to a specialist for further evaluation and additional treatment.

Prescribing

Prescribing is completely an independent function in the whole spectrum of refraction procedure. While the basic process of measuring refractive error is by and large straight forward, there are myriad complexities involved in prescribing refractive correction. Prescribing is not solely intellectually driven. It also involves a significant amount of critical thinking, clinical judgment and consideration of individual patient's unique needs and preferences. Most mistakes happen in prescribing, not in measurement of refractive error.

There may be a situation when symptoms that seem indicative of a refractive anomaly may actually stem from entirely different causes. Therefore, prescribing corrective measures should adhere to principles that ensure the safe and effective use of such corrections; the important among them are summarized below:

- Prescribe to treat patient's symptoms
- Avoid prescribing correction in case of asymptomatic patients.
- Avoid minor changes in refraction in the absence of symptoms.
- Be wary of malingering patients.
- Prescribe minimum minus and maximum plus to achieve the best corrected visual acuity.
- Smaller astigmatism in the absence of symptoms does not require correction.
- Larger astigmatic error should always be carefully prescribed as the wholesale correction of astigmatic error is considered more a negative practice.
- The prescription for small error should be decided in light of symptoms of binocular vision disorder.
- It is prudent to have an age-specific approach for prescribing refractive correction.
- A sudden prescription of high correction to a patient who has not previously worn correction is not advisable, and it is wise to prescribe under-correction which can be gradually strengthened over a period of time.
- Be very clear why you prescribe what you decided to prescribe.

Counseling

Patient counseling and follow-up with the patient is the last stage of clinical refraction when the examiner applies the psychotherapeutic procedure. Psychotherapy is the art of using words and a high relationship quotient with the patients as a part of the overall procedure to influence the patients' views of reality and to help them accept themselves as they are. Recognizing the psychosocial aspect of the patient's situation has an immense impact on the patient's well-being, and it requires the examiner to consider the patient as a whole and the context of the visit. When this is done as a part of practice protocol, the results are extraordinary and bring in very welcome

Chapter 6: Fundamentals of Clinical Refraction

outcome. The examiner connects meaningfully with the patient, understands their mental status, and then educates, motivates and empowers the patients to accept themselves "as they are" so that they can help themselves. The main goal is to enable the patients to make informed decisions about their vision care, improve their understanding of their ocular and visual conditions, and help them manage their vision effectively. Counseling covers a discussion on a range of topics, such as:

- ❖ Explaining diagnosis and prognosis
- ❖ Addressing patient's queries and concerns
- ❖ Providing different options for vision correction as solution
- ❖ Talking about cost involvement
- ❖ Professional recommendations
- ❖ Educating patients on adaptation and follow-up factor

In recent days due to development of technology, online therapy and availability of scientific research evidences, there has been a shift towards a more patient-centered approach in health care which emphasizes the importance of tailoring the treatments to meet the specific needs and preferences of the individual patient. Evidence-based counseling aligns with this approach by emphasizing the use of treatments that have been shown to be effective for specific population and conditions. It involves the integration of the best available research evidence with clinical expertise and patient values to provide optimal care. It allows the examiner to look beyond correction to incorporate prevention, protection and enhancement of vision into the practice. The approach requires that examiner stay up-to-date on the latest research findings and uses that information to inform the patients in their clinical practice.

METHODS OF CLINICAL REFRACTION

The clinical refraction is the art and science of neutralization of an individual's refractive error using a variety of tests in which the patient's responses help determine the lens prescription that produces the best possible image on the retina and prescribes the appropriate correction to provide good vision and ensure that the patient is able to adapt to it quickly and is able to use comfortably for a sustained period of time. A number of methods and tests are applied in the process to achieve the objectives. The methods and tests used may vary depending on the patient's age, medical history, and other factors. The examiner chooses the appropriate

Flowchart 6.4: Methods of clinical refraction.

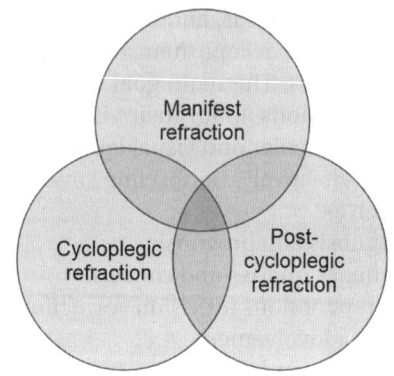

method and tests to provide an accurate assessment of the patient's visual function and refractive error to improve the patient's visual acuity. These methods can be classified under three broad categories to understand their application. They are outlined in the **Flowchart 6.4**.

Manifest Refraction

A refraction that is executed without using cycloplegic drops is also called manifest refraction. It is often called a "Dry refraction". Manifest refraction is the most traditional way of measuring the refractive error. The patient is involved in the process by being shown different choices, either using loose trial lenses or a phoropter.

Cycloplegic Refraction

A refraction done using cycloplegic drops to dilate the pupils and prevent accommodation is called cycloplegic refraction. It is often called "Wet refraction". The cycloplegic drop temporarily paralyzes the ciliary muscles that aid in focusing the eye. The method is most commonly used in children where accommodation is very strong and also in case of young adults who subconsciously accommodate during eye examination, making the results invalid. The method helps to determine patient's true refractive error.

Cyclopentolate 1% is used to paralyze the muscles by instilling 1 drop in each eye 6 times at 15 minutes' interval on the day of refraction. Refraction is done after 45 minutes of last drop. The younger patient may need stronger drops and /or more application of drops. In case of patients with light-colored iris less strong drop

Chapter 6: Fundamentals of Clinical Refraction

or fewer applications of the drop may be sufficient. Care should be taken with patients who have never been cyclopleged, or who are new to the clinic. They should be examined for narrow angles prior to instilling the drops. Also, it is important to enquire whether the patient is allergic to any of the cycloplegic drops before instillation.

Cycloplegic refraction is indicated in the following cases:
- ❖ When esophoria is present or latent hypermetropia is suspected
- ❖ A young patient with hypermetropic eyes
- ❖ Children below the age of 8 years

Only distance correction can be done after cycloplegia. Near vision is not examined as accommodation is being suspended. Near vision must be checked during manifest refraction prior to cycloplegia. Same visual acuity may not be achieved with cycloplegic refraction as dilated eyes lack the pinhole effect of small pupil. Therefore, cycloplegic refraction should be conducted after completing all other eye tests. Cycloplegic refraction indicates the magnitude of refractive error and non-cycloplegic refraction indicates the acceptability of the correction. Usually, cycloplegic refraction yields a little high plus correction. Prescription of lens power has to be backed with clinical decision. About 0.75 D should be subtracted from the net findings, if the complete cycloplegia has been achieved before the refraction.

Post-cycloplegic Refraction

Post-cycloplegic refraction refers to the refraction that an examiner chooses to perform after several days of wet refraction. The purpose is to see how much of the full cycloplegic refraction found on the previous visit can be accepted by the patient. It should be understood that post-cycloplegic refraction may not be indicated in all cases. In routine practice, after the preliminary examination, retinoscopy and subjective refraction are carried out both for distance and near vision, cycloplegic drops are instilled and retinoscopy is repeated after an appropriate interval. If the result of repeat retinoscopy agrees reasonably with the pre-cycloplegic refraction, post-cycloplegic refraction may not be necessary. Post-cycloplegic refraction is indicated only when there is a considerable discrepancy between the pre-cycloplegic refraction and cycloplegic refraction.

Refractive error can be measured objectively as well as subjectively; accordingly they are called objective method of refraction and subjective method of refraction.

Objective Refraction

Objective refraction is often used to determine the initial information pertaining to refractive error of the patient. There are mainly three methods of objective refraction—retinoscopy, keratometry and autorefractometry. The topic has been covered in detail in Chapter 10.

Subjective Refraction

Subjective refraction can be taken to understand as the verification of objective refraction. It is a sequential process for determining spherical and cylinder correction. At first, the spherical element of the refractive error is determined in such a way as to facilitate the accurate determination of any astigmatic element present. The refractive error may be only spherical, it may be only cylinder or it may be the combination of both known as spherocylinder error. The final phase of refraction involves refinement and balancing of measured error to ensure comfortable vision and optimal visual performance in real life. The topic has been covered in detail in Chapter 11.

All methods used to determine the static refraction during relaxed state of accommodation depends upon the fact that the fovea and the far point are conjugate foci, that is:

- Retina is imaged at the far point, and
- An object at the far point is imaged at the fovea.

In objective method, the image of the illuminated area of the retina is located and imaged by the examiner at the far point. In subjective method, the far point is seen by the patient to be imaged on his retina. In both cases the far point is brought to a suitable distance by adding to or subtracting from the refractivity of the eye by a lens system, if needed.

Both objective and subjective methods of refraction must be applied in all cases. The tests and techniques that can be applied under both the methods for clinical examination of refractive error are legion. It is nearly impossible for an individual examiner to know all of them. Law 1 of clinical refraction proposes to categorize all tests and techniques into three broad categories as given below:

- Entrance tests
- Core tests
- Refinement tests

The categorization is based upon the purpose of the tests and can be viewed as set tests that allow the examiner to initiate the

Chapter 6: Fundamentals of Clinical Refraction

whole process of clinical refraction, followed by measurement and refinement of refractive error.

Law 3 further states that every individual practitioner should decide a set under each of the above categories that may be employed to examine each of his patients. Based upon it, an organized flow of clinical refraction procedure for an individual practice may be proposed as shown by **Flowchart 6.5**.

Flowchart 6.5: Flow of clinical refraction.

Step-1 **ENTRANCE TEST**
- History taking
- Lensometry
- Visual acuity test
  - UCVA
  - Measure visual acuity with habitual correction
  - Pinhole acuity
- Objective measurement
  - Retinoscopy
  - Keratometry
  - Autorefractometry
- Assimilation of data and goal setting

Step-2 **CORE TEST**
- Dominant eye test
- Subjective refraction
- Determination of near addition
- Think and go ahead

Step-3 **REFINEMENTS TEST**
- Duochrome test
- Binocular balancing

STOP, PRESCRIBE AND COUNSEL

There are lots of advantages of following a sequential flow of process. These are:
- ❖ All action, movement, and thought follow inevitably from the previous one, like playing jazz.
- ❖ Your whole being is involved, and you are using your skills to the utmost.
- ❖ Feelings of personal control over the situation and the outcome
- ❖ You are able to recognize quickly the step where error has occurred.
- ❖ Spontaneous strong concentration and attention on even the smallest elements.
- ❖ It is an activity that you enjoy or feel passionate about.
- ❖ You are able to stretch your current skill level.
- ❖ You perform goal driven action plan.

CORRECTION OF REFRACTIVE ERROR

It is a long-established common practice to use the term "best corrected visual acuity" while correcting the refractive error. The best corrected visual acuity is normally measured in Snellen's fraction during clinical refraction. When a patient can read symbols or letters on the row designated 6/6 or 20/20 on the test chart placed at a distance of 6 meters or 20 feet in a clinical setting, it represents "normal acuity". The acuity score of 20/20 or 6/6 has been accepted as being normal or standard based upon the hypothesis that it is easy to recognize by most people at the respective distance. It is also considered optimum correction or full correction of refractive error. However, in most healthy eyes, the visual acuity does not truncate at 6/6 or 20/20, and the patient can even read beyond 20/20 or 6/6, which may be read as 20/16, 20/12.5, or 20/10, and in the metric system as 6/4.8, 6/3.8, or 6/3. The patient is able to adapt to it quickly. He is also able to use his vision comfortably and unconsciously for a prolonged period of time. He develops a positive feeling with his correction.

If letters of the 6/6 line become overly sharp or clear, resulting in discomfort or difficulty seeing, it may be coined as overcorrection. Other signs of overcorrection may include headaches, eye strain, blurred vision, or double vision. Overcorrection is a subjective term, as what is considered overcorrection for one person may not be the same for another. Undercorrection, on the other hand, occurs when

Chapter 6: Fundamentals of Clinical Refraction

the correction prescribed is not strong enough to fully correct the refractive error. The subject with healthy eyes is not able to read the 6/6 or 20/20 lines on the Snellen's test chart. Under-correction can also lead to symptoms of blurred or distorted vision and can cause symptoms such as headaches, eye strain, and difficulty seeing clearly at different distances.

The rule of thumb that is commonly followed while prescribing refractive correction is least minus for myopes and maximum plus for hyperopes to achieve the optimum correction. In other words, it can be translated to say that myopia is slightly under-corrected and hypermetropia is fully corrected. This is because we want to create a situation where the focus is just before the retina. Overcorrection in myopia will push the focus behind the retina, which will induce accommodation and ultimately lead to asthenopic symptoms. Similarly, under correction in hypermetropia will keep the focus behind the retina, which will also induce accommodation and eventually asthenopia. Constant over-accommodation may also lead to the development of convergent squint. It has also been observed that focus behind the retina creates stimulation for the posterior segment of the eye to elongate, which can increase the axial length of the eye. 1 mm increase in axial length leads to an increase in myopia by -3.00 D.

Overcorrection, for several reasons, remains the road less traveled, but it cannot be completely ruled out as it works well in cases of intermittent exotropia or exophoria, accommodative esotropia, convergence insufficiency, high anisometropia, and accommodative fatigue. The overcorrection is usually temporary and is gradually reduced over time as the patient's symptoms improve.

We would not like to prescribe a correction that brings the focus right onto the retina. This is because of the shape of the retina. Retina is not a flat structure. Due to its peripheral curvature, peripheral rays of light focus behind the retina, while the central rays focus on the retina. Most spectacle lenses also behave differently in their central portion and in their peripheral portion. Rays of light passing from the central portion of the lens focus on the retina, whereas rays of light passing from the peripheral portion of the lens focus behind the retina, known as peripheral defocus. Therefore, to avoid such a situation, the rule is followed.

The vision of people with astigmatism is characteristic. The image is not out of focus but is distorted. In an astigmatic eye, rays of light do not come to a point of focus. The image at the retina is never a point but is always either one of the two lines at the right angles when it is distorted or an ellipse when it is distorted and blurred, both of which have sizes that vary directly with the degree of astigmatism and with the size of the pupil. The aim of refractive correction is to eliminate the focal interval by using cylinder correction when the whole image becomes theoretically a point image, and then displacement of the stigmatic image to the point of the retina by a suitable spherical correction. A small amount of astigmatic correction may be avoided, whereas a larger amount of astigmatic correction may be tapered down to strengthen gradually over a period of time.

TRIAL FRAMING

Trial framing is an important process in the eyeglass prescription process, providing the patient with a real-world experience of how they feel about a new correction in a more natural environment. This process becomes especially significant when using a phoropter, as it may not simulate real-world conditions accurately. For those conducting trial frame refraction, the process is more straightforward, given that the lenses are already in the trial frame.

You could ask the patient to look around, you could ask the patient to walk around, if you are in a room, you could have them leave the room, go into a larger space, so you get a sense of how it feels for them to be wearing the new refraction, especially if it is a large change.

Trial framing is like putting up several combinations of trial lenses in the trial frame and asking the patient to look around in the open and larger environment, preferably non-clinical environment. It can be done monocularly as well as binocularly. During the process the patient may be asked to respond to how changes in trial lenses and the changes in axis of cylinder lenses affect his vision. The questions may be like:

- ❖ How does this feel?
- ❖ How do they look?
- ❖ See, if you notice any difference.
- ❖ With which one do you feel more comfortable?
- ❖ How does it compare to this? And then make a change.
- ❖ Is it comfortable?
- ❖ Is it clear?

The next important consideration is when should you trial frame? There is no hard and fast rule. As a clinician you can decide on

Chapter 6: Fundamentals of Clinical Refraction

case-to-case basis or you may go ahead with it in all cases. However, there are certain cases where trial framing should ideally be before taking a decision to prescribe the correction, for example:
- When there are significant changes in the correction?
- When does the patient's visual acuity not improve in spite of changing the correction?
- When the patient is very sensitive to small changes?
- When you want to compare with habitual correction?
- When the patient comes back for prescription check?

Trial framing is very useful technique which can be very effectively used after measurement of refractive error and before prescription of correction.

MULTIPLE CHOICE QUESTIONS

1. **Which of the following suggests the true objective of Clinical Refraction?**
   a. To prescribe a pair of lenses that ensure retina to be in conjugate with optical infinity.
   b. To prescribe a pair of lenses that provide the patient with clear and comfortable vision to which he adapts quickly, and which allows him to work for a longer period of time without any symptoms.
   c. To prescribe a pair of lenses that provides the patient maximum vision on Snellen's chart.
   d. To correct the refractive error.

2. **Which of the following is the reason for which it has been suggested to avoid dim light during clinical refraction?**
   a. Accommodation may not relax.
   b. Pupil will dilate which may alter the effect of wide beam aberrations.
   c. The examiner may find it difficult to observe a patient's reactions.
   d. All of the above.

3. **Which of the following is not always true about visual headache?**
   a. Visual headache occurs towards the middle or end of the day.
   b. Visual headache does not occur upon awakening in the morning.
   c. Visual headache often occurs in different pattern on weekends.
   d. Visual headache most often occurs towards the back of the head.

Chapter 6: Fundamentals of Clinical Refraction

4. The problem of double vision with the spectacle can be managed by:
   a. Spectacle frame fitting
   b. Placement of optical center
   c. Prism lenses
   d. All of the above
5. Which of the following is not true about diabetes and its effect on refractive correction?
   a. A rise in sugar concentration in blood causes myopic shift.
   b. A fall in sugar concentration leads to hypermetropic shift.
   c. Diabetes usually has bilateral effect on the refraction.
   d. None of the above
6. Uncorrected refractive error may lead to:
   a. Results in either under- or over-accommodation.
   b. May create unusual demand of either negative or positive fusional vergence.
   c. Creates decreased fusional ability as a result of blurred retinal images.
   d. All of the above.
7. What does spherical lens correct?
   a. Defocus
   b. Astigmatism
   c. Spherical aberration
   d. All of the above
8. What does cylinder lens correct?
   a. Defocus
   b. Astigmatism
   c. Off-axis astigmatism
   d. All of the above
9. Which of the following is indicated during clinical refraction?
   a. Accommodation results in a more myopic prescription.
   b. Visual acuity is measured binocularly for distance and near vision.
   c. A high minus lens over the non-examining eye of the patient with bilateral congenital nystagmus can reduce the nystagmus.
   d. Recent wearing of RGP lens has no effect on the clinical refraction.

ANSWER KEY

1. b	2. d	3. d	4. d	5. d	6. d	7. a	8. b	9. a

SELF-PRACTICE QUESTIONS

1. If the patient is symptomatic, how would you like to approach clinical procedures to determine refractive error of the patient? Explain in detail.
2. Describe the psychological explanation for patients complaining of non-adaptation to new lens correction.
3. What are the possible causes of double vision? What would be your sequential approach towards its remedy?
4. What do you understand by 'Goal of Clinical Refraction'? How do you set the goal for a given patient?
5. When is cycloplegic refraction indicated? What are pre-examinations that should be done before cycloplegic refraction? How much tonus allowance should be reduced during final refraction?

7 CHAPTER

Trial Lens Set

CHAPTER OUTLINE

- Spherical and Cylinder Trial Lenses
- Prism
- Pinhole Disc
- Stenopeic Slit
- Red and Green Filter
- Maddox Rod
- Occluder
- Trial Frame

A well-equipped clinical practice for eye and vision care should have a comprehensive set of test lenses to accommodate any necessary combination of spherical, cylindrical, and prism lenses for patient evaluations. A standard clinical refraction trial lens set typically includes a variety of lenses and assistive devices, each designed to perform specific tasks in the assessment and correction of vision.

SPHERICAL AND CYLINDER TRIAL LENSES

A comprehensive trial lens set, as shown in **Figure 7.1** contains a set of lenses that are designed to fit a standard trial frame and encircled by a metal rim for protection in spherical and cylinder powers. Spherical lenses are available with handle and cylinder lenses are without handle so as to expedite the rotation of cylinder lens for axis verifications. The set contains:

❖ A pair of plus spherical lens set containing trial lenses having back vertex power ranging from +0.12 D to +20.00 D
❖ A pair of minus spherical lens set containing trial lenses having back vertex power ranging from -0.12 D to -20.00 D

Chapter 7: Trial Lens Set

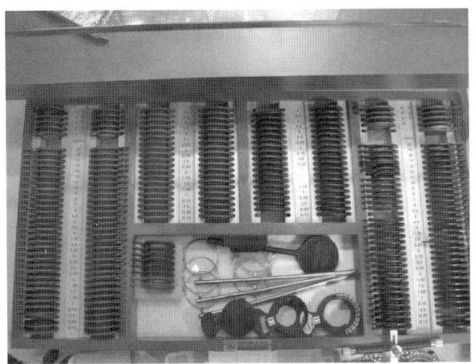

Fig. 7.1: The complete trial lens set.

- A pair of plus cylinder lens set containing trial lenses having back vertex power ranging from +0.12 D to +6.00 D
- A pair of minus cylinder lens set containing trial lenses having back vertex power ranging from -0.12 D to -6.00 D

The trial lenses simulate the effect of potential eyeglasses in the clinical environment. They are available in two types of mounting, one of them is commonly called as full aperture trial lens and another is called the small aperture trial lens. Small aperture trial lenses are light and thin and hence provide ease of manipulation to make quick changes. They are either surrounded by metal rim or plastic rim. Trial lenses are made in planoconvex and planoconcave form and are annotated with their back vertex power. Biconvex and biconcave lenses are not recommended for practical convenience reason.

PRISM

Prisms are triangular or wedge-shaped pieces of glass that displace the bundle of light towards the base (**Fig. 7.2**). When they are placed in front of the eyes, an object viewed through them appears to be displaced towards its apex. During the clinical refraction, they are employed to measure the presence and amount of any tropia or phoria. A standard trial lens set contains

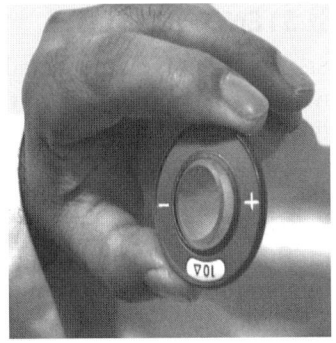

Fig. 7.2: Prism.

the following prism lenses measured in diopter 0.5Δ, 1Δ, 2 Δ, 3Δ, 4Δ, 5Δ, 6Δ, 8Δ, 10Δ, 12Δ.

PINHOLE DISC

Pinhole disc is a small disc with central opening as shown in **Figure 7.3** that eliminates peripheral rays of light to pass through. The optimal size of the central opening is 1.2 mm. Larger size pinholes do not effectively neutralize refractive error and smaller size pinholes significantly increase diffraction and decrease the amount of light entering the eye. Some trial lenses set also contain multiple pinhole discs which also serve the same purpose. The patient finds easier to use multiple pinhole disc as he does not require searching for a single tiny hole. The disc permits the examiner to differentiate between the reduced visual acuity caused by refractive error and that caused by some pathological changes within the eyes. In general, visual acuity that cannot be improved with pinhole disc cannot be improved by the use of lenses. Pinhole can be used to assess monocular diplopia. If a patient sees a single image when looking through a pinhole, it suggests that the double vision is caused by the refractive error.

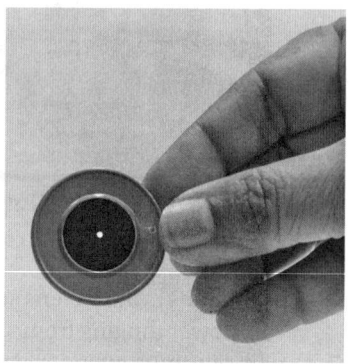

Fig. 7.3: Pinhole disc.
(*For color version, see Plate 1*)

STENOPEIC SLIT

Stenopeic slit is an elongated pinhole which is used to allow the light transmission in one meridian and is a useful tool for the correction of astigmatism **(Fig. 7.4)** The width of the slit aperture ranges between 0.50 mm to 1.00 mm and the length is 15 mm and is assumed to limit the light admission to one meridian.

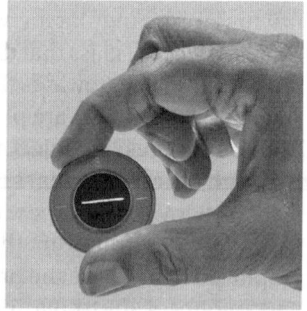

Fig. 7.4: Stenopeic slit.
(*For color version, see Plate 1*)

Stenopeic slit is also helpful in performing refraction as it facilitates detection of principal meridians. When slit is used for meridional refraction, only spherical trial lenses are used to correct the refractive error in different meridians. It is useful in performing refraction in cases of high astigmatism, refraction in low vision as well as in keratoconus patients.

Slit is also useful in measuring vertex distance to place trial frame properly. Stenopeic slit can also be used to differentiate the colored haloes caused by cataract or because of glaucoma. The test is known as 'Emsley-Fincham Stenopeic Slit Test'. Stenopeic slit is passed across the pupil. Haloes in immature cataract are broken into pieces while in glaucoma remains intact.

▌ RED AND GREEN FILTER (FIG. 7.5)

The standard trial lens set also contains one red and one green filter lens. Some trial lenses also contain yellow filter. These filter lenses are used to check overcorrection and undercorrection of refractive error. Under ordinary illumination conditions, the eyes are typically emmetropic for yellow light, slightly myopic for green light, and slightly hypermetropic for red light. This reflects the general tendency due to chromatic aberration, where shorter wavelengths (blue/green) focus in front of the retina and longer wavelengths (red) focus behind the retina. Yellow light, being in the middle of the visible spectrum, is often used as a reference point for emmetropia. With each eye occluded in turn, the uncovered eye views the best line first through the red filter, which is rapidly exchanged for green filter successively.

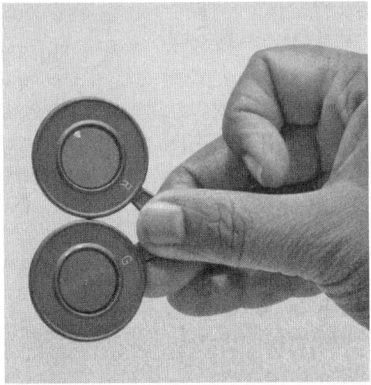

Fig. 7.5: Red and green filter. (*For color version, see Plate 2*)

The patient is asked to make a comparison of definition through the filter to notice the clarity of letters. If the patient states:
- No apparent difference between the two, it implies optimum correction is present. If the vision is clearer with red, the eye is slightly fogged. A small minus can be added until equality is demonstrated. Clearer vision with green filter indicates that the eye is hypermetropic and a plus lens can be added until equality is reached. If red and green appear clearer alternatively before any adjustment is made in the correction, this indicates accommodation is active. In such a case it is better to abandon the test. Yellow filter is sometimes used to break the confusion of the patient to identify correct observation.
- Red and green filters are also used to screen the macular functioning. If the patient can identify red and green color, macula can be taken to understand as functioning. They are great tools for Worth 4 Dot test to ensure eye teaming or to detect diplopia.

MADDOX ROD

Maddox rod is a group of either red or colorless parallel rods that together act as a cylinder (**Fig. 7.6**). The purpose of the Maddox Rod is to dissociate the two eyes and prevent the images from fusing. It accomplishes its function by changing the size, and shape of a point source of light. It is a useful tool to detect tropia or phoria.

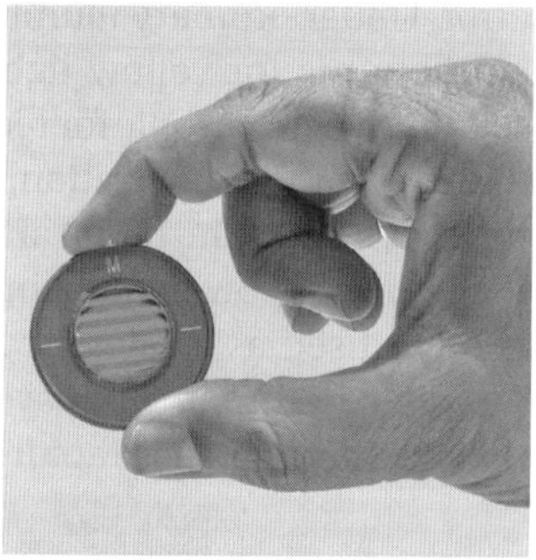

Fig. 7.6: Maddox rod.
(*For color version, see Plate 2*)

OCCLUDER

During a routine of examination, the practitioner often needs to check one eye's acuity compared to other. Examiner uses a set of special eye covers known as occluders. Occluders usually prevent the full penetration of light. There are also translucent occluders which create blurry effect over the eye (**Fig. 7.7**).

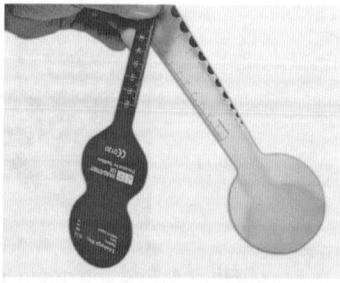

Fig. 7.7: Occluder.

TRIAL FRAME

A trial frame is used to put the trial lenses for refraction **(Fig. 7.8)**. Trial frames are usually with three cells which fit a spherical lens, a cylinder lens and also a prism. The front of the extreme front cell is marked with degree from 0 to 180 degree and also has hooks attached to it to provide an addition provision to place the 4th trial lens. While using the trial frame on a patient, it is important to fix the frame on patient's face so that it is stable and well centered. It can be adjusted from its earpiece and bridge to rest behind the ears and to alter interpupillary distance. Some trial frames also have an adjustment facility to alter its pantoscopic tilt. The new designs of trial frames have a thumbscrew mechanism on the side of the trial frame to rotate the front lens carrier. In practice the back cell of the trial frame is commonly used for spherical lenses. It may not very important for low correction but it is extremely important in case of high refractive error. Careful angling and adjustment of the trial frame is critical. It allows the patient to maintain the normal head and body posture better than refractor head, hence allowing a better judgment of the patient's near vision correction. It is essential that the trial lenses be angled perpendicular to and centered on the depressed line of sight to prevent the effect of oblique astigmatism.

Phoropters, also known as refractors are alternatives to trial lens set **(Fig. 7.9)**. All the lenses in the phoropters are inbuilt within the phoropter the help of motors. There are basically two types of phoropters —manual and automatic . Two spherical lens assemblies and two-cylinder lens assemblies are housed in the phoropter for each eye. Cylinder axis is altered by turning a knob for each eye that rotates the axis through meridian from 0 to 180°. Two cross cylinders, two rotary prisms, pinhole, stenopeic slit, occluders, red lens and

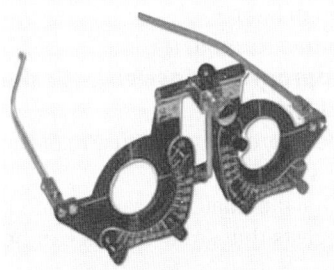

Fig. 7.8: Trial frame.

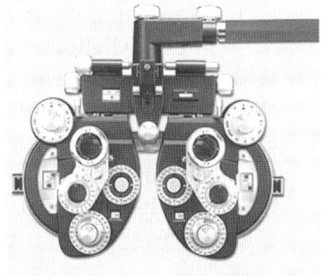

Fig. 7.9: Manual phoropter.

polarizing analyzer are also included on accessory post. The patient is asked to be seated behind the phoropter. Horizontal and vertical position of the lens apertures are determined by the mechanical arm adjustment suspending the phoropter. The adjustment knob for IPD and bubble device is used to adjust the geometric centers of apertures before the eyes. Pantoscopic tilt can be incorporated by adjustment of the swing connection between the phoropter and the mechanical arm. The light mounting provides illumination of the near test card.

Newer generation phoropters also provide additional feature to tilt during the course of reading to ensure natural reading posture. The only drawback of phoropter is the eyes of the patient is hidden behind the phoropter which means the practitioner cannot see patient's reactions and operational flexibility is less as it is fixed at one place. It is difficult to have eccentric viewing which may be a reason why it is not suitable for visually impaired patient. However, there are certain advantages of the phoropter. They can also measure phoria (natural resting position of the eyes), accommodative amplitudes, horizontal and vertical vergences, and many more.

MULTIPLE CHOICE QUESTIONS

1. **What is the standard size of central opening of the pinhole disc used in standard clinical trial set?**
   a. 1.50 mm
   b. 1.00 mm
   c. 1.20 mm
   d. 0.80 mm
2. **What is the application of Stenopeic slit used in standard clinical trial set?**
   a. To limit the transmission of light to one meridian only
   b. To block the transmission of light completely
   c. To allow complete transmission of light
   d. To filter the light that is transmitted through it
3. **Which of the following is an appropriate answer as to the clinical use of yellow filter in trial lens set?**
   a. It enhances contrast and is used to break the confusion of the patient to identify correct observation.
   b. It clears the vision that suggests that the small plus can be added.
   c. It reduces the contrast that suggests that small minus can be added.
   d. It facilitates Worth 4 Dot test to detect diplopia.

4. **Which of the following is not true about the Maddox rod?**
   a. The purpose of the Maddox rod is to dissociate the two eyes and prevent the images to fuse.
   b. It is used to measure phoria for distance.
   c. It can be used to measure cyclotorsion.
   d. It is used to check the overcorrection or undercorrection of refractive error.
5. **Which of the following is not the advantage of the phoropter?**
   a. Phoropter allows phoria measurement.
   b. Phoropter allows measurement of amplitude of accommodation.
   c. Phoropter allows eccentric viewing through lens aperture.
   d. Phoropter allows measurement of horizontal and vertical vergence.

ANSWER KEY

| 1. c | 2. a | 3. a | 4. d | 5. c |

SELF-PRACTICE QUESTIONS

1. Describe the different uses of Stenopeic slit.
2. What are the basic differences between trial frame refraction and phoropter refraction?

8 CHAPTER

Visual Acuity Test

> **CHAPTER OUTLINE**
> - Objectives of Visual Acuity Test
> - Factors Affecting Visual Acuity
> - Implications of Visual Acuity Test
> - Limitations of Visual Acuity Test
> - Designation of Visual Acuity
> - Visual Acuity Test Charts
> - Snellen's Test Chart
> - Visual Acuity Test Chart Formats
> - Clinical Assessment of Visual Acuity
> - Near Visual Acuity

Visual acuity is a time-dependent assessment of retinal health, specifying the examination date. This measure, associated with the sense of form perception, is gauged through various test charts in a specific environment. Among the four senses of visual perception, visual acuity particularly reflects the form sense.

The measurement of visual acuity involves determining a threshold, a process reliant on cone function, especially at the fovea. The fovea, characterized by a one-to-one relationship between cone cells, necessitates the stimulation of two cone cells with a one-cell gap to discern two separate objects. Measuring visual acuity requires establishing the minimum angle at which two objects are perceived as distinct entities. Thus, visual acuity quantifies the angular size of the object that an individual can effectively resolve.

OBJECTIVES OF VISUAL ACUITY TEST

Visual acuity test is a part of the comprehensive eye examination that in most cases forms the part of entrance tests applied in the entire battery of tests used for clinical refraction. The test also forms the basis for determining legal blindness in the United States and the rest of the world. It is applied at every presentation for varieties of reasons; the most common among them are as follows:

- ❖ Visual acuity test forms the part of diagnostic tests. Diagnostic tests are important at every step to improve patient care and for the purposes of diagnosing, monitoring, and prognosis.
- ❖ Visual acuity test is the part of baseline data. Baseline data is important because it allows the examiner to compare the behavior before and after the implementation of the treatment plan to determine if the interventions are working.
- ❖ A visual acuity test measures the progression of eye diseases. If reduced visual acuity is observed after refraction, further investigation is needed to determine the cause.
- ❖ Visual acuity test helps to evaluate the treatment. An improved and stable visual acuity indicates the positive side of a treatment plan on an easy-to-understand scale.
- ❖ As a screening test visual acuity test results suggest the presence or absence of refractive error and ocular abnormalities.
- ❖ Visual acuity test helps to estimate an individual's ability to perform certain tasks.
- ❖ Legally measuring visual acuity is mandatory for several statutory requirements. **Table 8.1** gives some very interesting information.
- ❖ Visual acuity is one of the important tests for a driver's license.

FACTORS AFFECTING VISUAL ACUITY

The visual acuity of an individual person depends upon a host of factors, which can be broadly grouped under physical factors and physiological factors, in addition to others. Physical factors may be

Table 8.1: Measured visual acuity and its implications.	
Measured visual acuity	Inferences
20/20 visual acuity	Desirable condition
20/70 visual acuity	Low vision
20/200 visual acuity	Legally blind
Visual acuity between 20/200 and 20/400	Severe vision loss
Visual acuity below 20/400	Profound vision loss

said to include those factors that directly or indirectly affect light and light transmission and thus influence the retinal image. Physiological factors are those that are individual-related. However, there are certain factors that overlap between the two groups. For example, light is a physical factor, but reflexes that control the size of the pupil, which in turn control the entry of light into the eye, are a physiological process. Therefore, segregating factors into two broader groups for the purpose of discussion may be limiting.

Flowchart 8.1 shows the common factors that may affect the visual acuity of an individual.

- ❖ The object size and the object distance are the most important factors that determine the visual acuity of an individual. The physical size of the object and its distance from the eye determine the visual angle. The bigger objects cast larger images on the retina than the smaller objects. The larger the object, the larger its visual angle will be. Closer objects cast larger images on the retina than objects lying at a far distance. Therefore, the closer the object is to the eye, the larger its visual angle will be.
- ❖ The ability of the eye to distinguish detail is dependent upon the intensity of the illumination falling upon the object. Although faint sources and movements can be perceived in comparative darkness, especially in the extrafoveal regions, we cannot recognize details in poor illumination. Attempts to do so or to carry out fine work under inadequate illumination lead to eye strain or headaches. Up to a certain limit, i.e., until the ceiling effect is reached, visual acuity increases with an increase in the

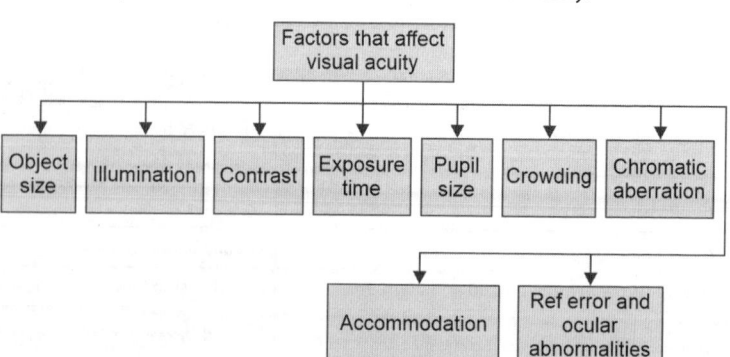

Flowchart 8.1: Factors that affect visual acuity.

luminance of the test object. Thereafter, the small variation in illumination does not improve the acuity.

- The contrast of the stimulus with its surroundings is also an important factor that affects the visual acuity of an individual. In general, greater contrast implies better visual acuity, and poor contrast implies poor visual acuity. In clinical practice, the contrast may be reduced because of the presence of glare in the visual field or because of light scatter within the eye itself, as found in cataracts.
- The exposure time to an object is also considered to affect the visual acuity of an individual. But there is less evidence available. However, the effect of observation time on visual acuity is of some practical importance, especially for dynamic visual acuity, i.e., when either the object or the observer or both are moving. In general, it has been accepted that dynamic visual acuity decreases when exposure time or the duration of the visualization of the object is shorter.
- The size of the pupil is an important factor affecting visual acuity. A large pupil implies that more light stimulates the retina and reduces diffraction, but resolution will be affected by aberrations of the eye. On the other hand, a small pupil will reduce optical aberrations, but resolution will be diffraction-limited. Therefore, a mid-size pupil of about 3–5 mm would be optimal, as this is a balance between the diffraction and aberration limits.
- The interaction effects of the two objects reduce visual acuity when the objects are too close together. The effect of crowding phenomena has often been seen in subjects with amblyopia or severe maculopathy. Crowding sets a fundamental limit on conscious visual perception and object recognition throughout the visual field.
- The use of monochromatic light as against white light should provide a clearer image because it should abolish the effect of chromatic aberrations.
- Form sense is a function of cones, and therefore, it is more acute at the fovea, where there are a higher number of cones that decrease very rapidly towards the periphery. In the periphery of the retina, the sensitivity of the cones decreases and that of the rods increases.
- Accommodation is essential for spatial resolution at various distances from the object. A young emmetrope with an accommo-

dative reflex can perform successful visual functions that require scanning in depth.
- ❖ Refractive errors, corneal curvature abnormalities, ocular media opacities, and axial length may affect visual acuity. Similarly, psychological factors like fatigue and malingering affect visual acuity.

IMPLICATIONS OF VISUAL ACUITY TEST

Visual acuity, a measure of central vision, is clinically evaluated under normal illumination using a specific test chart placed at an appropriate distance on a specific date and time. It gauges an individual's ability to discern the smallest recognizable letter, serving as a time-dependent indicator of retinal health.

Interpreting visual acuity test results is essential within the context of other findings. While each case may vary, a normal test result generally indicates:
- ❖ Presence of visual perception
- ❖ Stable tear film
- ❖ Clear cornea
- ❖ Clear crystalline lens
- ❖ Clear ocular media
- ❖ Intact retina, optic nerve, and visual pathway
- ❖ Total visual system, from the tear film to the occipital cortex is healthy.
- ❖ Both eyes are in alignment.

This comprehensive assessment provides valuable insights into the overall ocular health and functionality, allowing clinicians to make informed decisions regarding the individual's visual well-being.

LIMITATIONS OF VISUAL ACUITY TEST

The visual acuity test is so commonly used in clinical practice that it is often misunderstood as an indicator of visual status. But this is not precisely true because visual acuity only measures the health of a very small portion of the central retina on which the letters are projected. There are some limitations to the test, which can be seen in the following cases:
- ❖ Glaucoma is a condition where extensive and irreversible damage to the visual field occurs much before the visual acuity is

affected. When the visual acuity is blurred because of the optical factor of the eye, both the central and surrounding images will be equally blurred, but when the visual acuity loss is due to retinal factors, the letter chart acuity test does not detect anything about the surrounding retinal functions.
- ❖ The visual acuity test is conducted in standard room lighting conditions, which also limits the scope for conditions that require extra low illumination or extra high illumination.
- ❖ The visual acuity test is measured with high-contrast black letters on a white background. In real life, many activities have low contrast and are presented against a crowded background. A low-contrast test often gives additional information that a high-contrast test alone cannot provide.
- ❖ Contrast sensitivity can be affected by disorders of the outer retina, which prevent parts of the image from being detected, as can be seen in cases of macular degeneration. Neural factors may also interfere with vision processing, which may occur in the inner retina, optic nerve, or brain and visual cortex.

DESIGNATION OF VISUAL ACUITY

Visual acuity expresses the angular size of the smallest target that can just be resolved by an individual. There are several ways in which the clinicians specify the angular measurement, the common among them are shown in **Flowchart 8.2**.

Snellen's Fraction

Snellen's fraction expresses the visual acuity by using two factors, as given below:
- ❖ Test distance specified in meters or in feet as its numerator
- ❖ The distance at which letter subtends an angle of 5 minutes of arc as its denominator.

Flowchart 8.2: Different notations to designate visual acuity.

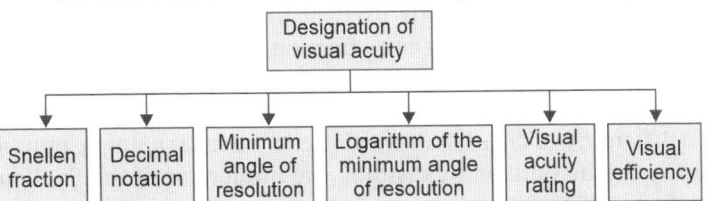

The visual acuity is given by the fraction:

$$\text{Visual acuity} = \frac{\text{Test distance}}{\text{Distance at which letters subtend 5 min of arc}}$$

The standard test distance used for measuring visual acuity is 20 feet which is usually the practice in the United States, while most other countries follow metric system, with 6 meters being the most common test distance. Therefore, a visual acuity measured as 20/20 denotes that the test distance was 20 feet and the smallest letters that could be read would subtend a visual angle of 5 minutes of arc when at a distance of 20 feet. Similarly, 20/200 denotes that the test distance was 20 feet and the smallest letters that could be read would subtend a visual angle of 5 minutes of arc when at a distance of 200 feet. When recorded in metric system as 6/6 would mean test distance was 6 meters and the smallest letters that could be read would subtend a visual angle of 5 minutes of arc when at a distance of 6 meters. Similarly, 6/60 denotes that the test distance was 6 meters and the smallest letters that could be read would subtend a visual angle of 5 minutes of arc when at a distance of 60 meters.

The acuity score of 20/20 or 6/6 has been accepted as being normal or standard based upon hypothesis of being 'easy to recognize'. However, the best acuity seldom truncates at this level. Most healthy eyes often exceed the standards which optometrists express as visual acuity of 20/16 or 20/12.5, or 20/10 and in metric system as 6/4.8 or 6/3.8 or 6/3.

Similarly, at lower level also it is possible to record visual acuity below 20/200 or 6/60 in which case the fraction may be read as 20/250 or 20/320 or 20/400 and in metric system 6/75 or 6/95 or 6/120. However, in reality, the biggest letter on an eye chart often represents acuity of "20/200" or '6/60' the value that is "legally blind."

Table 8.2 shows the Snellen's acuity at various distances.

Decimal Notation

Decimal notation is mostly used in the European continent. It effectively reduces the Snellen's fraction to a decimalized quantity as shown in **Table 8.3**.

Table 8.3 shows that the decimal notation does not indicate any test distance, nor does it indicate the letter size. It is a simple number which can be derived by dividing the numerator of the Snellen's fraction with its denominator.

Table 8.2: Snellen's notations as recorded at various test distance.

Snellen fraction at 20 feet	Snellen fraction at 6 meters	Snellen fraction at 4 meters
20/20	6/6	4/4
20/32	6/9.5	4/6.3
20/40	6/12	4/8
20/63	6/19	4/12.5
20/80	6/24	4/16
20/125	6/38	4/25
20/200	6/60	4/40

Table 8.3: Decimal notations.

Snellen fraction in feet	Snellen fraction in meter	Decimal notation
20/20	6/6	1.0
20/32	6/9.5	0.63
20/40	6/12	0.5
20/63	6/19	0.32
20/80	6/24	0.25
20/125	6/38	0.16
20/200	6/60	0.1

Minimum Angle of Resolution (MAR)

The angle at which two points are just perceived as two separate is the minimum angle of resolution. It is expressed in minutes of arc. The MAR relates to the resolution required to resolve the elements of a letter, thus 6/6 is equal to an MAR of 1 min of arc, as shown in **Table 8.4**.

The MAR in minutes of arc is equal to the reciprocal of the decimal acuity value.

Logarithm of the Minimum Angle of Resolution (LogMAR)

The logarithm of the MAR is simply $\log_{10}$ of the MAR. For a visual acuity of 6/6, the MAR is equal to 1 minute of arc, so the LogMAR equals $\log_{10}(1.0)$ equals 0.0 and as shown in **Table 8.5**.

Table 8.4: Minimum angle of resolution.

Snellen fraction in feet	Snellen fraction in meter	MAR
20/20	6/6	1.0
20/32	6/9.5	1.6
20/40	6/12	2.0
20/63	6/19	3.2
20/80	6/24	4.0
20/125	6/38	6.3
20/200	6/60	10

Table 8.5: LogMAR acuity.

Snellen fraction in feet	MAR	LogMAR
20/20	1.0	0.0
20/32	1.6	0.2
20/40	2.0	0.3
20/63	3.2	0.5
20/80	4.0	0.6
20/125	6.3	0.8
20/200	10	1.0

When visual acuity score is better than 6/6 or 20/20, the LogMAR value becomes negative. For example, for an acuity score of 20/16 or 6/4.8, MAR is 0.8 minute of arc and the LogMAR acuity is $\log_{10}(0.8)$ which is equal to -0.10. The logMAR scale is widely used in scientific publications where visual acuity values need to be depicted graphically to analyze trends or need to be averaged across population groups.

Visual Acuity Rating (VAR) (Table 8.6)

Another method for designating visual acuity is the Visual Acuity Rating, also known as 'Visual Acuity Score' (VAS). VAR provides a convenient scale to estimate visual abilities. The visual acuity rating is derived from LogMAR values:

$$VAR = 100 - 50 \, \text{logMAR}$$

Table 8.6: Visual acuity rating.

Snellen fraction in feet	LogMAR	VAR
20/20	0.0	100
20/32	0.2	90
20/40	0.3	85
20/63	0.5	75
20/80	0.6	70
20/125	0.8	60
20/200	1.0	50

On this scale, a score, 20/20 or 6/6 which corresponds to logMAR acuity of 0.0, equals VAR score of 100 and 20/200 or 6/60 which corresponds to logMAR acuity of 1.0 equals VAR score of 50. The VAR is equal 0 when visual acuity is 20/2000 or 6/600. The VAR is greater than 100 when the visual acuity is better than 20/20 or 6/6 like in case of 20/16 VAR equals 105. The VAR score changes by 5 for each size increment. There are 5 letters per size level, each letter carries VAR value of 1.

Visual Efficiency

In terms of minimum angle of resolution, a visual acuity of 6/6 is twice as good as 6/12 which often leads to imply that visual capacity in terms of fitness or capabilities reduces to one-half when acuity goes down from 6/6 to 6/12.

The visual efficiency (VE) scale was adopted by the American Medical Association (AMA) based upon the work of Snell and Scott Sterling. The visual acuity of 6/6 or 20/20 was rated as 100% and 6/60 or 20/200 was said to represent arbitrarily to 20%. Given these two benchmarks, the rest of the scale was designed as shown in **Table 8.7**.

Often for research and studies, visual acuity results frequently need to be averaged. LogMAR values can be averaged in the normal arithmetic way. Decimal acuity must not be averaged arithmetically. You could calculate the geometric mean, but best approach is to convert to LogMAR and then average. Even for Snellen fraction it is necessary to convert to LogMAR and then average.

Table 8.7: Visual efficiency.

Snellen fraction in feet	Snellen fraction in meter	VE% notation
20/20	6/6	100%
20/32	6/9.5	89.8%
20/40	6/12	83.6%
20/63	6/19	67.5%
20/80	6/24	58.5%
20/125	6/38	38.8%
20/200	6/60	20%

VISUAL ACUITY TEST CHARTS

Numerous test charts are available to measure visual acuity for different situations and for different population groups. Age is a primary criterion for an appropriate choice of test chart. There are objective and subjective methods of measuring visual acuity. Most tests are subjective in which the subject reads out the test chart, based upon which the observer records the acuity. The preferential-looking technique, visual evoked potential, and optokinetic nystagmus (OKN) testing have been attempted for the objective assessment of visual function which are commonly used for infants.

The following test charts are commonly used for the assessment of visual acuity for preschool children:
- Landolt 'C'
- Tumbling 'E'
- Sheridan Gardiner
- Stycar Visual Acuity Test
- Lea Symbol
- Kay Picture Test
- Allen Card Test

Snellen's test chart is the most widely used test chart in clinical practice for most patients and logMAR chart has been the recent introduction which is mostly used for research and studies. The principles and application of LogMAR test chart has been comprehensively discussed in author's another book titled "Low Vision Aids Practice". In this book, we will only discuss Snellen's test chart as this chart is mostly used for clinical refraction.

SNELLEN'S TEST CHART

Snellen's Test Chart (**Fig. 8.1**) has been named after the Dutch ophthalmologist Dr Herman Snellen is based upon recognition tests that determine the smallest letter that can be identified correctly. Dr Snellen proposed his optotypes in 1962 to measure visual acuity during clinical refraction.

Principle

The Snellen's chart uses letters as optotypes. The test not only requires spatial resolution but also recognition or naming of the target. It is for this reason careful letter choice and chart design are essential to ensure that letter recognition tasks are uniform for different letter sizes and chart working distances.

Optotypes

The optotypes on the test chart resemble block letters and are designed to be recognized and read as letters. Snellen letters are constructed so that the size of the critical detail, i.e., stroke, width and gap width subtends 1/5th of the overall size or in other words letters were so constructed that their constituent parts, i.e., limbs and spaces between them—each subtending a visual angle of 1 minute of arc as shown in **Figure 8.2** and the complete letter subtends a visual angle of 5 minutes of arc at the eye when viewed at a specified distance as shown in **Figure 8.3**.

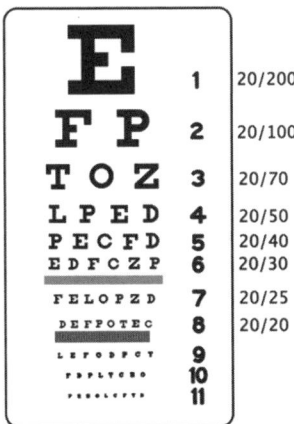

Fig. 8.1: Snellen's test chart.

Chapter 8: Visual Acuity Test

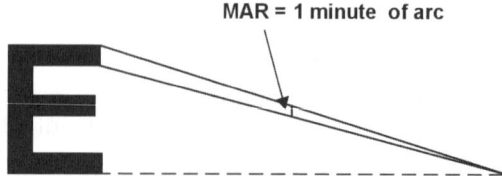

Fig. 8.2: Each limb of the letter subtends an angle of 1 minute of arc for a given distance.

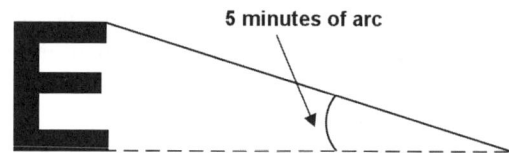

Fig. 8.3: The whole letter subtends an angle of 5 minutes of arc for a given distance.

The letters are not from any ordinary typographer's font. Most letters are designed to ensure:
- ❖ The thickness of the lines equals the thickness of the white spaces between lines and the thickness of the gap in the letter "C".
- ❖ The height and width of the letter is five times the thickness of the line.

Thus, most letters used in the test chart were alphanumeric capitals in the 5 × 5 grid **(Fig. 8.4)**.

There have been cases where letter widths of four units or six units have also been used but the height of the letter remains uniform.

The height of the Snellen's 6 meters letter can be calculated using the following notation:

1 minute of arc = h/6000 mm

where "h" is the size or height of the letter,

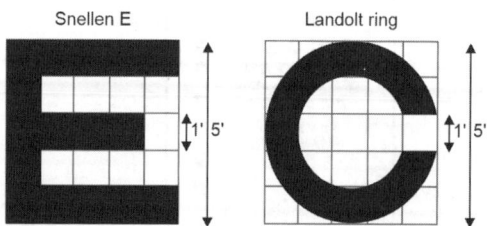

Fig. 8.4: 5 × 5 dimension of Snellen's optotype.

Taking the value from log table

0.000292 = h/6000 mm

Or, 0.000292 × 6000 = h

Or, h = 1.75 mm

Therefore, 5 minutes of arc 5 × 1.75 = 8.75 mm

On Snellen's test chart, 6/6 or 20/20 letter size subtends an angle of 5 minutes of arc which has a letter size of 8.75 mm. Snellen's fraction says that visual acuity depends on two factors:
1. Size of the letter seen
2. Distance at which it is presented

Since the test distance is fixed in the clinical environment, angular size of letter requires constant increase in size in proportion to distance as shown in **Figure 8.5**.

Therefore, the linear size of letter can be derived from the above equation which will be 87.50 mm for visual acuity score of 6/60 or 20/200 which will subtend an angle of 50 minutes of arc. **Table 8.8** shows the linear size of letter for various test distance.

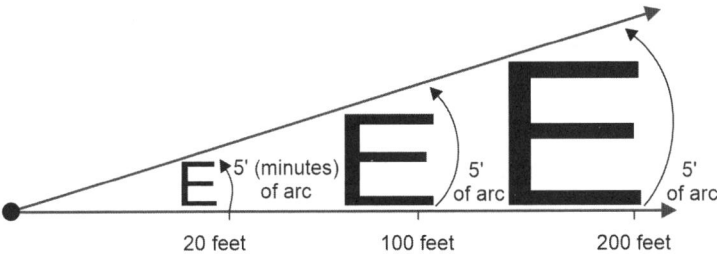

Fig. 8.5: Constant angular substance requires increasing size in proportion to distance.

Table 8.8: Snellen's test chart letter size.

Snellen's visual acuity test chart letters size		
VA in meters	VA in feet	Linear size of letter
6/6	20/20	8.75 mm
6/9	20/30	13.14 mm
6/12	20/40	17.52 mm
6/24	20/80	35.04 mm
6/36	20/120	52.50 mm
6/60	20/200	87.50 mm

Chart Design

The letters in Snellen's test chart are arranged in 11 rows starting from 20/200 or 6/60 to 20/20 or 6/6. There is only one letter in the top row and the number increases progressively in each size level with a maximum of eight at the smallest level (7 letters and 1 number). The size sequence in feet is 200, 160, 125, 100, 80, 63, 50, 40, 32, 25, and 20 or in metric units is 60, 48, 38, 30, 24, 19, 15, 12, 9.5, 7.5 and 6. Many modifications have been made in the original design and in practice the size of the test chart is further reduced to seven rows from 200 to 20 or from 60 to 6 in metric units. The number of letters per line and step size between the lines are variable, as is the horizontal and vertical spacing on the chart. There is also a marked difference in the legibility of different letters on the Snellen's test chart. However, it has been recommended to arrange the mixture of letters in each size level in such a manner so that the effect of difference in legibility is minimized. Two families of letters are mostly used Sloan's letters (5 × 5) and British letters (5 × 4). Sloan's letters are C, D, H, K, N, O, R, S, V, and Z and British letters are D, E, F, H, N, P, U, V, R, and Z.

Test Distance

The visual acuity can be measured in several ways—it can be measured either by varying the distance of the test target of a given size from the eye or keeping the test distance fixed, by presenting the test targets of gradually decreasing size. The latter is feasible in the clinical environment and also has an advantage that the visual acuity is examined at a fixed state of accommodation. In deciding the test distance, it is, therefore, critical that testing distance should be large enough not to stimulate accommodation. The accepted distance in Britain is 6 meters and in USA it is 20 feet. The light rays coming from the object are essentially parallel, and the rays are focused on the retina without effort, i.e., the eye is relaxed and focused on the object. If the gaze shifts to something closer, light rays from the source are too divergent to be focused without effort.

At 6 meters' distance, the letters on the line representing "normal" acuity subtend an angle of 5 minutes of arc, and the thickness of the lines and of the spaces between the lines subtends one minute of arc. There have been efforts to implement a reduced testing distance of 4 meters and to compensate for this change, a correction of -0.25 D is being added to the refractive findings.

In practical 20 feet distance is seldom seen, hence 'indirect' or 'reverse' test chart is placed over patient's head together with mirror at a distance of 3 meters or 10 feet. The mirror used has to be large enough to see whole of the chart and surroundings without moving the head. The mirror should not be framed with such a structure that stimulates accommodation.

Illumination

It is important to ensure adequate luminance for the visual acuity chart and overall room illumination. An increase in ambient room illumination reduces the pupil size. A smaller pupil increases the depth of focus and also reduces the peripheral light rays that enter the eye. Reduced pupil diameter produces less spherical aberration and other higher order aberrations. While illuminating the chart, care must be taken not to produce glare sources within the patient's field of view. In general, visual acuity measurements are made with the visual acuity chart at moderate photopic luminance, and typically, the general room lighting is standard. Bright conditions cause pupil constriction, which may have an adverse effect on visual acuity in cases of centrally located opacities or irregularities. On the other hand, more peripherally located optical defects, as often seen after refractive surgeries, might cause visual acuity reduction when illumination is reduced and the pupil dilates to expose the regions of optical irregularities. In some patients, especially those with retinal diseases, visual performance may be adversely affected by retinal luminance. Under these different circumstances, the clinician may choose to vary the illumination over a wide range to identify the patient's lighting dependencies. The general recommendation is to measure visual acuity in standard room illumination, which may vary between 400 and 850 lux. The rule of thumb is that contrast should be at its maximum and the charts should be illuminated well enough so that extra illumination will not improve visual acuity readings. Room illumination is important as the clinician needs to observe the patient's eyes and also control accommodation, as in dim light accommodation tends to shift towards different and individually characteristic resting positions.

Recording Visual Acuity

The visual acuity measured on Snellen's test chart is recorded as Snellen's fraction which expresses the visual acuity by using the following two factors, i.e., test distance specified in meters or in feet as its numerator and the distance at which letter subtends an angle of 5 minutes of arc as its denominator. The visual acuity is given by:

Chapter 8: Visual Acuity Test

$$\text{Visual acuity} = \frac{\text{Test distance}}{\text{Distance at which letters subtend 5 min of arc}}$$

Therefore, a visual acuity measured as 20/20 denotes that the test distance was 20 feet and the smallest letters that could be read would subtend a visual angle of 5 minutes of arc when at a distance of 20 feet. Similarly, 20/200 denotes that the test distance was 20 feet and the smallest letters that could be read would subtend a visual angle of 5 minutes of arc when at a distance of 200 feet. When recorded in metric system as 6/6 would mean test distance was 6 meters and the smallest letters that could be read would subtend a visual angle of 5 minutes of arc when at a distance of 6 meters. Similarly, 6/60 denotes that the test distance was 6 meters and the smallest letters that could be read would subtend a visual angle of 5 minutes of arc when at a distance of 60 meters.

When visual acuity is below the largest optotype, i.e., 6/60 or 20/200 on the chart, the reading distance is reduced until the patient can read it. And when the patient is able to read the chart, the letter size and test distance are noted.

If the patient is unable to read the chart at any distance, he may be tested to record the acuity in sequential order as given below:
- Counting fingers
- Hand motion
- Light perception

Counting fingers measures the ability of the patient to count fingers at a given distance. This test method is only utilized after it has been determined that the patient is not able to make out any of the letters, rings, or images on the acuity chart at any distance. The acuity measured would be recorded as 'CF 5,' which means the patient was able to count the examiner's fingers from a maximum distance of 5 feet directly in front of the examiner.

If the patient cannot pass the counting fingers test, the examiner moves his hand directly in front of the patient at a distance of 1 foot or less. This test method is only utilized after a patient shows little or no success with the counting fingers test. The results of the hand motion test are often recorded as 'HM' without the testing distance, as it is assumed that the hand motion test has been performed at a distance of 1 foot or less.

In case the patient fails to respond during the hand motion test, the examiner shines a pen light at the patient's pupil and asks the patient to either point to the light source or describe the direction that the light is coming from. If the patient is able to perceive light, the letters LP are recorded to represent the patient's acuity. If the patient is unable to perceive any light, the letters NLP (No Light Perception) are recorded. If NLP is recorded in both eyes, the patient is described as having total blindness.

Normal Values

The acuity score of 20/20 or 6/6 has been accepted as being normal or standard based upon hypothesis of being 'easy to recognize'. However, the best acuity seldom truncates at this level. Most healthy eyes often exceed the standards which optometrists express as visual acuity of 20/16 or 20/12.5, or 20/10 and in metric system as 6/4.8 or 6/3.8 or 6/3.

Testing Procedure

The patient is asked to sit comfortably on a chair at the designated distance from the chart, and monocular visual acuity is measured with one eye occluded. Usual practice is to start measuring the right eye's acuity first, followed by the left eye. Once the monocular acuity is measured, the clinician also measures binocular acuity, which is expected to be marginally better than monocular acuity or at least equal to the visual acuity of a better eye. Rarely, binocular acuity is poorer than the better of the two monocular acuities, which may happen in some cases of binocular vision disorder, nystagmus, metamorphopsia, and in monovision when the patient is unable to alternate central suppression from one eye to the other.

Some clinicians ask patients to read from the largest letter at the top of the chart through to the smallest that can be read. Most clinicians ask their patients to start reading at a size level that is expected to be a little larger than the patient's resolution limit. The patient is instructed to read the chart as much as possible. When reading letters close to the threshold limit, patients should be encouraged to guess.

There may be situations when some patients with macular function disorders or amblyopia miss many letters at different size levels. There may be a tendency to miss the letter at the start or end of rows. Some patients may name the letter sequence. The clinician may help such patients keep their bearings by pointing to individual letters. Eccentric viewing may help patients with macular scotomas achieve better acuity. Patients with amblyopia or macular disorders are likely to achieve better resolution if presented with isolated single letters rather than a series of letters in a row or chart.

▎VISUAL ACUITY TEST CHART FORMATS

An eye chart is probably the most recognizable item in an eye clinic. However, today's eye charts are more than just a printed image hung on a wall—some can be projected in a wide size for fast and efficient testing, while others are presented on an LCD screen in a variety of type sizes and contrast sensitivities to help meet the needs of different patient groups. In common, the visual acuity test charts are made in four different formats, as shown in **Flowchart 8.3**.

Printed Panel Charts

Opaque cards or plastic sheets are used to make printed panel charts. These are directly illuminated test charts and are usually large in size. Front lighting is easiest to implement. Portability and high contrast are the other two biggest advantages of printed panel charts. Test charts may be printed to be designed for low-vision patients, incorporating more rows at the lower acuity level. They may be designed to incorporate more rows at a higher acuity level or from a row of 6/60 to 6/5 for day-to-day clinical application. To predict the

Flowchart 8.3: Formats of visual acuity test charts.

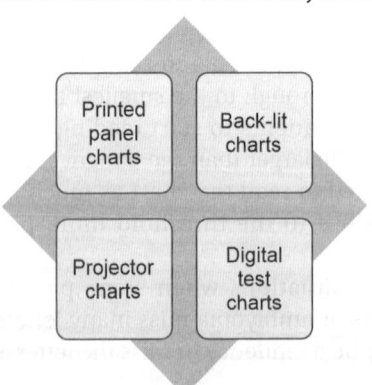

everyday performance of patients, a front-lit printed chart in a lighted room is most preferred.

Back-lit Test Charts

Back-lit charts are printed on translucent material and mounted on a light box that provides illumination from the back side **(Fig. 8.6)**. They are basically made in the form of vision drums along with other common tests like the fan and block test, the worth-4-dot test, the duochrome test, and a spotlight. Usually, they are heavy, and portability is always an issue with these types of charts. Aging of the backlight may adversely affect the contrast between letters and the white background in back-lit test charts. Back lighting of a translucent chart on a light box gives the most even and reproducible illumination.

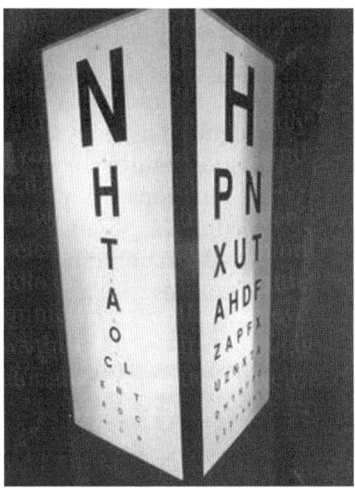

Fig. 8.6: Back-lit chart.

Projector Test Charts

An eye chart projector and screen gives practitioners access to a number of different chart types all in one device. Projector chart systems **(Fig. 8.7)** are usually arranged so that the distance from the patient to the screen is never varied. The projector is usually placed on top of the patient's head so that projector lens and the patient are equally distant from the projection screen. The print size on projector charts is given in angular terms.

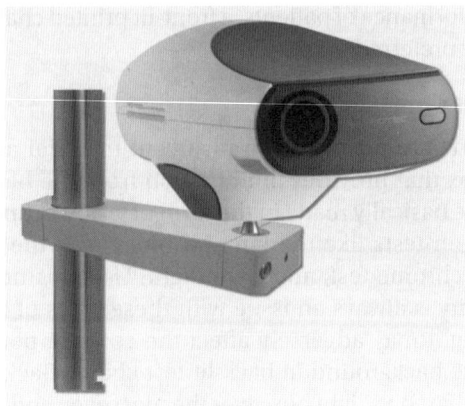

Fig. 8.7: Projector chart.

Digital Test Charts

The new digital acuity system features a wide range of popular optotypes, and test charts required in today's practice environment **(Fig. 8.8)**. The compact remote control is logically configured and provides direct access to all functions. They also provide means to vary letter sequences and stimulus parameters such as contrast, spacing arrangement, and presentation time. The test chart can be configured for various test distances with a click of a button.

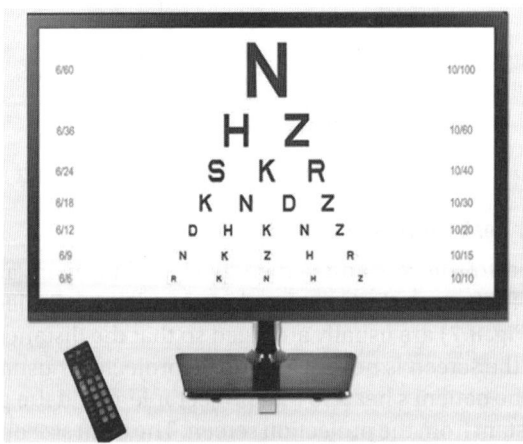

Fig. 8.8: Digital test chart.

CLINICAL ASSESSMENT OF VISUAL ACUITY

Visual acuity is a measure of the patient's ability to resolve the fine details. Distance visual acuity is used to assess the adequacy of the spectacle corrections and as an indicator of ocular health. Visual acuity is also used to check the individual's fitness to drive or enter into some professions like police, railway drivers, etc. There are four principal measures of visual acuity, commonly applied during refraction, shown in **Flowchart 8.4**.

UNCORRECTED VISUAL ACUITY

Uncorrected visual acuity, abbreviated as UCVA, refers to the measurement of acuity when no glasses or contact lenses are used and is most commonly measured immediately after history taking or objective refraction. This is an important measurement to know the current visual status of the eye, and it becomes a benchmark against which the benefits of using refractive correction may be compared. Care must be taken while measuring UCVA to ensure that the patient does not squint or reduce the palpebral aperture to reduce the blur created by defocus or optical irregularities. Measuring UCVA may not be needed in all cases. However, it should be regularly measured in the following cases:

❖ When the patient does not have any previous spectacles or his old spectacles are broken or lost.
❖ When a patient uses his spectacles selectively for some distance viewing task, the information of which has been obtained during case history.
❖ If the information is required for a report.

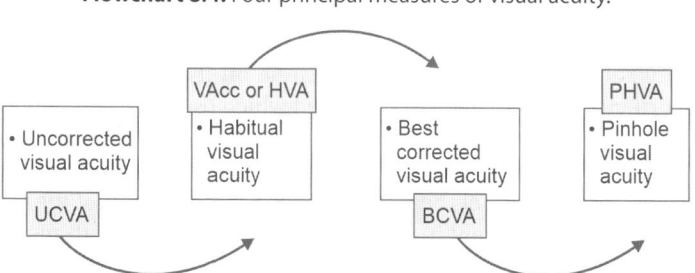

Flowchart 8.4: Four principal measures of visual acuity.

❖ When you suspect during refraction that the patient may not need the correction. This is usually possible in the case of young patients with low hypermetropia.

Habitual Visual Acuity

A well-taken visual acuity measurement is critical to ensure an accurate spectacle correction- just right .... not too strong....and not too weak. This implies that the examiner is looking for the finest detail that the visual system can resolve. Measuring the visual acuity with existing correction reveals information as to the possibilities of any improvements. Many a time the patient carries a perception that his acuity is better with his old correction than the new one. Recording the acuity with habitual correction provides opportunity to compare with the new correction and is also a strong indicator on which the subjective refraction may be initiated. It is recorded using the abbreviation VAcc, known as visual acuity with corrected correction or it may also be recorded as HVA.

Best Corrected Visual Acuity

Best corrected visual acuity refers to the measurement of the best vision correction that can be achieved using corrected correction after refraction has been completed and the new lens prescription has been prescribed. For example, if the UCVA measured for a patient is 20/200 but he can read 20/20 letters after correction, the BCVA would be recorded as 20/20. This implies that the patient's vision is normal using the prescribed correction. A person is considered legally blind if his BCVA is 20/200 or worse.

Pinhole Acuity

Pinhole restricts the light transmission through the hole as shown in **Figure 8.9**. Pinhole acuity can be measured if the visual acuity is worse than 20/30 and is a critical measurement to determine if the decreased visual acuity is correctable by lenses. When pinhole acuity is used, the size of the blur circle on the retina created by uncorrected refractive error is reduced which establishes that better visual acuity may be improved with refraction. Care must be taken in patients with keratoconus and cortical or posterior cataracts because it can channel the light through a better region of the eye's optics. No improvement in visual acuity measurement with pinhole

Chapter 8: Visual Acuity Test

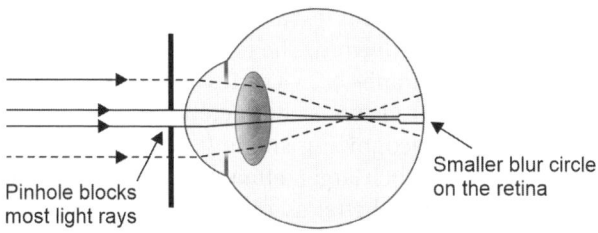

Fig. 8.9: Light transmitted through pinhole.

may indicate amblyopia, or an eye disease or some other disorder. If the acuity does not improve using pinhole, recording of acuity is done as "PH = NI" which means visual acuity not improved with pinhole. Pinhole acuity is applied only for distance. For near vision, the accommodation reflex comes into play, which is the eye's ability to adjust its focus when viewing objects at different distances. When performing tasks up close, like reading or working on a computer, the eyes need to accommodate to maintain clear vision. The pinhole test, designed to address optical issues, does not specifically evaluate the accommodative function needed for near vision tasks. Therefore, it may not provide a comprehensive assessment of the visual system's performance at close distances.

NEAR VISUAL ACUITY

Near vision is traditionally measured with a hand-held near vision test chart held in most cases at 40 cm. It is usually done to check the sufficiency of accommodation. The test for near visual acuity measurement is a test to assess the subject's ability to read progressively smaller print at his normal reading distance. The subject is asked to remain seated in the chair and with a good light on his shoulder, he is given a test chart or card to hold and read them. The near vision is recorded as the smallest type which he can read comfortably together with a note of approximate distance at which the card is held. The emphasis while reading test is on reading performance and not on optics. The objective is limited. Therefore, any reading sample—be it a letter text, word text, or continuous text—may be used, provided it is similar in style to newspaper and book print. Convention is to use the continuous text in the form of small paragraphs set in different sizes because in normal day-to-day life people mostly read continuous text arranged in different paragraphs, not just an isolated letter or word. The text material may be arranged in sentences or in paragraphs or in a series of unrelated words.

Reading text at near vision is completely a different perceptual process rather than recognizing single letter at distance vision. Reading tests require a much larger retinal area than letter recognition tests. They, thus, give us a better assessment of the parafoveal area. Moreover, reading is the function most patients list as their primary visual need.

If the test chart design and the luminance levels are comparable, near visual acuity score should be equal to the score of distance visual acuity, provided the eyes are accommodated or optically corrected to provide good focus for the retinal image. However, there is an exception, as patients with posterior subcapsular cataract whose pupil constriction at near vision tasks causes the pupil area to become more completely filled with the cataract so that the visual acuity becomes degraded.

Like distance visual acuity, there are several ways to designate near visual acuity. Some of them specify near visual acuity in terms of smallest print size read, while others only give in terms of smallest print size read together with test distance. **Flowchart 8.5** shows popular methods.

Sloan and Habel's M Units

Sloan and Habel introduced the M Unit as a measure of print size—a new notation for indicating the height of test letters. The print size is expressed by a number followed by 'M' denoting distance in meters at which it subtends an angle of 5 minutes of arc, for example, near acuity under this system is being recorded as 1.0 M or 2.0 M and so on. **Table 8.9** shows how the acuity is recorded.

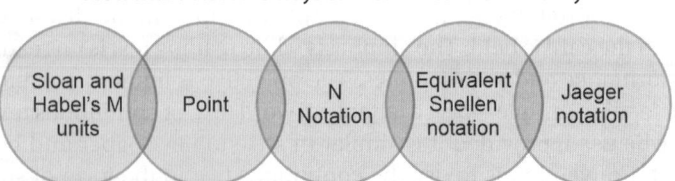

Flowchart 8.5: Five ways to record near visual acuity.

Table 8.9: M Unit as a measure of near visual acuity.

Print size	What does it express?
1.0 M	Letter size that subtends 5 min. of arc at 1 meter (6/6 @ 1 meter)
2.0 M	Letter size that subtends 5 min. of arc at 2 meters (6/6 @ 2 meters)
3.0 M	Letter size that subtends 5 min. of arc at 3 meters (6/6@ 3 meters)
4.0 M	Letter size that subtends 5 min. of arc at 4 meters (6/6 @ 4 meters)
5.0 M	Letter size that subtends 5 min. of arc at 5 meters (6/6 @ 5 meters)
6.0 M	Letter size that subtends 5 min. of arc at 6 meters (6/6 @ 6 meters)

Thus, the M number correspondence to the denominator of the Snellen's fraction. It implies, therefore, that the height 8.73 mm of 6 meters' letters on standard Snellen's chart is 6 M which means 1 M letter may be taken as 8.73/6 or approximately 1.45 mm. Regular newsprint is usually about 1.0 M in size. A patient who can read 1.0 M print size at a distance of 40 cm or 0.40 meter will have his visual acuity recorded as 0.40/1.0 M.

By using the M notation, near visual acuity can be expressed as a true Snellen fraction in which the numerator is the test distance in meters, and the denominator is the smallest size M-unit that can be read at that test distance.

Point

Point size is used in the printing industry to specify the size of the typeset print. One point is equal to 1/72 inch. 4/72 inch is equal to 1.45 mm which can be given an M-unit rating of about 1.0 M in newsprint style font. Near visual acuity is recorded as a point size with specific testing distance. It is handy to remember:

$$1.0 \text{ M units} = 1.45 \text{ mm} \approx 8 \text{ Points (Lower case)}$$

N Notation

In the United Kingdom, the N notation is used for recording near visual acuity. Near visual acuity is noted as N followed by a number with a specified test distance. The N indicates the size of the Times New Roman font. For example, N8 at 40 cm means that the smallest print size that the observer read was 8 point Times New Roman font tested at 40 cm.

Equivalent Snellen Notation

Equivalent Snellen notation, also known as 'Reduced Snellen Acuity' is used to express the distance visual acuity value that is mathematically equivalent to the near visual acuity, assuming a testing distance of 40 cm. Unfortunately, the standard test distance of 40 cm is not always used while measuring near visual acuity. At a testing distance of 40 cm, a 1.0-M size print would be noted as a 20/50 Snellen fraction equivalent. But this relationship does not hold good if the near visual acuity test distance is altered. The most appropriate method to assess and record near visual acuity requires usage of the M unit which allows for conversion to Snellen equivalence.

Jaeger Notation

In the US, Jaeger numbers are widely used. These numbers have no numeric meaning since they refer to item numbers in a printing house catalogue in Vienna in 1854. They cannot be used for calculations. The near visual acuity is recorded as print size and the test distance as J3 at 40 cm.

MULTIPLE CHOICE QUESTIONS

1. **What is visual acuity?**
    a. Visual acuity is the time-dependent measurement of retinal health, specified by the date.
    b. Vision with spectacle
    c. Vision with contact lenses
    d. All of the above
2. **In which year Dr Snellen proposed his optotypes to measure visual acuity?**
    a. 1862
    b. 1882
    c. 1872
    d. 1852
3. **Snellen's letters are so constructed that their each constituent part subtends an angle of:**
    a. 1 minute of arc
    b. 5 minutes of arc
    c. 1 second of arc
    d. 5 seconds of arc

Chapter 8: Visual Acuity Test

4. **What does the numerator of Snellen's fraction denote?**
   a. Test distance
   b. Size of the letter
   c. Angular measurement of visual acuity
   d. All of the above
5. **What does the denominator of Snellen's fraction denote?**
   a. Test distance
   b. Size of the letter
   c. Angular measurement of visual acuity
   d. All of the above
6. **What does the measure 20/20 indicate in Snellen's fraction?**
   a. 20/20 is being chosen as the measure of normal visual acuity based on 'easy to recognize' principle.
   b. 20/20 is the limit of threshold visual acuity beyond which no one can read.
   c. 20/20 is the limit where the average visual acuity is truncated.
   d. All of the above
7. **Which of the following is the most commonly used test for near visual acuity?**
   a. Jaeger card
   b. Confrontation test
   c. Snellen eye chart
   d. Hirschberg test

ANSWER KEY

| 1. a | 2. a | 3. a | 4. a | 5. b | 6. a | 7. a |

SELF-PRACTICE QUESTIONS

1. When a projected chart is used for measuring visual acuity, what are the problems that may result if an excess amount of overall illumination is used?
2. How would you like to record visual acuity using Snellen's test chart in the clinical set-up if a subject cannot see 6/60 at 6 meters distance?
3. Why is it important for the examiner to watch the subject's eyes during visual acuity assessment?
4. Describe when would you like to perform visual acuity assessment using pinhole and how would you do it?

5. What does 6/6 or 20/20 visual acuity mean? Can the visual acuity be better than 6/6 or 20/20?
6. Why 20 feet or 6 meters test distance is considered ideal for measuring visual acuity on Snellen's test chart?
7. What is the importance of room illumination while measuring a patient's refractive error?
8. When can you expect binocular visual acuity is poorer than better of the two monocular acuities?
9. Why is pinhole visual acuity test not applied for near vision distance?

CHAPTER 9

History Taking and Entrance Tests

CHAPTER OUTLINE

- History Taking
- Scripting an Effective Case History for Refraction
- Baseline Data Assimilation

HISTORY TAKING

Sir William Osier, a Canadian Physician considered the Father of Modern Medicine once said, "Listen to the patient, he is telling you the diagnosis."

History taking is one of the most important procedures in all healthcare examinations. It requires the finest skills in the interaction between a clinician and the patient. History taking influences the success of the treatment and management as planned. It provides important insights into how the patient has reacted to illness in the past as well as how he is most likely to react to current treatment. Unfortunately, with the advent of sophisticated diagnostic equipment, clinicians are undervaluing this important mode of clinical communication and relying more on the results of the diagnostic tests and equipment.

Case history for clinical refraction is also very important, and in most cases it is conducted at the beginning of the examination. The clinician asks a series of planned questions that reveal to the clinician the patient's perceptions about his ocular condition, visual functioning, concerns, stress, expectations, and feelings about the difficulties.

Objectives of Case History

Systematic and planned history taking helps the clinician achieve the following objectives during the extensive procedure of clinical refraction:

- ❖ History taking is the first direct interaction between the clinician and the patient. It helps the clinician break the barrier between him and the patient and helps the patient develop confidence in the clinician.
- ❖ History taking helps the clinician gather necessary information through a set of planned questions that allows him to set up the goal for clinical refraction together with the results of other methods of initial examination procedures.
- ❖ History taking is an opportunity for the clinician to educate the patient about his vision and visual system functioning, vision correction gadgets, and general ocular health.
- ❖ Senior and experienced clinicians use it as an opportunity to remove doubts and fears from the patient's mind and clear all myths that rule the patient's mind.
- ❖ History taking is also an opportunity for the clinician to get to know the patient as a person, to understand their lifestyle, their values, their beliefs, and their social and family history. By understanding the patient's context and background, the clinician can better appreciate the factors that may be contributing to their current health status. This can help the clinician tailor their treatment and management plan to the individual patient's needs, preferences, and circumstances.

Overall, history taking is a crucial component of the initial data gathering process during clinical refraction and an important tool for providing patient-centered care.

Who should Take the History?

The clinician who examines the patient must establish a direct practitioner-patient relationship and is the person who should always take the history. The case history should not be separated from the physical examination. It is during this short time that the 'trust and belief' factor is established, based on which the success of treatment and management plans depend. If an assistant or a receptionist takes the patient's history, it is more like a collection of biologic data, which may be used further for necessary reference if needed. But when the clinician himself takes the history, he may read the mental status of the patient and may also formulate the patient's symptoms into a differential diagnosis. An effective and successful treatment plan begins with the initial discussion between the clinician and the patient.

Traits of a Good Case History

An experienced and skilled clinician can often diagnose the outcome of the whole procedure of clinical refraction through a good case history alone, whereas the novice practitioner is frequently overwhelmed by the information gathered and is rarely able to use the information to link the different procedures of clinical refraction. A good case history for clinical refraction usually shows the following traits:

- ❖ The clinician must present himself in the most caring and empathetic manner.
- ❖ The clinician asks open-ended questions to assess the patient's reason for seeking care and to understand his visual needs and lifestyle. The questions must be probing to enable the clinician to dig deeper so that he can establish a link between symptoms and signs and relate the same to the results of different tests, which may be used to set up a link between the patient's visual demands and his visual efficiency.
- ❖ The clinician should directly put up some common symptoms of eye and visual problems to find out if the patient has experienced any of them. He may prepare a list of symptoms and ask the patient to tick them off. In such cases, he must follow up with a discussion to gain clarity of understanding.
- ❖ A comprehensive case history concludes with a summary of all the information gathered by the clinician, articulated in the clinician's own words. This is important for both the clinician and the patient, as the patient understands that the clinician has understood his concerns, and the clinician gets an opportunity to add anything that he might have missed.
- ❖ A good history does not look like a 'laundry list'. The clinician should leave time for spontaneous interaction, varying the sequence of questions depending on the situation.

Golden Rule of History Taking

History is a blend of art and science, and the right proportion brings out the best results from it. Therefore, the quality of interaction matters. A meaningful interaction between the clinician and the patient involves far more than a rigid question-and-answer session alone. The patient has to feel comfortable, and the clinician has to use all his social and scientific skills in an intelligent manner. The clinician should realize that he has to direct his objective principles of medical science in an artistic manner for the maximum benefit of the patient. Therefore, it is mandatory that, while taking history, he is careful about the following facts:

- Use the language that the patient understands. Make all the questions as simple and short as possible.
- Never assume that the patient understands the questions. If needed, clarify and re-clarify the questions.
- Do not expect that the patient will be able to answer you precisely. Often, he will answer in a way that he may not actually mean to convey. So try to read between the lines to be sure of what exactly he intends to convey.
- Always reiterate the patient's version or interpret what he said to clarify the understanding.
- Use simple and practical approaches to emphasize any important query.
- Make a legible record of important findings for future reference with a date.
- Check for contradictions in what the patient says.

SCRIPTING AN EFFECTIVE CASE HISTORY FOR REFRACTION

In an ideal situation, the clinician should begin interactions with the patient by asking appropriate questions, formulated in accordance with the laws of clinical refraction. It is not necessary to ask all the questions at the beginning of the examination; some questions can be reserved and asked during the examination process. Generally, the clinician may choose one or more questions from each of the following groups to establish a foundation for the diagnosis:

Group 1: Making a Connection

1. What is the purpose of today's visit?
2. What are your expectations?
3. How old are your current glasses? Is there any difficulty with them?
4. When did you have your eyes examination done last time? Did your lens prescription change or it was same?

Chapter 9: History Taking and Entrance Tests

The above set of questions are good enough to establish the reason for a patient's visit and kick off the communication between the patient and the clinician on which a foundation of free and effective communication can be established. Good communication or free communication between the patient and the clinician is always therapeutic.

Group 2: General Health Awareness
1. How frequently do you get your eyes examined?
2. How is your general health?
3. Do you have any history of blood pressure or diabetes?
4. Are you on any sort of medication or treatment?
5. Have you ever had any kind of surgery?

When patients are engaged with their own healthcare decisions, it can quickly improve even the most chronic condition. The purpose of the above set of questions is to understand the patient and his awareness about his own health. Achieving health and wellness embodies a holistic state where mental, physical and emotional conditions of the patient need to be in sync as they determine patient's responses.

Group 3: Ocular and Visual Condition
1. Do you have any history of any ocular treatment or surgery?
2. Whether the glasses are used only for distance vision?
3. Any separate glasses for near vision?
4. Any difficulties in bright sunlight?
5. Do you squint your eyes to see clearly?
6. Any difficulties in light/dark adaptation.
7. Any halos around the light, or flashes of light?
8. Itching, burning, tearing, irritation in eye?

The above question helps clinicians understand a patient's visual condition. Thoroughly investigating the patient's complaints about visual disturbances is critical to avoid missing red flags. The differential diagnosis for visual disturbance is very broad, encompassing both minor and serious pathologies.

Group 4: Understanding Occupation and Lifestyle
1. How do you spend your busy day?
2. How do you spend your leisure time?
3. What do you do? Please explain in detail.

4. Could you please describe your working environment briefly?
5. What are your hobbies?
6. Do you drive?
7. What are your specific visual needs?

Immediate dissatisfaction with vision correction in most cases is due to a failure to meet the primary occupational needs of patients. Therefore, it is crucial not only to identify key health and visual issues but also to discuss the patient's occupation, occupational needs, and leisure activities. Once the patient understands this, they are encouraged to talk in more detail about their visual needs. This builds trust in the clinician's understanding, and ultimately, the patient is more likely to listen to and follow the clinician's advice, as they now comprehend the limitations and advantages of different modes of vision correction.

Group 5: Family History

1. Do you have any family history of glaucoma?
2. Do you have any family history of blood pressure or diabetes?
3. Any family history of asthma and thyroid?

Knowledge of past and present family eye and systemic disorders can help save your vision. If there is a history of ARMD in your family, you have a greater than 50% chance of developing it. Research shows that having a family history of glaucoma makes you more likely to get the disease. The earlier the clinician can detect a condition, the better the chances are of preserving your vision. Individuals with no signs of any eye diseases need to know the importance of getting a baseline eye disease screening around the age of 40, when early signs of disease and changes in vision may be noticed.

Group 6: Educating the Patient

1. Do you always use spectacle?
2. Have you ever used contact lenses?
3. Is there anyone in your family who uses contact lenses? How is the experience?
4. Why have you not thought of using contact lenses?
5. Do you use sunglasses when you are outdoors?

The patient needs to know the different modes of vision correction that the clinician can provide and his areas of specialization. He also needs to understand that not all vision correction modes serve the same purpose. There is a need for in-depth discussion with the clinician based upon various factors so that the clinician can prescribe the appropriate mode or modes of vision correction. The patient needs to understand that only a professional clinician is the right person to suggest an appropriate mode of vision correction, and the clinician needs to make sure that he prescribes what is most appropriate for him based upon three factors: prevention, protection, and enhancement.

Group 7: Talking about Common Symptoms

1. Do you ever feel sandy or gritty sensation in your eyes?
2. Do you feel itching in your eyes?
3. Do you feel foreign body sensation?
4. Do you get mucoid discharge?
5. Do you have a dry mouth?

The questions listed under Group 7 are very important in today's context, as most patients report symptoms of dry eyes because of their working environment and occupational needs. It is important for clinicians to differentiate between dry eyes and ocular allergies because, in both cases, the patient's primary complaint is discomfort. The key to distinguishing is careful questioning while taking history. Asking the right questions and rephrasing when necessary will help the clinician have a diagnosis in mind even before he puts the patient on the slit lamp. There are some basic differentiating factors between the two conditions that can be elicited through effective questioning. Dry eye patients usually have mild itching, whereas those with ocular allergies tend to have intense itching. Working environments may cause dry eye symptoms; hence, time is the critical factor, whereas allergies are affected by seasonal variance or allergens that are not linked to time of day. A family history of eczema and asthma may indicate an atopic allergy, whereas the use of certain histamines may be associated with dry eye symptoms.

Additionally, the clinician may quickly check patient's response pertaining to the following queries to get more insights either during the procedure or at the beginning as a part of case history:

1. Feeling of eye strain, effect of glare.
2. Whether or not your eyes water?
3. Do you feel pain in and around eyes?
4. Whether or not he has any difficulties working on your computer?

For symptomatic patients the clinician needs to add the following additional set of questions for each symptom pertaining to time of onset, duration of symptom, severity, frequency, associated symptoms and what relieves the symptoms.

However, for non-adapting patients who re-visit the practice because the prescribed correction has not suited them, the objective of the clinical refraction is totally different. The situation is a little tricky and the clinician needs to think differently. The following set of questions may help:
1. What exactly is the difficulty with your glasses?
2. Is it for the first time you faced the problem or you had experienced before also?
3. How long have you used the new spectacle till today?
4. Is the severity of your difficulty the same from the date it started and now?
5. Is your lens type/frame type the same or changed? Was it your choice or it was recommended by someone?
6. Is there any change in your difficulty if you alter the position of your spectacle on your face or if you change your posture?

In case of children, it is not possible to have any feedback or visual complaints from the children, the clinician must rely on parental observation or guardian who accompanies them for examination, the detailed discussion is given in Chapter 20.

The case history is the beginning of the clinical refraction. The clinician must integrate the art and science of refraction and establish a good practitioner patient relationship, which is crucial to establishing mutual trust, understanding, and confidence. In fact, taking a history is not just trying to discover the patient's problems, it is like making an effort to understand the larger context. The author looks at history taking to include inquiry, insights, and identification, which he calls the 3I's of history taking. Inquiry relates to getting deeper into the patient's life. Insight is like connecting dots and looking at a situation from a deeper perspective. It is not an easy process. Identification stands for discovering the pain areas, the main problem, and gaining ground. Identification also includes observation, which must be connected to develop insights about the patient's ocular and visual condition so that the patient's life can be improved.

BASELINE DATA ASSIMILATION

Once the history taking is completed, the examiner initiates applying some basic tests to assimilate baseline data. He applies certain tests

that help him identify the present condition of his visual system. He also collects his habitual or previous corrections and measures how effectively it is working now for him. Finally, he also measures the refractive error objectively. To do this, conducts following tests:
- Lensometry
- Uncorrected visual acuity (UCVA)
- Vision with habitual correction (VAcc)
- Objective refraction

Lensometry

If the patient is already a user of spectacles, the lens power of the old spectacles should be found out using electronic equipment known as a lensmeter. The power of the old spectacle lens provides an important platform on which the refraction procedure can be initiated. Sometimes it is also used as an initial trial lens. It is an important factor to consider while making the decision to prescribe the new refractive correction. This is because a patient's visual system may have adapted to visual perception. A major change in prescription may alter the way the world is perceived, and therefore it has the potential to cause discomfort, visual disturbances, and even non-adaptation in some cases. It also helps to compare the refractive status of the patient's eyes during the counseling process. Hand neutralization is an alternate method that utilizes loose trial lenses of known power to find the power of unknown spectacle lenses.

There are two types of lensmeters: manual and auto lensmeters. While the manual lensmeter is operated by the user using some electrical or electronic devices involving human effort, skill, and knowledge of its operation, the automatic lensmeter works on its own without deliberation and connotes a predictable response. You simply put the lens on the lens aperture, center the lens well, and the exact lens power appears on the digital display screen. However, the use of a manual lensmeter requires training or a little experience.

Manual Lensmeter

Manual lensmeter **(Fig. 9.1)** is used to ascertain the spheric, cylinder and axis of an ophthalmic lens. It is also used to locate the optical center of the lens, determine the prism diopter in terms of base direction and the amount of prism present.

Chapter 9: History Taking and Entrance Tests

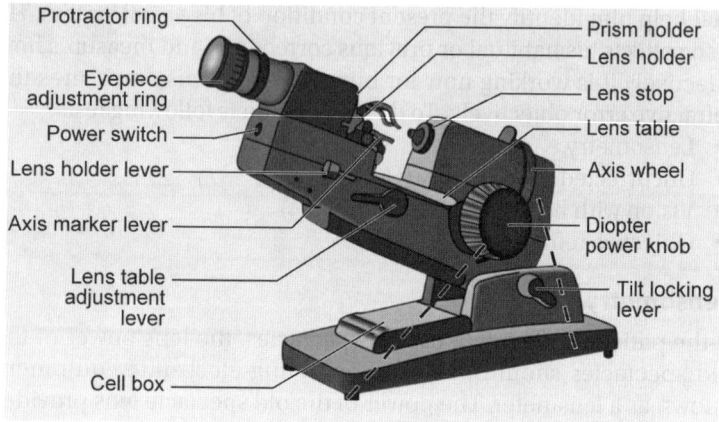

Fig. 9.1: Manual lensmeter.

Targets

Reticle inside the lensmeter is used for focusing the instrument with the help of eyepiece and to determine the prism power. The reticle is a permanently etched series of concentric rings. It also contains orientation lines for each lens meridian and a protractor scale. Each ring denotes one prism diopter.

The target consists of two sets of illuminated lines perpendicular to one another for reading the power of the lens. These lines are focused by the power wheel. They are a little thicker and closely spaced lines. Target types vary with different brands and different models of lensmeter. Three common types of targets that are most commonly found in different brands of lensmeter are given in **Figure 9.2**.

Figure 9.3 shows the pictorial representation of different types of targets.

Critical Factor

Lensmeter does not read lens prescription; it measures the powers of the lens in each meridian. In order to distinguish the sphere and cylinder lines for a particular lensmeter, with no lenses in place set the axis wheel at 180° and focus the lines. The vertically oriented lines are the sphere lines and the horizontally oriented lines are the cylinder lines. Keep the lensmeter in switch off condition and focus

Chapter 9: History Taking and Entrance Tests

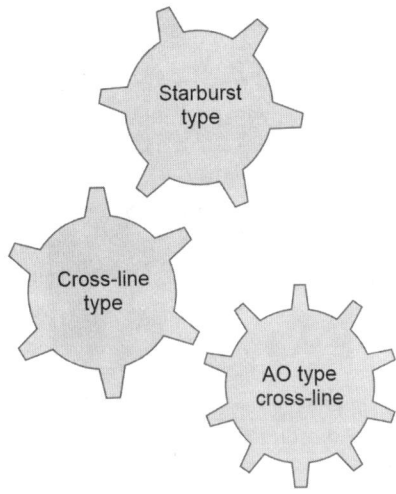

Fig. 9.2: Common types of targets found in lensmeter.

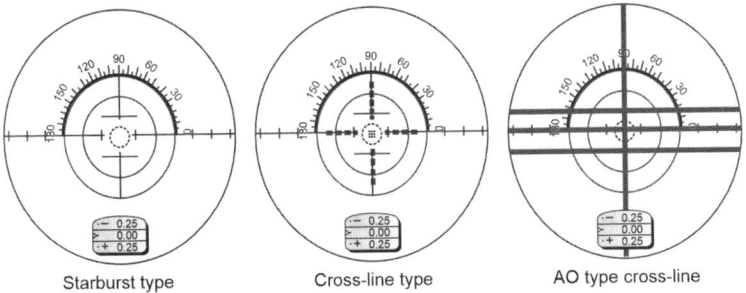

Fig. 9.3: Different types of targets.

the reticle with the eyepiece. Then switch on the instrument. At this time the power wheel should actually read zero diopter because there is only air in place. But often a small offset may be detected. Findings should be adjusted for any offset observed at this time.

Step-by-step Procedure

1. Sit right in front of the lensmeter and focus the black reticle with eyepiece. If it is not in focus, the reading will be erroneous. This is to be adjusted to accommodate the user's own refractive error **(Fig. 9.4)**.

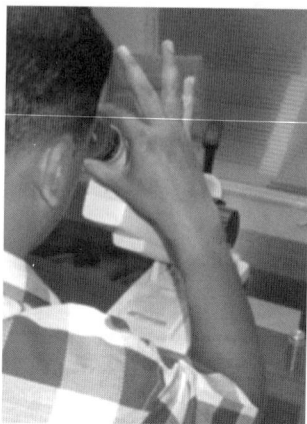

Fig. 9.4: Adjusting the eyepiece of the lensmeter.

2. Now switch on the lensmeter **(Fig. 9.5)**, set the axis wheel on 180° and bring the reading scale to zero and see whether the illuminated targets and the black reticle both are sharply in focus.

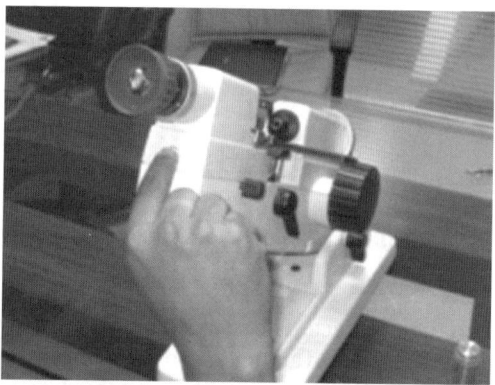

Fig. 9.5: Switching on the lensmeter.

3. Place the back vertex (ocular side) of the **(Fig. 9.6)** lens against the stop of the lensmeter on the platform or if the lens is fitted in a spectacle frame place the spectacle lens so that the temples of the frame is away from you. Make sure both front eye rims—right and left are in contact with the platform.

Chapter 9: History Taking and Entrance Tests

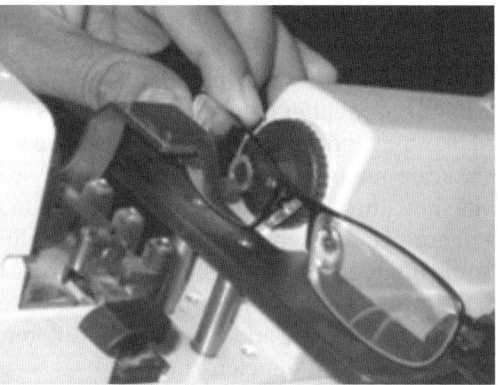

Fig. 9.6: Placing spectacle lens onto the platform.

4. Center the lens by moving it on the platform so that the illuminated target is aligned to the center of the reticle by moving the lens side to side or by moving platform up and down. If the lens also has prism correction, it will be difficult to align.
5. Rotate the power wheel to focus on the targets sharply and observe the two illuminated lines which are perpendicular to each other. If both the lines are in focus together, the lens is said to have only spherical power. The starburst ring is seen as a well-defined circular ring made of identifiable dots. The amount of spherical can be read on the power reading scale **(Fig. 9.7)**. Red letter shows minus power and the other shows plus power.

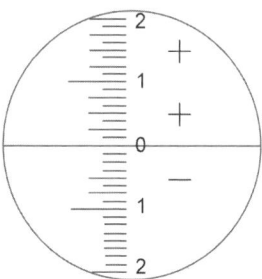

Fig. 9.7: Power reading scale inside the lensmeter.

6. If only one set of lines is in focus and the other is blurred, the lens is said to have cylindrical power. Since cylinder lens forms

the line image, the circular starburst ring made of dots is seen as oblong shape image made of well-defined lines which are focused twice on two principal meridians.
7. Cylinder power may either be plano-cylinder or spherocylinder. In case of plano-cylinder the spherical line will be focused when the power scale reads zero and cylinder line at some number which will show the amount of cylinder present in the lens. In case of sphero-cylinder lens, the spherical line will be focused first on some number which will show the spherical component and then the cylinder line at some other number which will show the summation of spherical and cylinder. The difference between the two will give the cylinder element.
8. The axis will be determined when the cylinder line is focused sharply. Orient the axis wheel of the lensmeter such that the cylinder lines are perfectly continuous together with the oblong illuminated image. Read the axis from the axis wheel. When the axis is not correctly positioned, the lines will appear "broken" or as if "gates were left open."
9. Axis can directly be determined by rotating the protractor ring. The black line when parallel to focused cylinder line will point at the axis on the protractor.
10. Before removing the lens, put the dot on the optical center of the lens using the ink marking device. While doing so, make sure the target should be right at the center of the reticle.
11. To ascertain the power of the multifocal lenses, following additional steps are needed:
    - Read and record the power of the distance portion as above.
    - Turn the lens around so that the ocular surface faces you. The bifocal segment power is measured with temples pointing towards you (FVP) when the lenses are fitted in the spectacle frame.
    - Raise the platform up and check the power through the near segment area.
    - Compare the spherical power through the near segment to the spherical power through the distance portion. The difference between the two is taken as the value of near addition power.
12. If the lens is ground with prism, it may be impossible to center the target within the reticle. Mark a dot at the point where the patient's interpupillary distance coincides. Align this dot at the center of the reticle. Read the position of the starburst circular

Chapter 9: History Taking and Entrance Tests

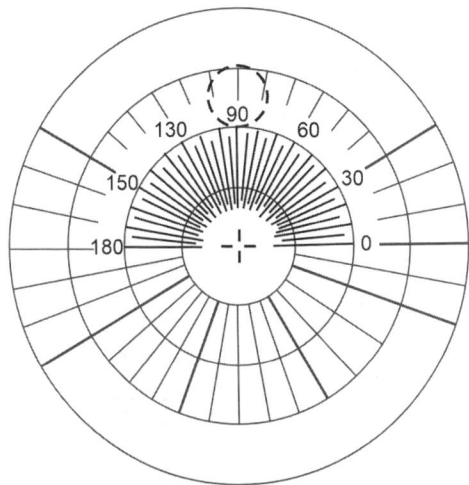

Fig. 9.8: Prism shifts the starburst circular ring position.

ring with respect to the number of circle in the reticle. Each circle denotes one diopter of prism **(Fig. 9.8)**.
13. Record the reading so derived.

Auto Lensmeter

Recently auto lensmeter has replaced manual lensmeter. **Figure 9.9** shows the different parts of the auto lensmeter.

LCD Screen

The LCD screen in a lensmeter serves as the display interface that provides the results of the lens power measurement. The user interface on the LCD screen is designed to be user-friendly, providing clear and concise information to the operator. It may include symbols or indicators for different measurement parameters.

Operation Switch

The operations switch in an auto lensmeter serves as a control mechanism to navigate through various interfaces and functionalities displayed on the screen. The switch allows users to access different menus and settings on the lensmeter. This is important for adjusting measurement parameters, configuring device settings, or accessing additional functionalities.

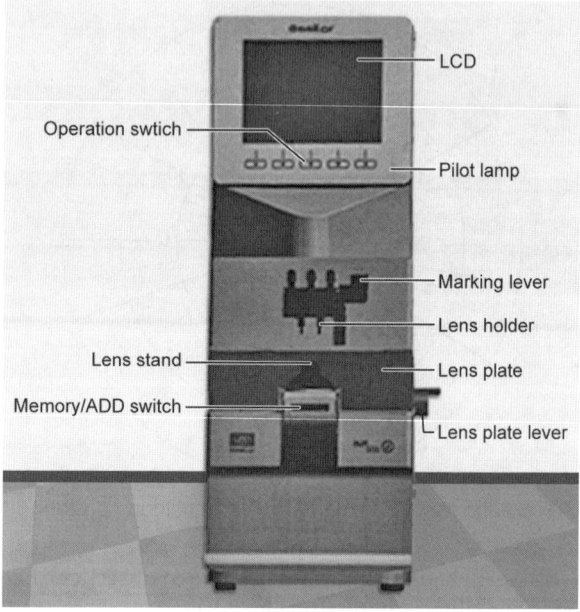

Fig. 9.9: Parts of auto lensmeter.

Pilot Lamp

The pilot lamp in an optical instrument is a crucial visual indicator that communicates the on/off state and power-saving mode, providing users with essential information about the operational status of the device.

Marking Lever and Lens Holder

The marking lever and lens holder are integrated. Marking lever is used to put the ink dots on the lens when it is pressed down. Lens holder fixes the framed lens on the lens stand by moving the lever up and down.

Lens Stand

The lens stand is a component of the lensmeter that provides a stable platform for positioning and measuring lenses. It is often equipped with a lens holder or clamps to secure the framed lens in place.

Lens Plate

The lens frame should be in contact with the lens plate, ensuring that the lens is stable and properly aligned for accurate measurements.

When measuring a framed lens on a lensmeter, accurate alignment with the cylinder axis reference, proper positioning for prism correction (if applicable), and stable contact between the lens frame and the lens plate are essential steps for obtaining precise and reliable measurements.

Lens Plate Lever
Lens plate lever is used to move the lens plate back and forth.

Memory/Add Switch
Memory/Add switch in an auto lensmeter plays a pivotal role in memory storage, freezing display values, and facilitating manual measurement for specific lens types, contributing to the overall functionality and efficiency of the lensmeter in diverse optical scenarios.

After pressing the Memory/Add switch, the lensmeter freezes the display, preventing any further changes to the measurement values. This ensures that the recorded values for the specific lens type (short focus, multifocal, or contact lens) are stored accurately for reference or documentation.

In the case of progressive lenses, the Memory/Add switch has a specific function related to manual measurement. It sets the near and far points on the measurement screen during manual measurement. Progressive lenses have distinct zones for near and far vision, and the switch aids in accurately defining these points for precise measurements.

Measurement of Uncut Single Vision Lens (Fig. 9.10)
The auto lensmeter measures the lens power quickly and automatically. The procedure for measuring lens power is as below **(Fig. 9.11)**.
1. Set the lens holder properly.
2. Clean the lens under lens stand.
3. Turn on the power switch, the display screen appears.
4. Place the lens on lens stand and then leave the lens holder softly on the lens, lens power is displayed on the screen.
5. Bring the cross cursor to the alignment mark by moving the lens.
6. The lensmeter may show 'Alignment Ok' on the screen. At this moment recheck the lens power as shown in the display screen. The alignment mark represents the optical center of the

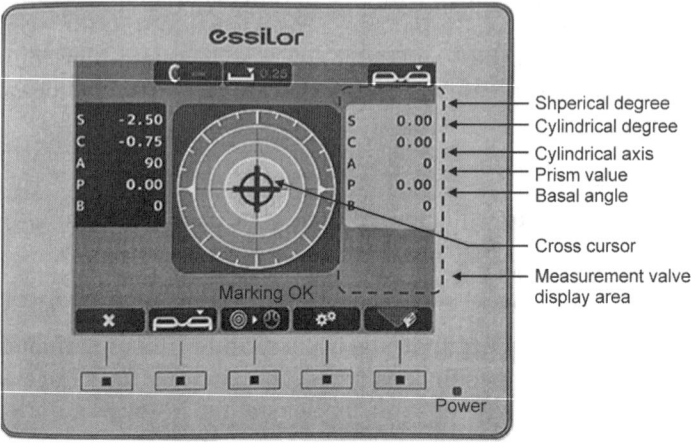

Fig. 9.10: Single vision lens measurement screen.

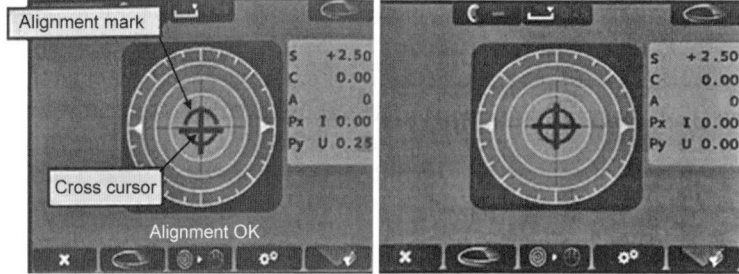

Fig. 9.11: Alignment mark and cross cursor.

lensmeter and the cross cursor represents the optical center of the lens.
7. If the lens power has cylinder power, rotate the lens to fit the axis direction.
8. Overlap the cross cursor and the alignment mark by moving the lens.
9. When they overlap, the instrument is ready to carry out marking.
10. Spherical, cylinder, axis and prism can be stored using Memory/Add switch.
11. The color of the measurement values are changed and fixed.

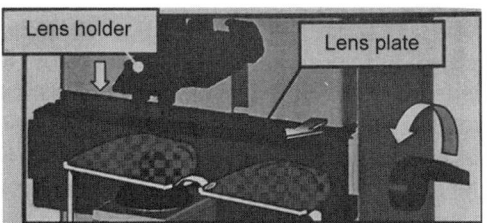

Fig. 9.12: Placing the framed lens on lens holder.

Measurement of Framed Single Vision Lens (Fig. 9.12)

In order to measure the lens power of framed lenses, follow the below steps:
1. Place the frame lens on the lens stand and lower the holder softly on the lens.
2. Move the lens plate so that the bottom of the lens touches the lens plate.
3. Specify the right or left of the lens.
4. Align the lens as explained above, but while aligning make sure that the bottom of the frame lens always touches the lens plate.
5. Also read the lens power on display screen.
6. Save the measurement values in memory by pressing Memory/Add switch.
7. Switch the lens to the other eye and follow the similar steps.
8. Switch the measurement to the left lens by pressing the respective switch.
9. At this moment the values of the right lens remain on the screen.

Measurement of Multifocal Lens

In case of bifocal lenses, follow the below steps:
1. Take the measurement of far point as explained above.
2. Press the Memory/Add switch. The lens power will be stored in memory.
3. Press the Memory/Add switch one more time, "Ad1" is displayed.
4. Now move the lens so as to center the near segment to the center of lens stand, near addition will be displayed.
5. Press the Memory/Add switch to store the value of near addition.
6. In case of trifocal, display "Ad2" by pressing the Memory/Add switch one more time. After that repeat the procedure as above after bringing the second near segment to the center of the lens stand.

Measurement of Progressive Addition Lens

In case of progressive addition lens, follow the below steps:
- ❖ Set the lensmeter to "AutoProg" mode. It allows the instrument to judge whether the lens is progressive or not.
- ❖ Switch to progressive lens measurement screen.
- ❖ Set the lens in the center region of the progressive zone.
- ❖ It starts autojudgment of the progressive lens. When the lens is identified as a progressive lens, the screen is switched to the progressive lens measurement screen.
- ❖ When the value of near addition power is small, the autodetection may not happen. In this case move the lens back and forth and right and left slowly. In such case you may need to take the measurement manually.
- ❖ The cross cursor appears when the progressive zone is found and the lens power appears on the screen.
- ❖ Now align the cross cursor with the alignment mark of the lensmeter and recheck the lens power. Distance power and near addition will appear simultaneously.

Uncorrected Visual Acuity (UCVA)

Monocular UCVA should be recorded immediately after history taking. Care must be taken to ensure that the patient does not squint or narrow the palpebral aperture to reduce the blur created by defocus or optical irregularities. Measuring UCVA without any lenses in front of the eye is an important step in evaluating visual function and providing appropriate eye care. It provides information on how well a person can see without any external corrective measures, such as glasses or contact lenses. By measuring UCVA, eye care the examiner can determine the baseline level of a person's visual function, which is important for assessing the degree of visual impairment and monitoring changes over time. This information can also guide decisions about the need for corrective lenses or other interventions to improve visual function. Furthermore, measuring UCVA can help diagnose underlying eye conditions that may be affecting a person's vision, such as cataracts or refractive errors. It can also be useful in assessing the effectiveness of treatments for such conditions.

Habitual Visual Acuity (HVA/VAcc)

Not only is measuring the power of previous spectacles important, but it is equally important also to measure the visual acuity with the same, as it provides the information that helps the clinician set up the goal for the clinical refraction. It must be measured for each eye separately at the beginning of the whole process. Measuring visual acuity with habitual correction is important for several reasons:

❖ Determining visual acuity with the individual's habitual correction provides a baseline assessment of their current vision with the existing prescription. This baseline is crucial for understanding the starting point and identifying any changes or improvements needed.

❖ Assessing visual acuity with habitual correction allows the clinician to understand the patient's everyday visual experience. This information can offer insights into the effectiveness of the current prescription and any challenges the patients might be facing in their daily activities.

❖ Comparing visual acuity with habitual correction to the visual acuity without correction helps identify changes in the refractive error. This is essential for making informed decisions about adjusting the prescription to address any alterations in the patient's vision.

❖ Understanding how the patient's vision functions with their habitual correction aids in optimizing the accuracy of the new prescription. It allows the eye care professional to fine-tune the prescription to meet the patient's visual needs and preferences.

Objective Refraction

Three common tests can objectively measure refractive error: the autorefractometer, retinoscope, and keratometer. The results from these objective methods, combined with the outcomes of UCVA and VAcc, are used to establish the goals for clinical refraction, taking into account the patient's history. For a detailed discussion on objective refraction, *refer* to Chapter 10.

MULTIPLE CHOICE QUESTIONS

1. Which of the following is not the part of history taking?
    a. Chief complaints
    b. History of past health
    c. Visual assessment
    d. Medication currently used
2. When recording a patient's ocular and visual history which one of the following types of information is not relevant?
    a. Details regarding difficulties in light/dark adaptation.

b. Details regarding history of any ocular treatment or surgery.
   c. Whether there is a family history of ARMD?
   d. Any difficulties in bright light.
3. When considering a systemic health condition of the patient for the purpose of refractive error assessment, which one of the following is an important consideration?
   a. Blood sugar level
   b. Hypertension
   c. AIDS
   d. All of the above
4. Which one of the following needs to be specifically asked about when enquiring about a person's lifestyle history for the purpose of refractive error assessment?
   a. Details regarding visual needs
   b. Hobbies
   c. Activities of busy day and leisure time
   d. All of the above

ANSWER KEY

| 1. c | 2. c | 3. d | 4. d |

SELF-PRACTICE QUESTIONS

1. A patient complains of significant loss of vision that he noticed recently. Outline a series of questions that you would like to ask as a part of history taking that will help you to elicit the characteristics features of the problem.
2. A patient complains of asthenomic symptoms after using the new correction. Outline a series of questions that you would like to ask as a part of history taking that will help you to elicit the characteristics feature of the problem.
3. How does information pertaining to previous lens prescription help in deciding the present prescription of vision correction?
4. During history taking what complaint or complaints would you expect to hear from a patient having (a) myopia (b) hypermetropia and (c) astigmatism.
5. List the patient reported symptoms that would cause you to suspect each of the forms of headache: (a) hypertension (b) eye strain.

10 CHAPTER

Objective Methods of Refraction

CHAPTER OUTLINE

- Objective Refraction
- Retinoscopy
- Autorefractometer
- Keratometry
- Assimilation of Initial Data and Goal Setting

OBJECTIVE REFRACTION

Objective refraction is the method to determine the refractive error of an eye without taking any responses from the patient, i.e., the patient is not asked to read anything and provide any input to the practitioner. This gives a good starting point for the subjective refraction for the regular patients and is the only technique for the patient whose subjective responses are absent, limited or unreliable. The refractive error is determined according to a set of criteria identified in advance by the examiner or by a preprogram instrument. The end point is achieved by the action of the examiner. There are several methods that can be applied to obtain an estimate of refractive error of a patient objectively. The most common of them are shown in **Figure 10.1**.

RETINOSCOPY

Retinoscopy has gained the recognition of gold standard and is an excellent objective method to determine the refractive status of the eye with respect to the point of fixation. If the point of fixation is at a close distance, it is called "Near Retinoscopy" or "Dynamic Retinoscopy" and if it is at a long distance, it is called "Static Retinoscopy". It also serves as first opportunity to view the internal

Chapter 10: Objective Methods of Refraction

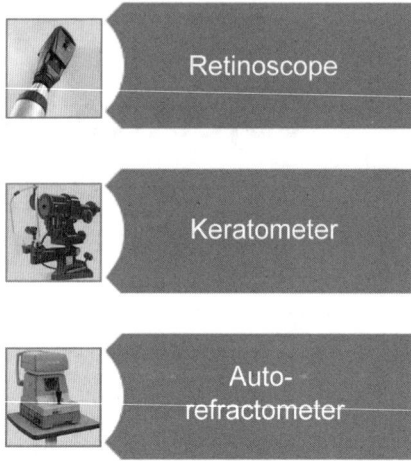

Fig. 10.1: Different types of equipment used for objective method of refraction.

structure of the eye. It is best done on undilated eyes with an exception of patients with pupil less than 2 mm and young patients with active accommodation. In case the retinoscopy is performed on a dilated eye, the practitioner should ignore the confusing reflexes seen at the pupil edge and pay attention to central reflex only. In order to determine the refractive status of the eye, it projects the light beam onto the retina through the pupil. When the light beam focuses onto the retina, the direction of light travel is reversed. The observer sees the light reflex coming from the pupil through peephole in the scope and determines the refractive error by observing the behavior of the reflex under certain condition. Thus, the results of the retinoscopy are not dependent upon the patient's response. The basic principles of retinoscopy for both static retinoscopy and dynamic retinoscopy are common.

Since the introduction of retinoscopy as a clinical procedure for eye examination, it has been performed as one of the very first procedures during the eye examination. It is a great tool to establish a strong basis for the refractive status of the eye on which subjective refraction can be followed. In addition, retinoscopy helps to detect the aberrations of the cornea and the crystalline lens. It also provides some clues in respect of opacities of ocular media. Retinoscopy is particularly very helpful tool with uncooperative or malingering patients, infants,

Chapter 10: Objective Methods of Refraction

deaf and in all such cases where language or communication creates difficulties during the process of refraction. Retinoscopy is ineffective in case of media opacities or corneal irregularities.

Parts of Retinoscope

The streak retinoscope **(Fig. 10.2)** is designed as a very compact hand-held instrument which has two main systems:
- Projection system, and
- Observation system

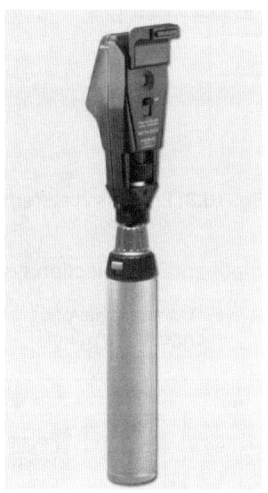

Fig. 10.2: Streak retinoscope.

Projection System

Projection system as shown in **Figure 10.3** projects the light beam through the pupil and illuminates the retina. It contains the components as shown in **Flowchart 10.1**.
- **Light source:** The light source contains a powerful halogen bulb and is at the bottom of the instrument. The streak retinoscope contains bulb with a linear filament to project a streak of light.
- **Condensing lens:** Condensing lens is a plus lens that lies in the path of light. It gathers the light emitting from the bulb and focuses them onto the mirror. The position of this lens in relation to the bulb can be changed by raising or lowering the focusing sleeve.

Chapter 10: Objective Methods of Refraction

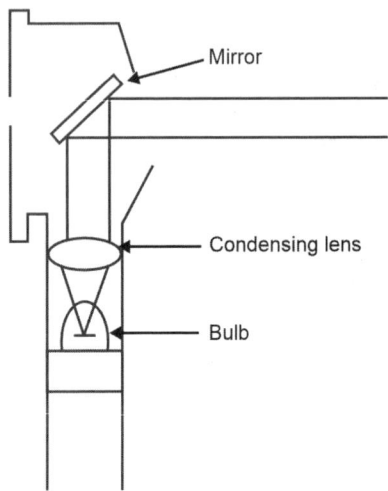

Fig. 10.3: Projection system.

Flowchart 10.1: Components of projection system of retinoscope.

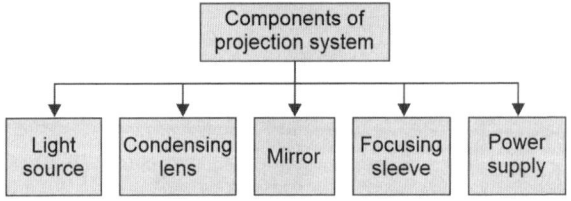

- ❖ **Mirror:** The mirror bends the path of light at right angle such that the light beam is projected onto the retina. It also facilitates reflected light from the retina to enter the examiner's eye.
- ❖ **Focusing sleeve:** Focusing sleeve varies the distance between the bulb and the lens. Changing the distance between the bulb and the lens is responsible for plane mirror effect or concave mirror effect. Sleeve up produces plane mirror effect and sleeve down produces concave mirror effect. Sleeve also controls streak rotation. Turning the sleeve rotates the bulb, which in turn rotates the projected streak.
- ❖ **Power supply:** Power supply needed to project the light beam may be generated either through battery or it may be electric operated.

Observation System

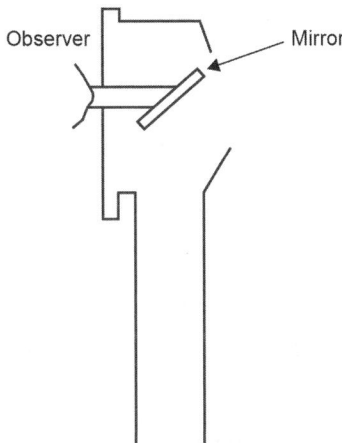

Fig. 10.4: Observation system.

Observation system **(Fig. 10.4)** lies towards the practitioner while using the retinoscope to observe the reflex. The system contains a peephole which allows the observer to see the retinal reflex from the pupil.

When the observer wiggles the scope while looking through the peephole, he sees the movement of streak projecting on the retina through the peephole. The rays of light emerging from retina are affected by the optical components of the eye. The manner in which they are affected tells us about the refractive state of the patient's eye.

Types of Retinoscope

There are two types of retinoscope:
1. Spot retinoscope
2. Streak retinoscope

Spot retinoscope has an ordinary light globe that gives a patch or spot of light. Streak retinoscope has a special light bulb with linear filament that gives a streak or line of light. This reflex appears as a red to red-orange glow with a slight shadow around it. The streak has both plano mode and concave mirror mode. The spot has a plano mode only. When streak is used in the plano mode, it is basically a spot with sides cut off. The streak retinoscope has less illumination and the optical phenomena that take place away from the center of the streak are obscured. It will be more difficult to observe subtle changes in color or brightness. Generally, this information is available with spot retinoscope. However, in practice streak retinoscope is more popular as it facilitates refinement of axis of cylinder correction. In all our further discussion, we will consider the use of streak retinoscope.

Principle of Retinoscope

Retinoscopy works on the concept of Far Point which is an important aspect of visual optics **(Fig. 10.5)**. The concept states that the "far point" is the point in the space at which the object must be placed along the optical axis so that its image is focused on the retina when the eye is not accommodating. It is the farthest point from the eye at which the object is kept so that one can see it clearly when the accommodation is at rest. The meaning, therefore, is that the object has to be brought to a point conjugate to the retina in order to be seen clearly by the unaccommodating eye. Accommodation is needed only when the object is brought closer to the eye than the conjugate point. A myope has the far point at a finite distance from the eye. High myopes have closer far point than the low myopes. In hypermetropic eye the far point always lies behind the retina. The far point of an emmetropic eye is at infinity.

The aim of static retinoscopy is to find the position of the paraxial far point of the eye. The refractive components of the eye apply vergence to the emerging rays of light. Using the plane mirror, the outgoing light rays leave the eye according to the nature of refractive error. In emmetropia rays of light leave parallel, in hypermetropia the outgoing rays of light are diverging and in myopia the emerging rays

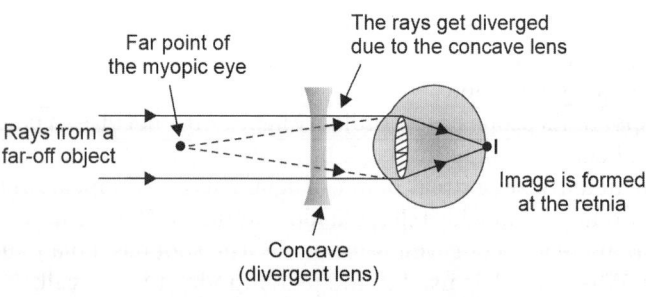

Fig. 10.5: Far point principle.

are converging. When the practitioner looks through the peephole, he sees those emerging rays as retinal reflex in the patient's pupil. Sweeping the streak across the pupil moves the reflex. If the movement of reflex is in the same direction of the streak, it is called "with motion reflex" and is because of the fact that the rays of light have not yet converged to a far point. If the reflex moves in the opposite to the streak, it is called "against motion reflex" and is because the rays have come to a focus and then have diverged. So, we see "against motion reflex". Simplifying the concept, if the observer sees against motion reflex, he is beyond the Far Point. If you see with motion reflex, the Far Point is beyond him.

Working Distance

The working distance while doing retinoscopy is the distance between patient's eye and the practitioner's position as shown in **Figure 10.6**. It is an important factor which may range anywhere between 40 cm to 100 cm. Usually, we choose to hold the retinoscope either at 66 cm away from the patient or 50 cm if your arms are short. The closer distance provides bright reflex, but distance error is high, whereas larger distance provides dim illumination but distance error is low.

When the neutrality is reached, it implies that the patient's retina is in sharp focus. If you were 6 m away from the patient, the lenses needed to neutralize the reflex would be the same as the person's

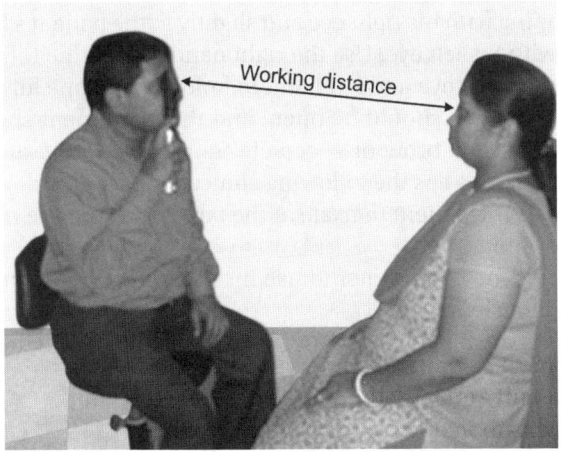

Fig. 10.6: Working distance.

refractive error. But this is impractical. That is why a shorter working distance is chosen. When we choose a shorter working distance, we need to compensate the results of the retinoscope for the working distance.

For a working distance of 66 cm we subtract the retinoscopy results by 1.50 D and for 50 cm, we subtract the retinoscopy result by 2.00 D.

Room Illumination

Retinoscopy should ideally be done in a dimly lit room. In total dark, accommodation is not completely at rest. Complete darkness also creates problem in movement and handling the correcting lenses and is absolutely not advised when there is gender difference. Dim light facilitates ease of movements and also allows the patient to fixate at suitable target.

Patient and Practitioner Posture

The patient should sit on the patient's chair upright in front of the practitioner at the same level. He should keep looking at the fixation target at the distance to keep his accommodation at rest. A light usually provides the most suitable fixation target. If nothing is available 6/60 letter of the illuminated vision drum is suitable. He should also wear the trial frame to facilitate the use of correcting lens.

The practitioner should sit before the patient on his chair. He should move slightly to the patient's right as shown in **Figure 10.7** while scoping with his right eye and slightly to the patient's left while scoping with his left eye. Use the right hand to hold the retinoscope for patient's right eye and left hand to hold retinoscope for patient's left eye. Both eyes should be open, and the instrument should rest firmly against the brow or spectacle frame **(Figs. 10.8 and 10.9)**. Using both hands has the following clinical implications:
1. It allows the patient to fixate at the target with the eye not under observation.
2. It allows the practitioner to use his other hand for handling the correcting lenses.
3. Helps maintain horizontal and vertical alignment with the patient.

Projecting the Light Beam

In order to move the projected streak **(Fig. 10.10)**, he needs to wiggle the scope. The streak is always moved perpendicular to its axis, i.e.,

Chapter 10: Objective Methods of Refraction

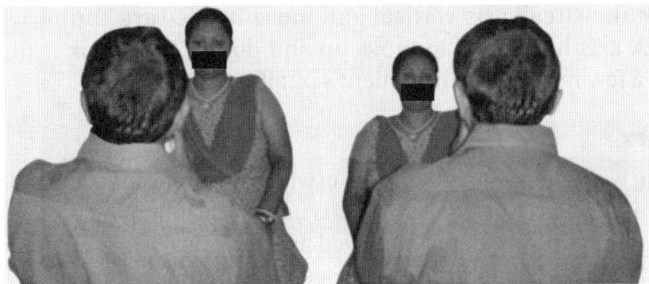

Fig. 10.7: Practitioner and patient posture.

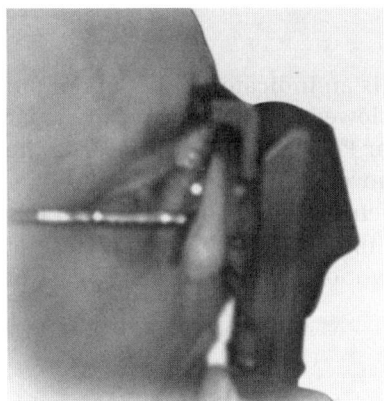

Fig. 10.8: Using brow rest with spectacle.

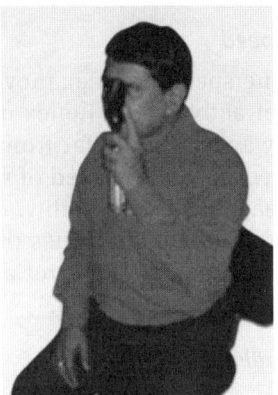

Fig. 10.9: Practitioner posture with retinoscope.

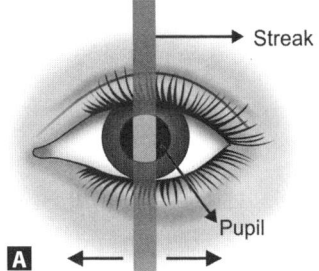
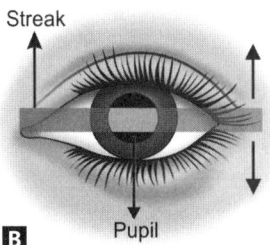

Figs. 10.10A and B: Projecting streak. (A) Streak vertical; (B) Streak horizontal.

place the streak axis vertical and move it sideways and place the streak axis horizontal to move up and down. The streak is moved only a few mm across the patient's pupil.

Reflex

When we project light on the retina with the retinoscope, the retina is illuminated as if it were a luminous body. The emerging rays of light from the retina are being observed as a retinal reflex in the patient's pupil while looking through the peephole in the retinoscope which moves if we sweep the streak across the pupil. The moving reflex is analyzed to determine the refractive error under the three categories as shown in **Figure 10.11**.

Speed

The speed of reflex movement is an indicator of the amount of refractive error. Reflex moves slower when the neutrality is far away or you are far from the Far Point. As you get closer to the neutrality, the speed of reflex movement becomes rapid, and on reaching the neutrality, no movement is seen, i.e., the pupil fills completely. It implies that fast moving reflex is seen in case of smaller refractive error and slow-moving reflex is seen in case of large refractive error.

Brilliance

The brilliance of the reflex also indicates the amount of the refractive error. A bright reflex is being seen when you approach the neutrality and a dull reflex is being seen when you are far away from the

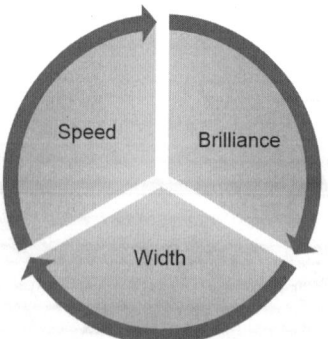

Fig. 10.11: Three aspects retinoscopy reflex.

neutrality, i.e., away from far point. This implies larger errors have a dull reflex and smaller errors have a bright reflex. The brilliance of reflex is also different in case of "with motion reflex" and "against motion reflex". It is comparatively dull in case of against motion reflex at any comparable distance from the far point.

Width

The change in width of the reflex band **(Figs. 10.12 and 10.13)** is noticed as you approach neutrality. It is narrow when you are far away from the neutrality and is widest, i.e., entire pupil fills up, when the neutrality is achieved. The width of the band increases gradually from narrow to wide as you approach the far point.

Spherical and Astigmatic Reflex

The spherical refractive error show different characteristics than the astigmatic reflex. Reflex in spherical error has the following features:

- ❖ The reflex will appear similar in all the meridians.
- ❖ The reflex will not show "Break phenomenon".
- ❖ Similar brilliance and width are seen in all meridians.
- ❖ Speed of movement of reflex is same in all meridians.
- ❖ As the streak is rotated, the reflex stays aligned with the streak in all meridians.
- ❖ Reflex will be neutralized in all the meridians by the same lens power.

The astigmatic reflex has the following features:

- ❖ The retinal reflex will appear different in different meridians.
- ❖ The reflex will show "Break phenomena" and will be aligned to the streak only in two principal meridians.

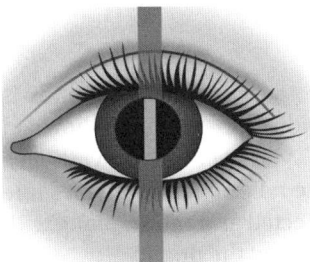

Fig. 10.12: Appearance of streak narrow.

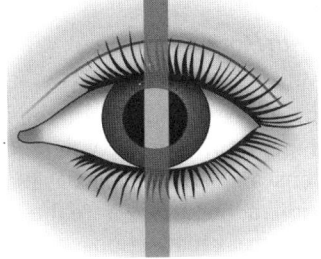

Fig. 10.13: Appearance of streak wide.

- In each principal meridian, the reflex will show different brightness and width.
- The reflex may have different movement in each of the principal meridians. Their speed may also differ.
- The reflex will be neutralized in each of the two principal meridians by different correcting lens.
- Occasionally unusual reflex may be seen.

Movement of the Reflex

The concept of retinoscopy is based on the movement of the reflex observed within the pupil. While attempting to estimate the refractive error, the retinoscopist tries to understand the movement of the reflex. During the process he may observe one of the several types of movement of the reflex as shown in **Flowchart 10.2**.

Flowchart 10.2: Different types of movement of reflex.

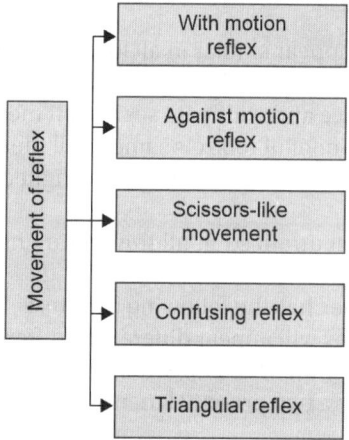

With Motion Reflex

When the retinoscopist wiggles the retinoscope and the reflex is being seen as moving in the same direction as the streak as shown in **Figure 10.14**, it is "With motion reflex". This is neutralized with plus lenses when the sleeve is moved up. The reflex appears at the same side of the pupil where the streak is projected and moves along with the streak to disappear at the opposite side of the pupil.

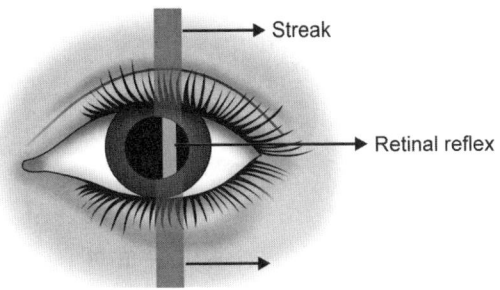

Fig. 10.14: With motion reflex.

Against Motion Reflex

When the retinal reflex moves in the opposite direction of the streak as shown in **Figure 10.15**, it is "Against motion reflex". This is neutralized with minus lenses when the sleeve is positioned up. The reflex first appears at the side of the pupil opposite to the streak and moves in opposite direction across the pupil to disappear at the side of the pupil opposite the streak.

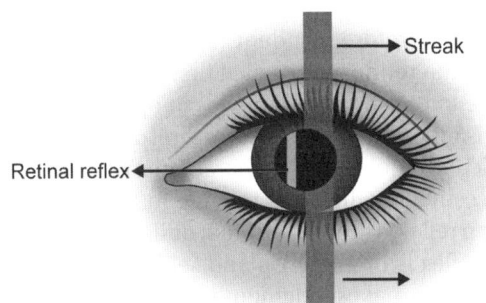

Fig. 10.15: Against motion reflex.

Scissors-like Movement

Scissors-like movement **(Fig. 10.16)** seems to split and move in opposite direction like the blades of the scissors. This is often seen in distorted corneas and large pupil. Scissors movement is difficult to work with while doing retinoscopy. The retinoscopist should attempt to align with the intercept by rotating the streak. If he fails, he should concentrate on the central reflex.

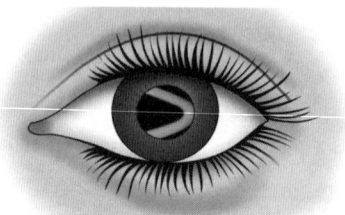

Fig. 10.16: Scissors-like movement.

Confusing Reflex

In irregular astigmatism, all sorts of distorted shadows may be observed which may move about in a confusing manner. In such cases retinoscopy results are not reliable and are used to guess the approximate values.

Triangular Reflex

Conical cornea shows triangular shadows with their apex at the center of the cone which appears to swirl round as the streak is moved **(Fig. 10.17)**.

Neutralizing using "against motion reflex" poses quite a lot of problems. It is, therefore, prudent to avoid it. In case of "against motion reflex" the retinoscopy reflex first appears at the side of the pupil opposite to the streak and moves in opposite direction across the pupil to disappear at the side of the pupil opposite the streak. This makes it difficult to quantify the characteristics of the reflex. Speed is difficult to estimate when it is moving in the opposite direction. Against motion reflex is more aberrated, dull, and difficult to evaluate. With motion reflex is bright, crisp and seldom confusing. Brilliance also reduces which makes judgment process difficult. This, in turn, makes it hard to see the width clearly.

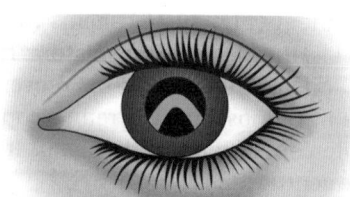

Fig. 10.17: Triangular reflex.

Correcting Lens

While doing the retinoscopy our job is to find a correcting lens that brings the far point to the peephole of the retinoscope. The lens that does so is known as correcting lens and is the measure of the refractive error. Since the plus lens converges the emerging rays, they will pull in the far point towards the eye and minus lens diverges the emerging rays; they will push the far point away from the eye. Hyperope, will therefore, take plus lens and myope will take minus lens. This can be done either with the help of trial lenses or with lens rack.

Neutralization

Retinoscopy is done with the aim of ascertaining the refractive error of the eye and this is achieved by neutralizing the movement of the reflex seen within the pupil. Neutralization in this context is the process to neutralize the movement of reflex with suitable correcting lens. Neutrality is the state arrived while neutralizing the moving reflex that shows no movement of the reflex within the pupil during sweeping the streak and the pupil is completely filled up with the red glow **(Fig. 10.18)**. Neutrality implies that the far point of the eye is at the peephole of the retinoscope. The correcting lens that neutralizes the reflex is the measure of the refractive error, ignoring the working distance and this is the endpoint of the retinoscope.

It is important to note that neutrality is not a specific point that is easily identified. Rather it is a range of uncertainty between perceptible "with" and "against" motion reflex. It is, therefore, prudent to bracket midway between just noticeable with and against motion. Neutralization is difficult to achieve with "against motion

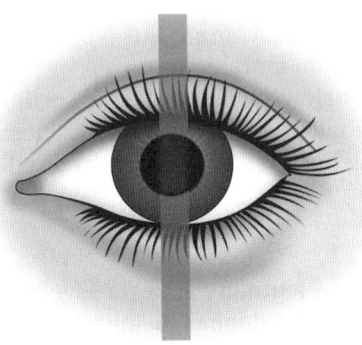

Fig. 10.18: Pupil is filled with glow.

reflex". It is therefore good to over-neutralize when you see against motion reflex to ensure that you see "with motion reflex", and then simply reduce 'with' until you reach neutral. Always use a plane mirror while neutralizing. The rule is look for the "with" and then follow it to neutrality.

Interpreting Neutrality

The neutrality achieved during retinoscopy is not a specific point. It is a zone of uncertainties between with and against movement, created by spherical aberration and other factors. The size of zone varies with pupil size and the working distance. It increases in direct proportion with the size of pupil and is narrow with small pupil whereas wider with large pupil. The width of the zone also varies because of working distance: narrow when working at a closer distance than that of a longer distance.

Usually, neutrality is achieved first at the center of the pupil and then at the periphery. Neutralization of peripheral reflex needs more minus. Therefore, it is prudent to concentrate on central pupillary reflex while scoping the patient with dilated pupil. At times, there are following doubts within the zone of neutrality:

- Nature of movement–WITH or AGAINST.
- WITH in the center and AGAINST in the periphery
- Presence of movement

It is wise to not to get into these uncertainties and make judgment just ahead of where the zone of doubt begins, i.e., stay in a little plus.

How to be Sure about Neutrality?

The practitioner can apply three methods:
1. Move closer with your scope and see "WITH" motion movement and then move away from the working distance and see "AGAINST" motion movement.
2. Go above and below the neutral lens to set the limits.
3. Verify the neutrality with sleeve down position. If it is neutralized with sleeve up position, it will be neutralized with sleeve down position also.

Pseudoneutrality

Many a time pseudoneutrality appears as a full motionless reflex which suggests that the endpoint is being reached. In order to be sure about it, simply lean in 10–15 cm, if the reflex does not change, we are not near neutrality. Try stronger lens to see if there is any change in the reflex.

Estimating Cylinder Axis

There are four important phenomena that help finding the axis. All of them are the results we observe from the off-axis reflexes and oblique motion you observe when the streak is not on the cylinder meridian. These are shown in **Flowchart 10.3**.

Flowchart 10.3: BWIS phenomena that help find the cylinder axis during retinoscopy.

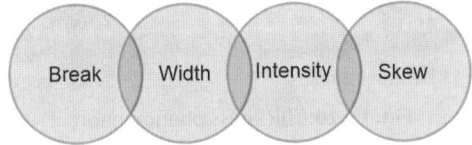

Break Phenomena

When the intercept and the reflex are not aligned, it forms a broken line which can be seen simply by rotating the streak to either side of the astigmatic reflex **(Fig. 10.19)**. It disappears when the intercept and the reflex are aligned, i.e., when the streak is on the axis. For example, if the axis is 90°, rotate the streak to about 15° on either side, i.e., from 75 to 115° to observe the break phenomena. Break is most marked at the extremes of the arc and it decreases as you approach the axis. Observing break proves effective in case of large cylinders, but it provides no help in dealing with small cylinders.

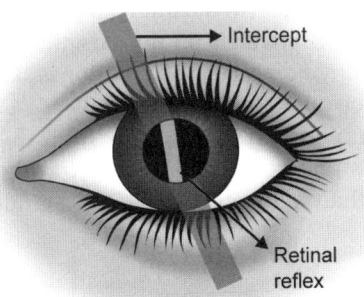

Fig. 10.19: Break phenomenon.

Thickness Phenomena

When you rotate the streak to either side of the correct axis, the thickness (width) of the reflex varies. The reflex appears narrowest when the streak aligns with the axis and wider when it is off aligned (**Fig. 10.20**). Observe the variation in the width of the reflex using your other eye.

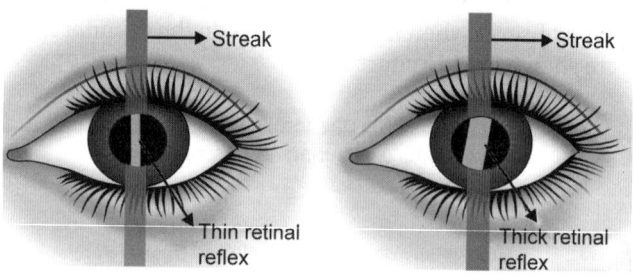

Fig. 10.20: Thickness phenomenon.

Intensity Phenomena

The brightness of the reflex changes slightly as we rotate the streak about the cylinder meridian. The reflex is brighter when the streak is on the correct axis. This phenomenon is not very useful in small cylinder.

Skew Phenomena

Skew phenomenon is very useful in case of low cylinders. In order to observe the skew phenomenon, we do not rotate the streak, instead we wiggle the streak to either side of the apparent axis perpendicularly and compare the motion of the reflex with that of intercept. The retinal reflex moves parallel to the intercept when the streak is on the proper axis. When the streak is off the axis, the reflex and intercept move in different directions, i.e., their motion is skewed (**Fig. 10.21**). The concept can be put in other words as:

If we streak a meridian that is away from the meridian of the correct axis, the streak reflex will tend to travel along the correct meridian rather than follow the streak. This guides us back to the correct meridian.

Straddling the Axis

When both the principal meridians are neutralized in case of astigmatism, the axis of the cylinder can be verified by streaking

Chapter 10: Objective Methods of Refraction

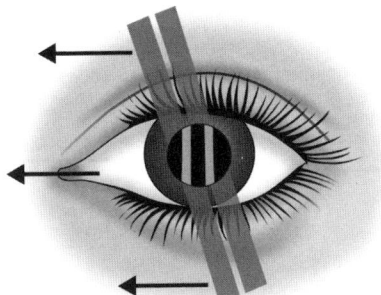

Fig. 10.21: Skew phenomenon.

the meridians 45°on either side of the meridian believed to be the axis of the cylinder. Streaking the 45°on either side, the streak reflex will widen and degrade in sharpness on both the sides equally. This confirms the correct axis. The thinner image on one side gives a guide to correct the axis towards which the axis of the cylinder lens should be rotated.

Retinoscopy Results

The retinoscopy results provide gross refractive error. These results are to be recorded on a cross chart as meridian values. In order to arrive at the net retinoscopy results, compensation has to be done for the chosen working distance.

For example, take for example 90° meridian is neutralized with +2.00 Dsph and 180-degree meridian is neutralized with +3.00 Dsph at a working distance of 66 cm. Record this as meridian values on a cross chart as shown in **Figure 10.22**.

Subtracting the values by 1.50 D, the resultant result is shown in **Figure 10.23**.

Therefore, the lens power derived from the net retinoscopy result would be +0.50Dsph/ +1.00 Dcyl X 90°.

Step-by-step Procedure

Retinoscopy, if done following the sequential steps, can be completed very fast with good results. The following steps in the given order may be followed:
1. Ask the patient to sit on patient's chair and instruct him to look at the fixation target.

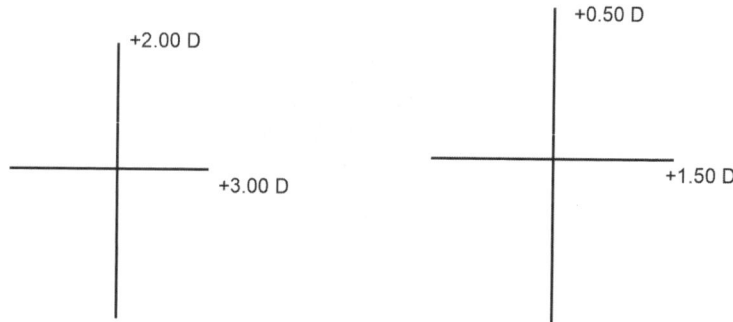

Fig. 10.22: Cross chart for recording retinoscopy results.

Fig. 10.23: Compensated values of retinoscopy results.

2. Reduce the room illumination and assume your own sitting posture.
3. Set the focusing streak to plane mirror mode and fix up the distance between you and the patient in such a position that enhances the reflex.
4. Project the light beam onto the patient's right eye.
5. Now we need to make four fast decisions:
   - Whether the eye is spherical or astigmatic,
   - Then we decide whether the eye is myopic or hypermetropic
   - Next, we locate the principal meridians, and
   - Finally, we estimate the lens power needed to neutralize these meridians.
6. Now in order to determine whether the refractive error is spherical or astigmatic, rotate the streak through 360° to look for the break, thickness and skew phenomenon or changes in brightness of the reflex within the pupil as explained earlier.
7. If the error is spherical, observe the reflex for 'With' or 'Against' motion and add plus or minus to reach neutrality.
8. Neutralize the 'With' motion reflex with plus lenses while keeping the sleeve up position and 'Against' motion reflex with minus lenses.
9. While neutralizing the 'Against' motion reflex, over-neutralize a little and then come to an end point from the with motion reflex.
10. In order to determine astigmatic error, first identify two principal meridians and then neutralize each meridian separately.

11. The simplest method is to neutralize both the meridians with spherical lens to find out the meridian values. Note down the results on a cross chart.
12. In case of hypermetropia, neutralize the least plus meridian first with plus spherical lens and then rotate the streak to opposite meridian and add more plus lens to neutralize.
13. In case of myopia, neutralize the most minus meridian first and note down its value on the cross chart.
14. This will result in 'With' motion reflex in the other meridian. Add plus spherical lens to neutralize the same and note the value on the cross chart.
15. Now subtract 1.50 D from both the meridian values, if retinoscopy was conducted at a working distance of 66 cm.
16. Elicit the lens power from the meridian values and put the same into the trial frame.
17. Hold +1.50 D spherical in front of the trial lenses and verify the neutralization in all four major meridians.
18. Recheck the neutrality with sleeve down. It should also show neutrality.
19. Repeat all the above steps for the other eye.

This is one of the methods for neutralizing the refractive error with retinoscope. However, some practitioners may be more comfortable using cylinder lenses in case of astigmatic eyes. The entire procedure can be summarized with **Flowchart 10.4**.

Nonrefractive Uses of Retinoscopy

Retinoscopy may be performed before ophthalmoscopy, and thus it may serve as first chance to view the internal structure of the eye. The appearance of retinal reflex may be altered under certain conditions which may provide a clue to diagnose certain ocular abnormalities. For example:

1. The reflected light from retina retro-illuminates the lens, iris and the cornea. The opacities in the lens and the cornea around the pupil can be seen as dark areas against a red background.
2. Keratoconus distorts the reflex and produces a swirling motion.
3. Retinal detachment involving the central area will distort the reflecting surface and hence the reflex observed may have grayish appearance.
4. A tight soft contact lens will have apical clearance in the central area which will distort retinal reflex.

Chapter 10: Objective Methods of Refraction

Flowchart 10.4: Step-by-step procedure for retinoscopy.

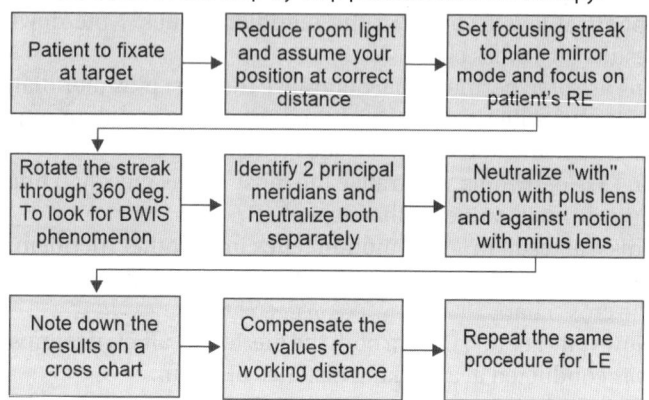

Heine Beta 200 Retinoscope

Heine Beta 200 is one of the most popular retinoscopes available which is made by HEINE OPTOTECHNIK GmbH and Co.KG. It has a single control sleeve which is a control ring to adjust the vergence of light beam. The control ring also provides streak rotation. The streak retinoscope can be changed to spot retinoscope simply by changing the bulb. The salient features of this retinoscope are as under:

1. The retinoscope has two different types of brow rests which can be changed according to the user's preference **(Fig. 10.24)**. The detachable brow rest is more convenient for spectacle wearer practitioners.
2. The single control ring is used to rotate the streak image 360°. When the control ring is positioned down, it gives divergent beam or concave mirror effect and when the control ring is positioned up it provides parallel beam or plane mirror effect.
3. Parastop limits the upward travel of the control ring and is designed to simplify precise selection of the parallel beam.
4. Two optional attachments are available with the retinoscope—one near fixation card for dynamic retinoscopy **(Fig. 10.25)** and another detachable orange filter for light sensitive patients.
5. The internal polarization filter eliminates strong light and internal reflections without reducing brightness.

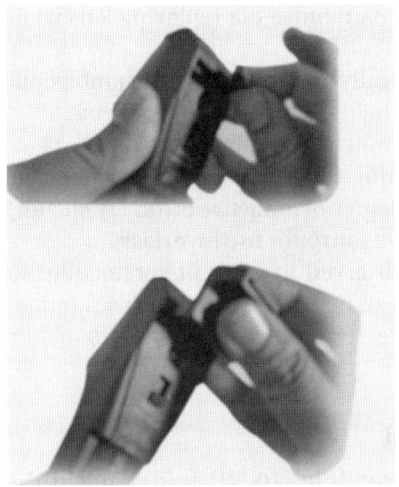
Fig. 10.24: Brow rests.

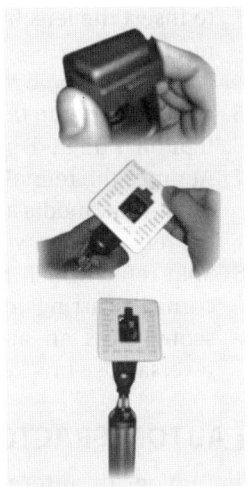
Fig. 10.25: MEM card.

To sum up retinoscopy is very useful and can be used to quickly measure long or short sightedness, astigmatism or a difference between the two eyes and the results can be quickly linked to visual acuity tests results. Retinoscopy can be done over the spectacle or if the participant wears contact lens, it can be done over contact lenses also. The another advantage of using retinoscopy is signs of pathology can often be detected, which cannot be ignored. However, keeping an understanding of the following helps a lot while performing retinoscopy:

1. Make sure that the trial lenses used are clean and centered properly.
2. In cases of media opacities, try to work around the opacities by moving off-axis. It may be needed to work closer to obtain a brighter reflex.
3. In a young hyperope, retinoscopy results often show more plus than eventual subjective refraction due to high accommodative tonus. Patience is the key in such situations. Keep asking the patient to fixate at target and keep sweeping the beam across the pupil. Also try fogging retinoscopy in such cases. Fogging retinoscopy can be done by putting higher plus lenses in front of the eye than expected retinoscopic results. Ask the patient to look straight ahead at the distance target without making effort to see clearly and perform retinoscopy. Care should be taken

to insert the lens first and then remove the replacing lens while reducing plus.
4. Dull retinoscopic reflex is usually observed in case of amblyopia.
5. Moving closer to the patient helps in high myopic patients.
6. If pupil is dilated, be sure to watch the center of the reflex.
7. At times the retinal reflex is not visible. This happens with small pupil, hazy media and high degree of refractive error. Try eliciting the retinal reflex with concave mirror or use mydriasis.
8. Split reflex which may be observed in cases of keratoconus or corneal scarring are difficult to neutralize. In such cases retinoscopy gives an approximate result. So do not try to obtain reversal, use bracketing technique.

■ AUTOREFRACTOMETER

The advent of autorefractometer **(Fig. 10.26)** has changed the scenario of eye examination procedure. Today many practitioners have started relying more on autorefractometer for its speed and accuracy. Autorefractometer uses infrared light to determine the refractive status of the eye. Multiple readings are taken and the system computes the amount of refractive error on the basis of different readings taken and gives a print out of the results. The human observation and judgment involved during retinoscopy are being replaced by the logic function of the computer from the beginning till the endpoint, making the examiner more machines dependent rather than relying on his own judgment.

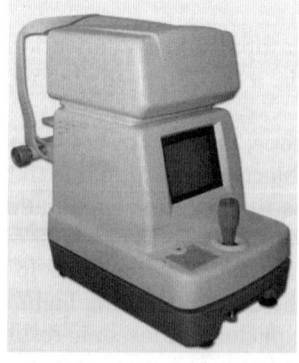

Fig. 10.26: Autorefractometer.

Chapter 10: Objective Methods of Refraction

Autorefractometers have made the objective method of refraction automated, more repeatable, reproducible, faster, user-friendly and also patient-friendly. The examiner takes several measurements of a patient and each measurement is assigned with reliable coefficient in the form of a single digit number which helps the examiner judge the accuracy of the measurement.

Components of Autorefractometer

There are three main components of autorefractometer shown in the **Figure 10.27**.

Light Source

Almost all automated autorefractometers use near-infrared radiation (NIR) at wavelengths between 780 nm and 950 nm as the primary source of electromagnetic radiation to determine the refractive error. There are two basic reasons:
1. NIR are efficiently reflected back from the fundus. There is a little loss of radiation before and after reflection by the fundus, if the eye is free from any pathology.
2. NIR is essentially invisible to the visual system. So, the patient does not experience any photophobia, the pupil of the eye does not constrict and the accommodation system is unaffected.

All autorefractometers make use of visible light for the supply of fixation target, but no autorefractometer uses visible light to determine refractive error.

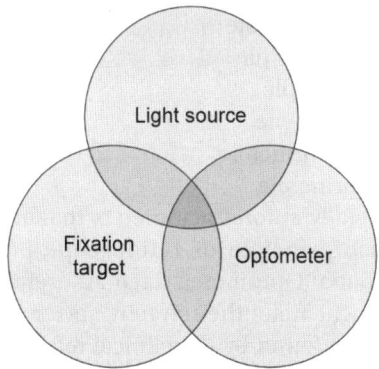

Fig. 10.27: Components of autorefractometer.

Fixation Target

All autorefractometers provide fixation target. The fixation target is provided along the same optical axis as the NIR primary source so that when the patient looks at the target, the secondary NIR source is created on the fundus at the fovea. The fixation target is most likely to be blur initially because it will not be located at the far point of the eye, the dioptric position of the fixation target is adjusted by the instrument to make dioptric position of the fixation target coincident with that of the far point plane. The patient perceives the target to be clear during this process and perhaps even clearer at the end of the measurement.

Optometer

An optometer is an instrument used to determine the refractive state of the human eye. The optometers need to be aligned to the patient's eye so that accurate refractive measurements can be made. This accurate alignment is possible by restricting the range of head and eye movement possible by using head rest to limit the range of head movement and enable the system to track the eye movement. Most autorefractometers use automatic Badal Optometer. Badal Optometer provides an optical system that moves towards or away from the eye without changing the magnification of the retinal image, but allows the change of optical vergence.

Calculation of Refractive Error

The refractive error is calculated by analyzing how the patient's eye influences the infrared rays. The following design principles are commonly used in most autorefractometers for analysis:
- ❖ The Scheiner disc principle
- ❖ The retinoscopic principle
- ❖ The best focus principle
- ❖ The knife-edge principle
- ❖ The ray-deflection principle
- ❖ The image size principle

Most commercially autorefractometers that are available either use Scheiner Disc principle or retinoscope principle coupled with automated Badal Optometer. Each autorefractometer design is programmed to calculate the refractive error on the basis of an empirical calibration found by the clinical refraction of the patient extending over the instrument's dioptric range. Accommodative fluctuations may affect spherical more than cylinder power. The resolution of the cylinder power is the function of the automated refractor's measurement system and it is essentially fixed. The resolution of axis of cylinder power, however, depends on the magnitude of cylinder. As cylinder power increases, the ability to determine the cylinder axis is enhanced.

Autorefractometers are designed to calculate the refractive state of the eye at the plane of the cornea. The desired refraction at spectacle plane is calculated by vertex distance compensation range provided by the individual Autorefractometer.

Clinical Use of Autorefractometer

The following steps in the given order may be followed for the effective use of autorefractometer:
1. Make the patients sit comfortably on patient chair.
2. Ask him to put the chin-on-chin rest and head against forehead rest.
3. Instruct him to keep the head as still as possible and to keep the eyes open between blinks. Most autorefractometers automatically discard readings that is obstructed by blink.
4. The patient should be relaxed and should be fixating at the target of the eye being tested even when the target is blurred.
5. The examiner, then aligns the instrument on the center of the entrance pupil with the help of joystick and actuate the button to capture the reading.
6. Usually autorefractometer takes a few seconds to capture the reading.
7. It may be necessary for the examiner to track the eye with joystick after actuating the button in case the patient is unable to maintain fixation.
8. When the examination is completed for one eye, a similar process is repeated for the other eye.

Limitations of Objective Autorefractometer

Although autorefractometers are very useful in most situations, there are certain situations where they fail to provide reliable measurement of refractive error. It must be remembered that results of objective autorefractometer should not be used as the final refractive correction without further confirmation. They should only be used to determine an initial objective refraction before the performance of subjective

refraction. The practitioner must keep in mind the various limitations of autorefractometers and be wary of conditions that may produce invalid results, for example:
- ❖ Ametropia outside the range of Autorefractometer
- ❖ Autorefractometer often fails with small pupil below the minimum size.
- ❖ Often autorefractometer fails to control accommodation adequately.
- ❖ Anterior segment abnormalities resulting in opacities, cloudy ocular media, distorted pupil and irregular astigmatism caused by corneal irregularities such as keratoconus, corneal trauma and postrefractive surgical corneas are the cases where the measurements are not reliable.
- ❖ Posterior segment abnormalities resulting in a poor fundus reflex, such as retinal detachment, staphyloma and retinopathies.
- ❖ Young patients with active accommodative system may produce more minus than revealed in retinoscopy or subjective refraction.
- ❖ Certain geriatric and pediatric patients are difficult to measure with autorefractometer because of inability to keep the head in position and the eyes fixated.
- ❖ During the automated objective refraction, the clinician will not be able to identify latent hypermetropia, pseudomyopia and various other accommodative abnormalities, nor will the clinician be able to reasonably estimate the extent to which the accommodative system has altered the spherical portion of the refractive end point.

Since the objective autorefractometers are designed to determine refractive error for distance, the accommodation system of the eye has to be at rest, with usual amount of tonus for distance vision. An auto-fogging mechanism is provided in the most sophisticated Autorefractometer. Most autorefractometers use spherical focusing to bring the monocular fixation target to approximate plane of the far point.

The use of internal fixating target provides strong cues for proximally induced accommodation. This internal fixating target is composed of color photographs of outdoor scenes, with a prominent central feature in the distance. Accommodation is most relaxed when a prominent feature is of low spatial frequency, when the visual scene has wide band of spatial frequencies for observation and when the patient identifies it as one typical scene at distance.

KERATOMETRY

Keratometry is an instrument used to measure the front surface curvature of the cornea. The readings provide information as to the corneal astigmatism which may be used as baseline cylinder correction needed for the patient. The other uses of Keratometry are:
- Keratometry is of great importance for fitting contact lenses.
- Keratometry can be used for calculating the power of intraocular lens to be implanted.
- Keratometry is useful to monitor pre- and post-surgical astigmatism.
- Keratometry is helpful equipment for qualitative assessment of corneal integrity.

General Principle of Keratometry

Keratometry is based on the principle of convex mirror optics. It is based on the fact that the anterior surface of the cornea acts as a convex mirror. The size of image formed by cornea varies with its curvature. The greater the curvature of the cornea, smaller is the image size. Therefore, from the size of the image formed by the anterior surface of cornea, i.e., first Purkinje image, the radius of the curvature of cornea can be calculated. However, it is difficult to measure the reflected image directly, because it is constantly moving as a result of microscopic eye movements. To overcome this problem, the principle of doubling is applied by using suitable prism midway in the observation system that forms a second image of the target and the effect of eye movement is nullified as both images move with the eye.

Keratometry measures the radius of curvature of very small portion of central cornea. The reflected image formed is very small in size and lies in anterior chamber of the eye, it is inaccessible for direct measurement. That is why a telescope is used to magnify the reflected image and forms the second image of the mire which is accessible for measurements.

Types of Keratometry

There are two types of keratometry available:
1. Two-position keratometry
2. One-position keratometry

Two-position Keratometry (Figs. 10.28 and 10.29)

The two-position keratometry requires rotation about the axis to measure each of the principal meridians. Javal-Schiotz keratometry is two-position keratometry. Javal-Schiotz Keratometry is based on the principle of variable object size and constant image size. The mires have variable separations and are mechanically arranged so as to allow the radius of curvature of the surface to be read from their separation.

One-position Keratometry

One-position keratometry does not require rotation about the axis. Simultaneous doubling of perpendicular pairs of mires is produced by doubling devices in each of the corresponding meridians. Bausch and Lomb keratometry is a one-position keratometry. The object in the B and L keratometry is the circular mire with two plus and two minus signs. A lamp illuminates the mire by means of a diagonally

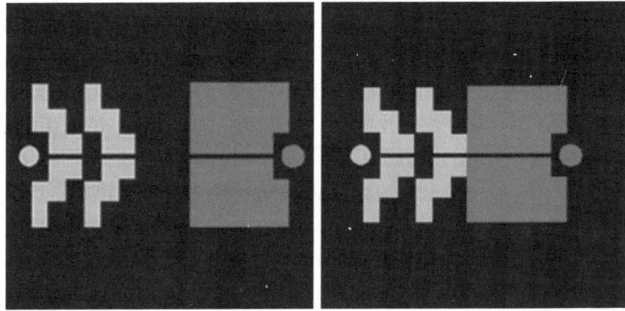

Fig. 10.28: Two-position keratometry.

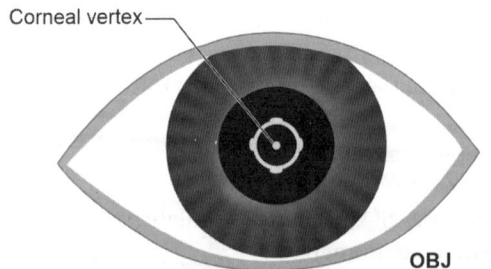

Fig. 10.29: One-position keratometry.

placed mirror. Light from the mire strikes the patient's cornea and produces a diminished image behind it. This image becomes the object for the remainder of optical system.

Estimation of Total Corneal Power

Keratometry gives only anterior corneal radius—it cannot measure posterior radius. The total corneal power reading is only an estimate. And this estimate is reasonable because the anterior cornea carries so much of the total corneal power. To do this, Keratometry uses a fudge factor in the index of refraction to account for the posterior corneal power and also to allow 45.00 CD to equal 7.50 mm radius of curvature.

Therefore, instead of calibrating the instruments for the true refractive index of the cornea (1.376) which would give a reading of the front surface power, a lower refractive index is assumed. Most instruments use 1.3375.

Axis of the corneal astigmatism can be measured by rotating the Keratometry tube until the left mire and the focusing mire plus signs are not staggered but rather perfectly in line as shown in the figure. For moderate to high corneal astigmatism, this is simple. To verify alignment for low astigmatism, the focusing mire can be thrown slightly out of focus, and the left mire plus sign should line up exactly between the doubled plus.

An estimation of corneal astigmatism can be done by measuring the curvatures of the cornea at two principal meridians and recording the values as under:

Flat K Values: 44.00 D @ 180 or 7.80 mm @ 180

Steep K Values: 45.00 D @ 90 or 7.70 mm @ 90

Estimated Corneal Astigmatism: 1.00 D @ 180°

However, the amount of astigmatism derived by Keratometry may differ from that of spectacle refraction. It may be more than the spectacle refraction, or less than the spectacle refraction or may be same.

ASSIMILATION OF INITIAL DATA AND GOAL SETTING

With objective assessment of refraction completed, the clinician has following data in his hand:

1. The context for the visit
2. Chief complaints and visual needs, as derived from case history
3. Uncorrected visual acuity
4. Habitual correction
5. Visual acuity with habitual correction
6. Results of objective refraction

The examiner analyzes entire data against their expected values individually and collectively. These data not only reveal the current state of the visual system but also provide insights into potential changes in refractive correction. The examiner establishes a connection between the patient's habitual correction and the objective measurements of refractive errors, recalling visual symptoms and reassessing visual needs. Through the application of clinical judgment and experience, the examiner sets clear goals before engaging in subjective methods of refraction.

Goal setting is a crucial step, allowing the examiner to execute an organized flow of processes with appropriate tests for a quicker and more accurate measurement of refractive error. It is essential to emphasize that subjective refraction should not rely on blindly changing trial lenses within the trial lens set. Instead, the clinician should gather clues from data collected during various entrance tests.

This phase holds paramount importance in the entire clinical refraction procedure. The practice of estimating refractive error by simply adding plus spheres to the highest possible consonant or minus spheres to the lowest possible consonant with good vision, followed by attempting all plus or minus cylinder lenses through all meridians, is not only farcical but also impractical. A thoughtful and strategic approach, based on comprehensive data analysis and goal setting, is imperative for the success of the subjective refraction process.

MULTIPLE CHOICE QUESTIONS

1. **Which of the following statements is true with regard to objective methods of refraction?**
    a. The examiner makes the measurement to determine the refractive error without enlisting patient's response.
    b. Patient's response is very critical during objective refraction.
    c. The method of objective refraction can be applied as a means to verify the refractive error as determined subjectively.
    d. During the objective refraction sophisticated test charts are used to determine the refractive error.

Chapter 10: Objective Methods of Refraction

2. **Which of the following is true regarding retinoscopy?**
   a. Accommodation is stimulated when the patient looks at the light from retinoscope.
   b. The power of the working distance lens is proportion to the working distance in meters.
   c. Movement of the reflex slows as the neutralization point is approached.
   d. 'With motion' with plain mirror retinoscope implies 'add minus' and 'Against movement' with plain mirror retinoscope implies 'add plus'.
3. **Retinoscopy is done on a -0.50 D myopic patient at a distance of 1 meter. Movement of the image will be:**
   a. Move with the mirror
   b. Move against the mirror
   c. No movement of the image with mirror
   d. Image can move to any side.
4. **When using the plane mirror technique during retinoscopy, which of the following is not true?**
   a. 'With' movement is neutralized with a plus lens.
   b. 'Against' movement is neutralized with a minus lens.
   c. 'With' movement always indicates hypermetropia.
   d. 'Against' movement always indicates myopia.
5. **What is the amount of lenticular astigmatism when the keratometry readings of the cornea are 44.00 D @90° and 42.00 D @180° and the manifest refraction is -6.00/-4.00 @90°?**
   a. -4.00 Dcyl @90°
   b. -4.00 Dcyl @180°
   c. -2.00 Dcyl @90°
   d. -2.00 Dcyl @180°

ANSWER KEY

| 1. a | 2. a | 3. a | 4. c | 5. d |

SELF-PRACTICE QUESTIONS

1. What are the possible errors that may happen while performing retinoscopy?
2. In which of the situations spot retinoscopy may be more helpful than streak retinoscopy?
3. Explain the advantages and disadvantages of autorefractometer.

11 CHAPTER

Subjective Methods of Refraction

CHAPTER OUTLINE

- Subjective Refraction
- Challenges Faced during Subjective Refraction
- Methods of Subjective Refraction
- Delayed Subjective Refraction
- Determination of Near Addition
- Jackson Cross-cylinder Test
- Refraction Using Stenopeic Slit

SUBJECTIVE REFRACTION

Subjective refraction is the method to determine the refractive error by applying a technique of comparing one lens against another, using changes in vision as the criterion, to arrive at the dioptric lens combination that provides the maximum visual acuity. The procedure is highly dependent on the patient's response, as they are constantly asked to distinguish the difference between changes in acuity with every change of trial lens. The subjective methods of refraction are usually applied after the baseline refractive error has already been determined using one or more objective methods of refraction and a goal has been set for the end results of clinical refraction. The starting lens for subjective refraction may be any of the following:

❖ The results of an objective method of refraction, or
❖ The patient's habitual correction, or
❖ As set goal for the end result of clinical refraction.

In his professional practice, the author consistently selected the initial set of trial lenses based on the specific goals he aimed for the patient to achieve by the end of the clinical refraction procedure. This approach proved immensely beneficial, significantly reducing the need for frequent changes in trial lenses, minimizing confusion, and maximizing overall patient satisfaction.

Subjective refraction may be performed using loose trial lenses and trial frames, or phoropter, also known as refractor. Phoropter provides a significant advantage by permitting rapid change of spherical and cylinder power lenses by rotation of knobs. But there are some associated concerns with the use of phoropter. There is a difference between vertex distance, pantoscopic angle, and face form wrap that may render them a little less effective for higher correction. The patient's face is completely hidden behind the phoropter, because of which the clinician's interaction with the patient may be reduced and he may not be able to watch his responses. The small size of the lens aperture increases the propensity for proximal accommodation relative to a trial frame and prevents a realistic duplication of the real-life environment as created by the trial frame. It also hinders binocular vision while conducting near vision test as the eyes do not lose the benefits of convergence that occurs during downgaze, especially when the pupillary distance of the patient is large. The trial frame and loose trial lens resonates real-life visual circumstances better than the phoropter.

Two appropriate conditions are very important for subjective refraction:
1. Test distance
2. Room illumination

They have been discussed in detail in Chapter 8. The distance at which subjective refraction is normally carried out is 20 feet, or 6 meters. It may be direct or indirect, using a mirror hung on the opposite wall with a reversed test chart placed above the patient's head. The distance of 6 meters to infinity represents approximately the depth of focus in the eye, so that the rays of light that enter the eyes suffer so little divergence that for most purposes they may be taken as parallel, i.e., as if coming from infinity. In fact, the vergence at 6 meters is equivalent to about 1/6th of a dioptre, or 0.166 D, which is negligible and is very close to the zero vergence associated with rays of light coming from infinity.

There have been several efforts to use reduced testing by adjusting the size of the letters to achieve the same effect. However, if the gaze shifts to a target closer than 20 feet, the light rays from the target are too divergent to be focused without accommodative effort. To counteract the effect, the researcher has reduced the letter size so that it does not stimulate accommodation.

In deciding the test distance, it is critical that the distance be large enough not to stimulate accommodation. The accommodation is at rest, and the crystalline lens of the eye is thin. The refraction is performed at a fixed state of accommodation.

With the introduction of technology, many efforts have also been made to employ virtual reality, i.e., to create a non-existent environment where all visual cues can be controlled and manipulated. Although virtual reality is intended to be an analog for the real world, it does not always accurately represent our experiences of the natural world. Therefore, how much they can be successfully employed in clinical refraction is an area for more research as of now.

The room's illumination is another important factor that must be controlled. The subjective refraction should be carried out in room illumination similar to that encountered by the patient during normal use of refractive correction, unless the correction will be used primarily in dim or dark surroundings. Room light should be enough to allow normal pupil size and retinal adaptation. Dim light should ideally be avoided as the pupil dilates, which may increase the effect of wide beam aberration created by peripheral rays of light. In dim light, accommodations may not be relaxed. Also, there is a possibility of overcorrection, especially in myopia, because of the increased effect of spherical aberration with increased pupil size. However, the patient reporting difficulties in night vision may be refracted in low illumination. Either the patient may be asked to wear a dark filter or the test chart may be illuminated using a torch light. A few minutes should be allowed for the retina to adapt to the dark before initiating the procedure. The duochrome test is always done in dim light because of the principle of chromatic aberration.

■ CHALLENGES FACED DURING SUBJECTIVE REFRACTION

While performing the clinical procedures, the examiner often faces certain challenges. These challenges may have differential impact on the outcome of the procedure. Some of the common challenges are:

- ❖ The end result is highly patient dependent as the conclusion is arrived at when the maximum acuity is achieved which depends upon patient's judgment and opinion.
- ❖ The ability to discriminate between dioptric changes varies greatly from one individual to another, some individuals being more sensitive to changes of as small as 0.12 D, while others may not be able to notice difference in blur to changes of as much as 0.50 D. In such cases the clinician's judgement to final prescription may be adversely affected.
- ❖ Intelligence, the patient's psychological condition, his state of mind during refraction, his previous experience and expectations; all these may prevent perfect correlation of the subjective findings with the true refractive status of the eye.
- ❖ Some individuals are poor observers and are unable to respond adequately to forced choice presentation of lenses. Patients may complain that trial lenses are changed very fast, hence they find it difficult to differentiate between the two lenses. Some patients complain that there are too many changes of trial lenses that confuse them, while some patients memorize the test charts.
- ❖ Malingering patients may mislead by intent who deny the presence or absence of vision for no obvious organic reason. Handling malingering patients is little tricky. The examiner has to decide whether he is dealing with a sick hysteric or a willful cheat. Using neutralizing lens combination, filter lenses, changing test charts or changing the distance of the test charts, use of pinhole may help catch those patients. The examiner can suddenly drop an object to see whether the patient reacts reflexively or not. Vertical prism dissociation test can also help. A 6.00 D base down prism is placed in front of the good eye and 20/20 line of Snellen's Chart is projected. If the patient is able to see letters of two lines with equal clarity, it establishes good vision in the affected eye.
- ❖ Often examiner himself creates trouble for him during refraction. This is often seen when the examiner puts the trial lens without cleaning thoroughly. Some patients lose their temperament and become irritated when they find it difficult to read what is written on the test chart.

These challenges can easily be handled by the examiner if he is endowed with a capacity for taking pains. A professional attitude and the keenness to deliver excellence are the two simple elements that can help the examiner go a long distance.

METHODS OF SUBJECTIVE REFRACTION

Broadly speaking there are four methods which are most commonly practiced in the clinical practice for subjective refraction, they are shown in **Figure 11.1**.

Manifest Monocular Subjective Refraction

Manifest monocular subjective refraction is the most commonly used method of subjective refraction. It is invariably the first choice. Each eye is examined separately; usually the right eye is examined first in most cases. The procedure starts with the patient sitting on a chair at a distance of 6 meters from the illuminated test chart (**Fig. 11.2**) and the examiner assumes his position. The following sequential process is followed:
1. Put the trial frame on the patient's face and center it properly.
2. Place the opaque disc in front of the left eye and start with right eye.
3. Put the first selected trial lenses in the trial frame. The selection of first trial lenses may be based on the results of objective refraction or previous correction or as set goal, depending upon individual preference.
4. Begin altering trial lenses. The alteration of trial lenses should be done swiftly and the patient should be asked to report improvement in distinctness only.
5. Start with changing spherical lenses in the trial frame for one of greater or smaller power. There is no hard and fast rule about

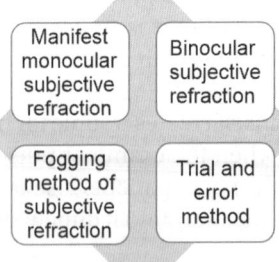

Fig. 11.1: Four methods of subjective refraction.

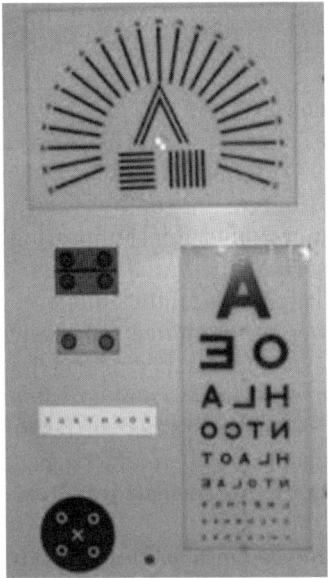

Fig. 11.2: Vision chart.

the steps in which the change is made. There are several factors that may be considered to decide the steps, for example—acuity obtained with the first trial lens and power of spherical lens. In most cases the changes are at the step of 0.25 D or 0.50 D. The initial sphere is achieved when the best possible acuity is achieved by using most plus or least minus lens.

6. When the best vision is attained with the spherical trial lens, attention is directed to cylinder lenses. This is done in two steps —first the axis of cylinder is determined and then the amount of cylinder is measured.
7. Cylinder axis is determined by rotating the cylinder lens through different axes on either side. Jackson Cross-cylinder test for the purpose.
8. After the correct axis is determined, the cylinder lens is altered to determine the amount of cylinder. A continuous check on cylinder axis should be monitored throughout subjective refraction each time the cylinder lens is changed. Jackson Cross cylinder test may be applied for the purpose.
9. Care must be taken in case of small degree of astigmatism as indicated by objective refraction. If the patient finds little

difference in acuity on rotating cylinder, the astigmatic correction may not be necessary and the best sphere by itself can be the end result.
10. When the cylinder axis and cylinder amount have been finally determined, the spherical should be checked again by changing in a step of 0.25 D. Stop at most plus or least minus with best achieved acuity. Make a note of the visual acuity. In majority of cases the examiner should aim at improving the acuity to 6/6 on the Snellen's test chart, in normal subjects.
11. Repeat the similar process for the other eye.
12. Once the two eyes are examined separately, the opaque disc is removed and the patient is asked to read the test chart with both eyes open before applying the refinement tests. At this stage the examiner must look at two immediate responses:
    a. Binocular visual acuity should be better than monocular visual acuity, if the corrected acuities are approximately equal.
    b. An immediate response of the subject to the new correction.

Flowchart 11.1 summarizes the complete step-by-step procedure of manifest monocular subjective refraction.

Flowchart 11.1: Step-by-step procedure of manifest monocular subjective refraction.

```
Ask the patient      →   Keep checking        →   When cylinder is
to sit                   axis with every          finally determined,
                         change of cyl            check spherical
                         lenses                   again
    ↓                        ↑                        ↓
Put trial frame          Direct your              Try and attain
on patient's             attention to alter       6/6 acuity
face                     cylinder lens
    ↓                        ↑                        ↓
Cover the                Try and achieve          Repeat the
left eye                 best possible            same process
                         vision with              for LE
                         spherical lenses
    ↓                        ↑                        ↓
Place the first      →   Begin altering       →   Remove opaque
trial lenses in          lenses in front          disc and check
front of RE              of RE at small           with both eyes
                         steps                    open
```

Binocular Subjective Refraction

There are certain situations when binocular subjective refraction is preferred to manifest monocular subjective refraction. These situations are listed below:
- ❖ Hyperopic anisometropia
- ❖ Antimetropia
- ❖ Latent hyperopia
- ❖ Pseudomyopia
- ❖ Aniso-oxyopia, the condition in which visual acuity between two eyes are different.
- ❖ Unilateral reduced acuity due to disease or physiological factors.
- ❖ Unilateral amblyopia, in which vision of the better eye supports to stabilize the accommodation of amblyopic eye. Also, in binocular condition fixation of the amblyopic eye is steadied by the simultaneous fixation of the non-amblyopic eye. Degree of eccentricity diminishes under binocular condition compared with when amblyopic eye fixates on its own.
- ❖ Conditions where significant horizontal and vertical phorias, cylophoria are present.
- ❖ When there is latent nystagmus, binocular refraction has been found to be lessening the extent of eye movements in nystagmus compared with monocular subjective refraction.

Binocular subjective refraction is the clinical procedure in which subjective refraction is performed monocularly under binocular viewing condition, i.e., both eyes of the patient remain unoccluded, viewing the common target. Each eye is refracted in the presence of stimuli for peripheral fusion, but the central portion of the test chart is seen monocularly. All procedures that are applied for monocular subjective refraction are performed in a similar manner except that both eyes of the patient are open.

The first step in applying binocular subjective refraction is to ensure monocular viewing under binocular vision condition which is achieved in one of the following ways:
1. By fogging the eye that is not under test
2. By using septum
3. By applying polarizing technique

The following process can be followed:
1. Slightly blur the central vision in the eye not under test. It suspends foveal vision such that the eye is refracted under condition of binocular vision with peripheral fusion.

2. Start subjective refraction in the other eye following the technique of manifest monocular subjective refraction technique using initial lenses as selected.
3. Fogging method may also be applied to control the accommodation in both eyes in which case both eyes are fogged initially to at least +0.75 D, which is maintained in untested eye. Unfogging is done only in the eye under test till spherical equivalent is placed at the retina.

Most practitioners ignore the fact that the difference may range from subtle to profound between the outcomes of monocular and binocular subjective refraction. As a result of which monocular subjective refraction overwhelmingly prevails. However, in a day-to-day life the vast majority of people see the world using both eyes together. It is because of this reason arguments have been put forward in favor of binocular subjective refraction. Binocular subjective refraction has the advantage of determining the refractive error when the eyes are used in their normal state, i.e., binocularly. The unoccluded two eyes provide more realistic and real-life scenarios. It allows assessment of the performance of each eye as it actually contributes to the binocular perception, and of the sensory and motor efficiency with which the two eyes function together in day-to-day life.

In binocular vision condition accommodation and vergence function are more constant and coordinated because they are in habitual state. The accommodative system is more stable and relaxed for distance viewing as a response for one unified image and peripheral vision in the process helps hold accommodation steadily. This is the most important aspect of binocular subjective refraction which ensures additional control of accommodation. The fusion attained during binocular vision condition incorporates all of the patient's binocular efforts including horizontal and vertical phorias. This is the only method that assists in determining if there is any effect of cyclophoria in deciding the cylinder axis.

There are advantages of binocular refraction over monocular refraction, though there are patients who cannot be refracted binocularly. These may be summarized as under:

- ❖ Accommodation is suspended with a plus sphere and tied to convergence.
- ❖ No separate binocular balancing is needed. This saves quite a lot of time.
- ❖ With both eyes the impact of latent nystagmus reduces.

The results obtained from binocular subjective refraction technique is very much similar to what is expected of monocular subjective refraction with a little difference in spherical value as it may contain additional +0.25 D. In case of patient having cyclophoria, the cylinder axis may be found to be different by as much as 5°.

Fogging Method of Subjective Refraction

Fogging method of subjective refraction involves a build-up plus power until the patient's visual acuity is reduced by one or two lines. Fogging is followed by defogging, when the plus power is reduced until there is no further improvement in visual acuity. Spherical plus lenses are used to create artificial myopia and the entire focus is brought in front of the retina to create a situation where any attempt to accommodate will further blur the vision, which induces accommodation relaxation.

Indications

Fogging method of refraction is indicated in the following conditions:
- Latent hypermetropia
- Pediatric patients
- Young patients who have excessive accommodation
- Patients with asthenopic symptoms
- When over minus correction is suspected
- Case of ocular deviation and amblyopia

Clinical Significance of Fogging

Cornea and crystalline lens determine the refractive state of the eye. While the power of cornea is fixed, the power of crystalline lens varies because of accommodation. The fluctuation in refractive state may result in prolonging the process of refraction and in a situation if the ametropia is not adequately corrected, it may lead to asthenopic symptoms. Proper accommodation control is, therefore, the most important factor in the refraction process. Fogging can help determine hypermetropic conditions and proper lens prescription, which can attenuate symptoms in some patients.

Steps-by-step Process

Broadly, there are two steps as shown in **Flowchart 11.2**.

Flowchart 11.2: Fogging and defogging.

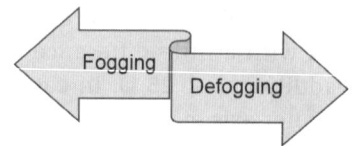

Occlude one eye preferably left eye and fog the eye under test preferably right eye with plus sphere which is higher than the results of the objective refraction in case of hypermetropia and with low plus in case of low myopia. However, no plus lens is needed in high myopia. While fogging care should be taken not to over-fog or under-fog. Under-fogging allows the patient to continue to accommodate and over-fogging using too much plus spherical power may push the strum conoid too far in front of the retina into hypothetical vitreous which may unnecessarily prolong the defogging process.

Once fogging is done, start defogging gradually. While defogging care must be taken to put the new plus lens first and then remove the one from the trial frame, if plus lens used; and for minus lens, remove the minus lens first and then put the new one.

Also, be careful not to allow too much time between removal and insertion of lenses. Removing the fogging lens to replace it with another one should be done as quickly as possible without causing the patient any discomfort. This can be achieved by keeping the replacement lens ready in hand while removing the fogging lens.

The patient should be asked to read the optotypes on the examination chart stepwise from the largest to the smallest possible.

The sequential process of measuring refractive error follows the below sequential process:
1. Obtain the best visual acuity using spherical lenses only, i.e., best vision sphere. It is assumed that the best vision sphere will put the circle of least confusion on the retina and the patient will report the acuity which is 6/9 or more.
2. Now ask the patient to look at the Fan Chart for astigmatic correction and ask which line or group of lines appear clearest and darkest. This gives an approximate direction of the cylinder axis.
3. If no line or set of lines appear to be black, there are two possibilities—either the patient may not need any astigmatic correction or the eye is excessively fogged. In case the patient

Chapter 11: Subjective Methods of Refraction

identifies any one line or group of lines as darker than the rest, align the Maddox Arrow with the same.

4. Now direct the patient's attention to Maddox Arrow. Ask the patient if both the limbs of the arrow are equally blurred. Rotate it away from the black limb towards the blur limb until both limbs appear equally blurred. This gives the axis of the astigmatic correction. Care must be taken to ensure that the patient's head is upright.
5. Then direct the patient's attention to two blocks. The patient will report that one of the two blocks is clearer and darker than the other. Add minus cylinder at the appropriate axis until the second block becomes as clearer as the first one. If this is not quite possible, over add cylinder lens by -0.25 D to get the reversal. Once the reversal is achieved, you may reduce the additional cylinder lens added and go one step down. Remember it is always better to undercorrect than to overcorrect, leaving the initial block clearer than the other.
6. Finally, with corrected sphere and cylinder divert the attention of the patient to Snellen's chart to refine the spherical. Do not continue reducing plus unless you are very sure that they really need it to see clearly. Similarly, do not go on adding minus as well, it will not make the letters clearer, rather letters will become smaller and darker black. The goal is to find "maximum plus to best acuity" or "minimum minus to best acuity".
7. A simple fogging with +0.50 Dsph and then defogging at the step of 0.25 step may be applied at this stage.

It is quite likely that defogging another 0.25 D may also yield 6/6 acuity. The defogging process ends when the examiner notices that reducing the plus power does not improve visual acuity. For some acuity charts, one can stop the defogging process once the patient has correctly read all the letters on the smallest line, as long as that chart reaches a minimum of the 20/20 line. A clinical judgment is critical to decide the final correction.

The complete step-by-step of fogging method subjective refraction can be described in **Flowchart 11.3**.

Trial and Error Method

Although trial and error method of clinical subjective refraction is not recommended in professional clinical practice, it is often practiced by experienced practitioners as a quick-fix method or by untrained

Chapter 11: Subjective Methods of Refraction

Flowchart 11.3: Step-by-step procedure of fogging method of refraction.

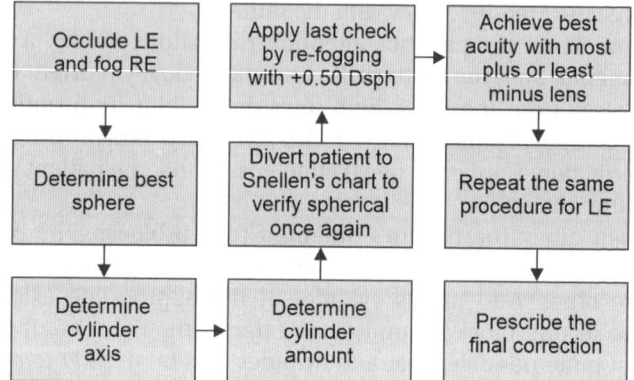

individuals who have learnt the art of examining the eyes for lens prescription by dint of their experience in opticianry. In fact, it should not have been mentioned as a method of subjective refraction in this book. Since the author saw many individuals practicing this method, he took a bold step to include so that readers can discern the difference.

When an untrained individual examines the eyes, most prescriptions will have spherical correction. Cylinder corrections will be seen very rarely. However, if the cylinder correction is prescribed, it is mostly either at 90 degree or 180 degrees. Past lens correction is used as the baseline correction. In the absence of previous lens correction, random changes of trial lenses are made to achieve the best possible acuity. Low cylinder correction is almost always avoided and high cylinders are rarely prescribed unless used before.

Some individuals perform spherical overrefraction on patient's habitual glasses, presenting choices "over" each lens. One eye may be occluded or may not be occluded. First minus and plus lenses are put in front of glasses randomly at the step of 0.25 Dsph or 0.50 Dsph to determine whether to continue with adding plus lenses or minus lenses. Based upon the patient's response the refractionist continues changing lenses till 6/6 acuity is achieved. The patient is invariably taken outside the clinic and is asked to check the vision in natural condition with both eyes open in most cases.

When trial and error method is adopted by an experienced practitioner, it is more of an intellectual procedure based upon his clinical judgment and experience. Based upon the results of the objective method of refraction, patient's symptoms and the preliminary assessment of the eye the practitioner decides the goal of the clinical refraction and uses the same as the first trial lens and in one or two lens change, he decides the final lens prescription for the patient. He may also verify axis of cylinder by rotating cylinder lens by a few degrees on the either side as given by the objective refraction.

The method can be refined to include Bichrome Test to find out initial or working sphere. The patient may be asked to look from the green side to the red side and then back to green side and indicate which side has the clearer letters or both the sides are equally clear. Red side clearer indicates the need of minus spherical and green side clearer implies the need of plus spherical. Keep changing the spherical lens until both side's letters are equally clearer. Introduce an additional 0.25 D minus spherical power. Then the patient is "into the green". Now check the visual acuity on the Snellen's Chart. At this stage Jackson Cross-cylinder may be applied to hunt cylinder correction.

DELAYED SUBJECTIVE REFRACTION

Delayed subjective refraction is a non-cycloplegic method of maximizing the relaxation of accommodation after determining the correction of refractive error. The objective of the test is to relax the patient's accommodation and subsequently stimulate the acceptance of plus while determining the refractive error. The technique may produce a greater plus acceptance than was indicated by routine manifest subjective refraction.

When
- ❖ When you want to detect latent hyperopia.
- ❖ When the patient is suspected to have accommodative spasm.

What You Need
- ❖ Near test chart
- ❖ Distance test chart

Set-up
- ❖ Room light on
- ❖ Head lamp focused on near test chart
- ❖ Target distance for distance test chart 20 feet/6 meters
- ❖ Target distance for near test chart 40 cm

How

Delayed subjective refraction is performed after the routine refraction has been completed with near addition determination, if the patient is presbyope.

In case of non-presbyope
- Patient's both eyes open.
- His full distance correction is placed in the trial frame.
- Ask the patient to hold the near test chart at 40 cm.
- Keep the best distance correction in trial frame.
- Room light on and head lamp focused on reading test target.
- Ask the patients to focus on letters one or two lines larger than his near visual acuity.
- Make sure that the letters are clearer at the beginning of the test.

  If it is not clear, add plus spherical power at the step of +0.25 D at a time in front of both eyes until patient reports that the letters are clear. This becomes the tentative near prescription.
- Now add plus sphere lenses binocularly at the step of +0.25 D until the patient reports the first sustained blur. The patient notices that letters are not as clear as they were initially, even if the patient can read.
- Note the total plus added so.
- Keeping the plus lenses in the trial frame, now ask the patient to look at distance chart.
- Isolate the line of patient's best distance acuity, but not smaller than 20/20.
- The patient should report that it is blurry.
- Now reduce the plus binocularly at the step of 0.25 D until 6/6 line is read clearly.
- Confirm the end point with duochrome test.
- If more plus remains, it is the measure of latest hyperopia that may help such patient.
- Record the result as 'Delayed Subjective' followed by lens prescription and visual acuities.

In case of presbyope
- If the patient is presbyopic, the only difference is instead of putting only distance correction, you also put the tentative near addition in front of distance correction.

  Record the result as 'Delayed Subjective' followed by lens prescription and visual acuities.

DETERMINATION OF NEAR ADDITION

The eye must always accommodate for near objects. However, the ability of eyes to accommodate for near objects decreases with the age and this is because of decrease in amplitude of accommodation. An addition of plus power over and above distance power correction becomes inevitable to bring the near object into focus on the retina. The extra lens power prescribed is called 'reading addition' or 'near addition'.

Since the condition brings in changes in the near vision as the age increases, most practitioners formulate their own loose relationship between the age and the amount of near addition that would be needed by the patients as shown in **Table 11.1**.

But the near addition should never be prescribed by referring to any of such table. Each patient should be tested individually and prescription of correction should be based on individual patient needs, providing him most serviceable and comfortable, not necessarily the clearest vision at his habitual reading distance.

It is customary to start with a near addition of +0.75 Dsph to distance correction as the first correction to a patient showing the early symptoms of difficulties with reading newsprint in the dim illumination or during nighttime. As the patient ages and finds his ability to accommodate shrinking gradually, he may need an increase in prescription of near addition. On an average an individual accommodation declines and around the age of 52–55 years of age, he may need the near addition of +2.50 Dsph over his distance correction. Thereafter, in general not much change is required in near addition. Usually the same near addition is prescribed in both eyes. Unequal and very high near addition (above +3.50 D) indicates the presence of medical lesion or condition causing poor visual acuity in

Table 11.1: Different near additions at different ages.	
Age	Near addition
40 years	0.75 D
42 years	1.00 D
44 years	1.50 D
46 years	1.75 D
48 years	2.00 D
50 years	2.25 D

one or both eyes. The patient with cataract may need a near addition prescription of +3.50 Dsph or +4.00 Dsph. Even higher addition may be considered as visual aids.

The second important criteria while prescribing near addition is the reading distance. Usually a distance of 40 cm is considered an ideal reading distance for most presbyopes. But the best practice is to prescribe the near addition at his habitual reading distance. In any case if the near point is closer than 28 cm, it is rarely tolerated by the patient. If for any reason the patient needs to work at a very close distance or the demand for fine work requires a higher near addition, the convergence may be added with prism as well as accommodation with sphere. In all cases except for specific purpose correction the goal is to prescribe the near addition at not only his habitual reading distance but also some 12–15 cm further away to ensure that the patient can read satisfactorily not only at his habitual reading distance but also at a range of distances. This is also a good way to avoid over-correcting near addition. Remember it is good to under-correct than to over-correct so that the patient has no difficulties with accommodation and convergence and at the same time he has a range of vision, instead of fixed distance vision. This is very important because most people need to work at multiple near viewing distances. For example, a woman may hold her books at 50 cm while reading but she may be new to look at 40 cm while sewing and at 60 cm while chopping vegetables.

The test for near addition is usually done with both eyes open. However, in certain cases as mentioned below it may be executed monocularly, however, binocular verification must be done before writing the prescription for near addition:
- ❖ Anisometropia
- ❖ Amblyopia
- ❖ Cataract and other pathological condition

The optical correction for a presbyope is the sum of the refractive correction for distance correction plus the power of the near addition. It is, therefore, important to consider the change in net reading power while prescribing the near addition to a patient, instead of only near addition value. This is because a large increase in net plus spherical in near vision in a hyperope may bring in near point too close to the eyes and can also reduce the range of vision. Chapter 17 describes the different methods that may be applied to perform the test for near addition.

JACKSON CROSS-CYLINDER TEST

Jackson cross-cylinder (JCC) test is performed to achieve the following two objectives:
1. To refine cylinder power and cylinder axis
2. JCC can also be used to hunt for astigmatic error.

Refine Cylinder Axis

Verify cylinder axis before verifying cylinder power. Follow the below steps:
- Occlude one eye.
- Ask the patient to read the line which is one line above the best vision line.
- Place the JCC with its handle in line with the axis line of the cylinder lens in the trial frame (**Fig. 11.3**) and call it a Position 1.
- Now flip the JCC and call it a Position 2.
- Ask the patient to compare the images in two positions. However, before asking do not forget to remind the patient that the vision may not be as good as you notice earlier with your original lenses.
- If the patient reports no improvement of vision in the two positions of the JCC, the axis of cylinder in the trial frame is correct.
- If the better image quality with any of the two positions of JCC is reported, rotate the axis of trial frame cylinder lens in the direction of the similar cylinder component of JCC.

Reference is the cylinder lens in the trial frame

Refine Cylinder Power

- JCC will either increase or decrease the cylinder power in the trial frame.

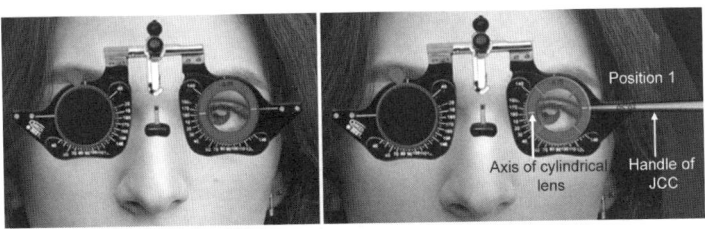

Fig. 11.3: Cylinder axis verification using JCC.

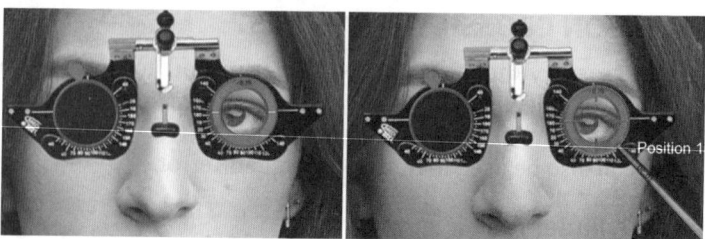

Fig. 11.4: Verifying cylinder power using JCC.

- Align the JCC axis with the cylinder axis in the trial frame **(Fig. 11.4)**.
- Flip the JCC and ask the patient to compare the clarity of images in two positions.
- If the patient reports no improvement in the two positions, the power of the cylinder in the trial frame is correct.
- If the patient reports better image clarity with any of the positions, the cylinder power in the trial frame is replaced with new cylinder power.
- Add minus cylinder when the patient says red axis line of JCC is aligned with minus cylinder lens in the trial frame.
- Add plus cylinder when the patient says green axis line of JCC is aligned with the plus cylinder lens in the trial frame.

> Throughout the JCC power check, maintain the spherical equivalent. For example, for every increase in minus cylinder of -0.50 D, add +0.25 D to the sphere or take away -0.25 D spherical. For every decrease in minus cylinder of - 0.50 D, add -0.25 D to the sphere.

Hunting Cylinder

- Use the spherical correction to achieve the best visual acuity with spherical correction **(Fig. 11.5)**.

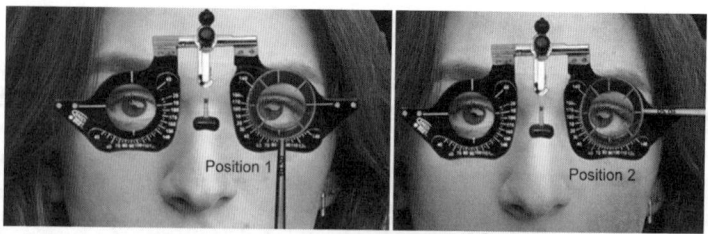

Fig. 11.5: Hunting cylinder using JCC.

Chapter 11: Subjective Methods of Refraction

- Use JCC to determine whether the patient needs the cylinder correction or not.
- When there is no cylinder lens in the trial frame, place the JCC at 90° and 180° to determine the presence of cylinder.
- If no preference is reported at two axes, it implies that the patient may not need cylinder correction.

REFRACTION USING STENOPEIC SLIT

Objective
Stenopeic slit is used to determine the refractive error in each of the meridians individually. It is a very useful method for high astigmatic patients. It is also a useful technique for patients with irregular astigmatism.

Stenopeic slit can also be used like the pinhole to diagnose the potential visual acuity of the patient.

Test
The stenopeic slit consists of rectangular aperture ranging from 0.50 to 1.00 mm in width and up to 15 mm in length. It is assumed to limit the admission of light to one meridian. Stenopeic slit can be used to find the two principal meridians and thereafter determine the refractive error in each of the meridians individually.

Illumination
Refraction is done in full room illumination.

Test Distance
Once the primary meridians are located, the test is done at a standard distance of 20 feet.

Patient Position
The patient may assume an unusual posture to look through the slit aperture.

Step-by-step Procedure
1. Occlude the left eye.
2. To begin with, the patient's right eye is fogged and then gradually defogged until the best possible visual acuity is attained.
3. Now place the slit before the eye being tested **(Fig. 11.6)** and slowly rotate while the patient's attention is towards the chart.

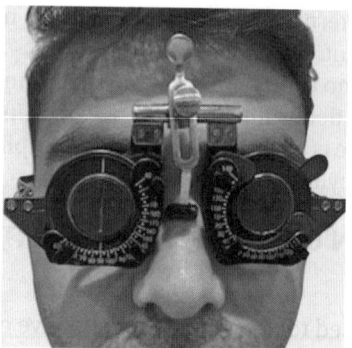

Fig. 11.6: Placing slit for refraction.

4. The patient is instructed to notify if at any position the visual acuity improves or better than other position.
5. If such a position is found, it is refined and bracketed by slight rotation of the slit on either side.
6. To be sure, rotate the slit by 90° to opposite meridian to compare the acuity. If astigmatism is significant, the second position should reveal poorer acuity than the first one. The disparity of acuity relates to the magnitude of the cylinder correction.
6. Correct the better acuity meridian first with spherical lens and then correct the opposite meridian again with spherical lens. (**Fig. 11.7**).
7. Achieve the best possible acuity in both the meridians separately and then remove the slit from the trial frame (**Fig. 11.8**).

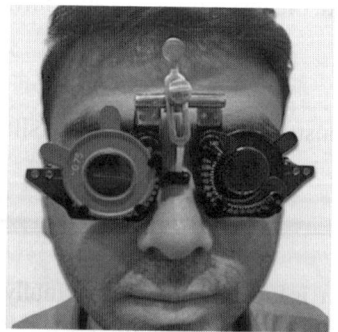

Fig. 11.7: Only spherical lens is used to correct meridian values.

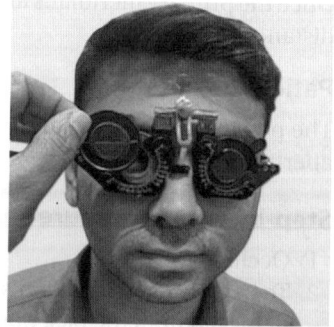

Fig. 11.8: Removing the slit.

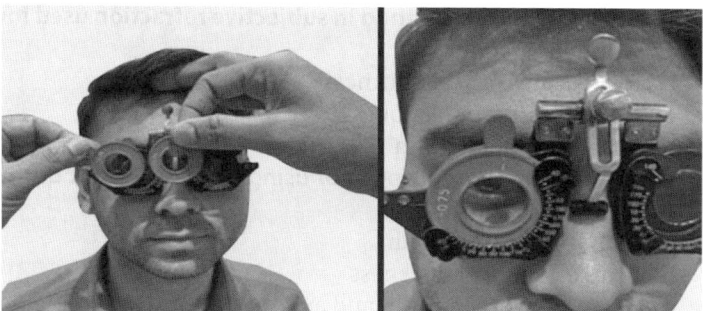

Fig. 11.9: Transforming the meridian values into sphero-cylinder form.

8. Transform the meridian values so derived into sphero-cylinder form and refine the same **(Fig. 11.9)**.
9. Record the results in the sphero-cylinder form with best corrected visual acuity.
10. If the patient has irregular astigmatism, record the results for major meridians separately as given below:

Stenopeic Slit Refraction
RE -2.50 D at 160, -4.50 D at 110
LE -3.00 D at 170, -5.50 D at 80

It is clear that subjective refraction is critical to the overall procedure of clinical refraction. It not only measures the refractive error of the patient but also assesses their tolerance to correction. The appropriate environments in terms of illumination and test distance has a significant impact on results. Most procedures take a long time and are patient-dependent, which implies that there is scope for research and development to introduce quicker, more flexible and less patient-dependent procedures.

MULTIPLE CHOICE QUESTIONS

1. **Which of the following statements about binocular refraction is not true?**
   a. It is better for patients with latent nystagmus.
   b. It reduces errors related to cyclophoria.
   c. It is better when visual acuity is grossly different in two eyes.
   d. It suspends accommodation well.

Chapter 11: Subjective Methods of Refraction

2. **What is the fogging method in subjective refraction used for?**
   a. To induce myopia
   b. To measure corneal thickness
   c. To relax accommodation
   d. To assess retinal health
3. **What is the primary purpose of using a stenopeic slit during refraction?**
   a. To measure axial length
   b. To assess corneal thickness
   c. To refine cylinder power and axis
   d. To evaluate color vision
4. **What is the primary function of the Jackson Cross-cylinder (JCC) in subjective refraction?**
   a. To measure axial length
   b. To assess color vision
   c. To refine cylinder power and axis
   d. To evaluate corneal thickness

ANSWER KEY

| 1. c | 2. c | 3. c | 4. c |

SELF-PRACTICE QUESTIONS

1. What is the difference between binocular balancing procedure and binocular subjective refraction?
2. What are the criteria for determining the end point in subjective refraction? What are the important considerations that you must think over before making a new lens prescription?
3. What is JCC? Explain the optical basis of cylinder power determination with JCC.
4. Why is it recommended to use minus cylinder during the fogging method of subjective refraction?

12 CHAPTER

Refinement Tests

CHAPTER OUTLINE

- Duochrome Test for Spherical
- Tests for Binocular Balancing

The last part of the measurement of refractive error is the application of end point techniques. The objective is to refine the results of the subjective refraction before prescribing. First, the results of the subjective refraction are refined monocularly using the Jackson cross-cylinder test for the cylinder axis and cylinder amount, if the cylinder correction has been done without using it. Once the cylinder correction is refined, the examiner proceeds to refine the spherical correction monocularly using the duochrome test for the spherical end point. If the patient is truly binocular, not suppressing vision in any eye or having a squint, monocular refinement of refractive error is followed by an attempt to equalize the accommodative effort exerted by the two eyes. Hence, the next step is to spherically equalize or balance the corrections of the two eyes.

Two clinical tests that are most commonly applied for the purpose are shown in **Flowchart 12.1**.

DUOCHROME TEST FOR SPHERICAL

Aim
The test is performed to refine the spherical correction or to determine the spherical end point of the refractive error after the subjective refraction is completed.

Chapter 12: Refinement Tests

Flowchart 12.1: Two tests commonly used for refinement of refraction correction.

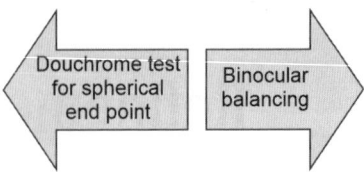

Illumination

The test has to be done under complete darkness as it reduces veiling luminance and dilates the pupil, thereby increases the chromatic aberration, making the test more effective.

Position

The patient should be asked to sit with face upright and the results of subjective refraction should be in the trial frame in front of his eyes. The patient is, sighting at distant chart.

Test Distance

The test has to be done at the usual distance of 20 feet.

Principle

The test makes use of chromatic aberration present in the human eyes. Near the end point, an eye that is residually myopic by a small degree of spherical, sees black letters having a red background to be sharper and darker, with more defined borders. Letters on the green background appear slightly fuzzy and less dark with less defined border. An eye that is residually hyperopic by a small degree of the spherical power sees the letters on the green background sharp, darkened and more defined. An emmetropic eye sees the letters on both sides of the chart to be equally sharp, dark and defined.

Green light of 535 nm tends to focus 0.20 D before the retina and red light of 620 nm tends to focus behind the retina.

Color blindness does not invalidate the test because chromatic aberration is present even in color blind subject.

Critical Factor

It is important to control the accommodation by slight fogging. Add +0.25 Dsph lens monocularly before asking the patient to notice the difference between letters of two backgrounds. The idea is to take the patient in a position where he reports that the letters on the red background appear to stand out better. This should occur in only one or two increments of plus sphere unless the eye is over minus.

Normative Data

The test is very sensitive to even a small change of 0.25 DS. The plus sphere is reduced until letters on the both backgrounds appear equally distinct. Or the next reduction of only 0.25 D makes letters on the green background more distinct. Ideally, spherical end point should be decided when the letters on the red background are comparatively sharper.

Limitations

Although the test is very effective but its applications are also limited as may be seen in the following cases:

- ❖ Test may be ineffective when the pupil is exceedingly small. Therefore, over 55 years of age when the chromatic aberration of the eye drops markedly, the dioptric interval of the red and green may reduce further.
- ❖ Red and green wavelengths of different charts may bring in disparity in results.
- ❖ Aging of bulb, faded or dirty charts may adversely affect.
- ❖ Yellowing of crystalline lens in cataract tends to reduce transmission of shorter wavelength, it may alter the patient's preference for one color or visual acuity is not adequate to discern a difference.
- ❖ The instruction to the subject is to emphasize the sharpness, darkness and definition of the black letters and not their background.
- ❖ If the error is over 1.00 D, or the vision 6/9 or worse, the results may be unreliable. The red and green only have a 0.50 D difference in focus.

TESTS FOR BINOCULAR BALANCING

Aim

The test is performed to equalize the stimulus to accommodation for the two eyes.

Test

The two most common procedures which are normally used for binocular balancing of refractive correction are given in **Flowchart 12.2**.

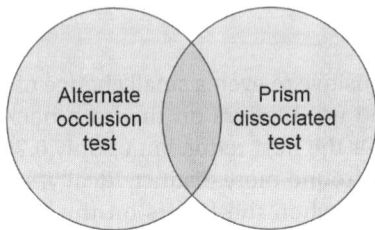

Fig. 12.2: Two methods of binocular balancing tests.

Illumination

The test has to be done under standard room lights.

Patient Position

The patient is asked to sit upright with monocular correction in the trial frame and both eyes open.

Test Distance

The test is performed at a distance of 20 feet.

Critical Factor

If balancing is not possible, leave the patient at a point which produces least difference. The dominant eye is left with a little clearer vision.

Indications

The test is performed in the following cases:
- When visual acuity in both eyes is nearer to 20/20.
- When both eyes visual acuity is equal.
- The test is not effective for amblyopia.

Procedure of Alternate Occlusion Test

1. Ask the patient to keep both eyes open.
2. Begin with the results of monocular subjective refraction.

Chapter 12: Refinement Tests

3. Ask the patient to look at a line three lines above BCVA, i.e., 20/50.
4. Fog both eyes with +0.75 Dsph.
5. Alternately occlude each eye and ask the patient with which eye he sees better.
6. Add +0.25 Dsph to the better eye and continue until each eye sees equally blur or clearer when vision switches to other eye.
7. This is the end point.
8. In order to confirm, add +0.25 Dsph before both eyes and repeat the test. If balance is correct, both eyes will lose equal amount of acuity.
9. Now both eyes are in perfect balance.
10. Subtract 0.75 Dsph from each eye.
11. Do this while the patient is viewing the full chart with 20/20 at bottom.

Procedure of Prism Dissociated Test

1. Ask the patient to keep both eyes open.
2. Begin with the results of monocular subjective refraction.
3. Fog both eyes with 0.75 Dsph or 1.00 Dsph.
4. Isolate a line of letters (pref. 20/40 or 20/50).
5. Put 3 prism dioptre base up over right eye and 3 prism dioptre base down over left eye.
6. Make sure that the patient sees same line as two—one on top of other.
7. Instruct the patient to compare two lines.
8. Images of both the lines should be equally blurred.
9. Add 0.25 Dsph to better eye and continue until each eye sees equal blur or clear vision switches to the other eye.
10. This is the end point
11. Now both eyes are in perfect balance
12. Subtract the original fogging lens power from each eye.

MULTIPLE CHOICE QUESTIONS

1. **What is the dioptric difference between the red and green targets on a duochrome target?**
    a. 0.25 DS
    b. 0.50 DS
    c. 1.00 DS
    d. 2.00 DS

Chapter 12: Refinement Tests

2. Which of the following statements about duochrome test is true?
   a. Smaller pupils enhance the accuracy of the test.
   b. The brightness of the colors is more important than the distinctness of the rings.
   c. Cataract will tend towards favoring the rings on the red background.
   d. Accommodation will favor the rings on the green.

ANSWER KEY

1. b   2. c

SELF-PRACTICE QUESTION

1. Explain the significance of binocular balancing during clinical refraction. How does it impact the patient's visual experience?

13 CHAPTER

Prescribing and Counseling

CHAPTER OUTLINE

- Prescribing Considerations
- Factors that Influence Prescribing Decision
- Fundamental Rule for Prescribing Correction
- Counseling

The measurement of refractive error and prescribing of refractive correction are two distinct functions and are always unique for every individual. While the basic process of measuring refractive error is by and large straight forward, there are myriad complexities involved in prescribing refractive correction.

The Law 2 of the clinical refraction says that there are broadly three different reasons why an individual visits an eye clinic for vision correction. **Table 13.1** shows the three reasons.

In all these cases the examiner is driven by different objectives. While the mechanics of measuring the refractive error may be same in all three cases, the considerations for prescribing refractive

Table 13.1: Why patients visit practice for clinical refraction?	
Classification of patients	*Purpose*
Routine examination patients	Visit to practice as a part of routine care
Symptomatic patients	Symptoms that are troubling him in his day-to-day life
Non-adaptation cases	Having dissatisfaction with the prescribed correction

correction must vary to meet the requisite objectives. The clinician must think judiciously and prescribe appropriately.

PRESCRIBING CONSIDERATIONS

There are four factors that form the part of important considerations before prescribing the refractive correction. These factors are shown in **Flowchart 13.1**.

Vision

The process of vision ideally operates as a subconscious function, meaning that individuals should naturally and effortlessly perceive a clear and sharp visual environment without conscious effort. When it comes to prescribing refractive correction, the primary consideration is to restore this subconscious visual experience. It is important to understand that a patient can read 6/6 line on the Snellen's test chart with several combinations of spherical and cylinder lenses. It is the examiner who chooses the most appropriate one. Despite the patient's ability to achieve a clear vision on the test chart, it is the examiner who evaluates and selects the most appropriate combination of lenses. The choice involves considerations beyond achieving a specific acuity level; it includes factors such as optimizing visual comfort, addressing specific refractive errors like astigmatism, and ensuring that the correction aligns with the patient's unique visual needs and daily activities.

The goal is to provide a refractive correction that not only meets the basic requirement of clear vision on the test chart but also enhances the overall visual experience. This may involve refining the prescription based on the patient's subjective feedback, adjusting for factors like binocular vision, and considering the demands of the patient's lifestyle. In essence, the examiner's expertise is crucial in translating the objective measurement of visual acuity into a

Flowchart 13.1: Important factors to consider while prescribing refractive correction.

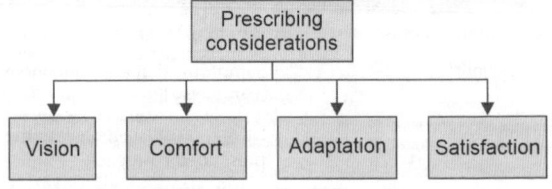

Chapter 13: Prescribing and Counseling

tailored and effective prescription. By choosing the most appropriate combination of lenses, the examiner ensures that the patient experiences optimal vision in a way that is comfortable, efficient, and aligned with the subconscious nature of the visual process.

The rule of thumb that is commonly followed is prescribing least minus for best correction in myopia and maximum plus to achieve the best correction in hypermetropia. The understanding is—myopia is little undercorrected and hypermetropia is fully corrected.

A change in spherical correction can lead to changes in magnification. Positive spherical correction brings in positive change in magnification and negative spherical correction brings in negative change in magnification. Magnification is also associated with change in apparent image size which ultimately has an impact on the spatial localization of the object. A magnified object looks closer, whereas a minified object appears farther. The phenomenon ultimately leads in issues related to adaptation. Plus lens has contrast lowering effect whereas minus lens makes the letters sharper and darker. Plus lens creates pincushion effect and minus lens creates barrel distortion which may bring in unpleasant optical effects.

The vision in astigmatism is characteristic. The image is not out of focus but distortion of image is produced. In the majority of cases small amount of astigmatic error does not give rise to visual symptoms, hence considered physiological. It is usually not prescribed but in case it produces symptoms of eyestrain, even a small amount of astigmatic correction should be prescribed. An important practical consideration is in relation to altering cylinder axis; extreme caution should be exercised while changing the cylinder axis especially in the patient who has no optical or visual complaints. Too often changing a cylinder axis to theoretically correct position leads to a complaint of spatial disorientation as well as asthenopic symptoms. A care should be taken to ensure symmetry of astigmatic correction between two eyes not only with respect to amount of correction but also to the direction of the axis, excluding the cases of anisometropia.

Prescribing near addition to presbyope is probably the trickiest for which no rule can be firmly laid down. The nature of the task for which the near vision correction is required must be analyzed in each individual together with established visual habits and fineness of the near objects and decision for prescribing correction should be taken based upon their habitual reading distance. The focus is more on comfort and depth of field, rather than clarity of vision.

The equal retinal image is not produced on the two retinas in case of anisometropia. The consideration of dominant eye becomes an important factor for prescribing correction. When prescribing correction for anisometropia, the clinician may consider emphasizing the correction in the dominant eye to ensure clearer and more comfortable vision. This helps optimize the visual experience for daily activities.

Comfort

Visual comfort is the subjective reaction of a patient to his refractive correction. It often transpires when there is a correct relationship between the visual task, the environment in which it is performed, and the person performing it. An individual expects seamless and comfortable vision at any point in the day, regardless of any deleterious factor that has the potential to incapacitate him from performing the task. Visual comfort is something that is the most important guiding factor to prescribe a correction. The reasons are simple. What is not comfortable to use is never used; it is just discarded, and the objective of prescribing is not achieved.

While considering visual comfort before prescribing refractive correction, it is important to consider the human factor. A person may live placidly and comfortably with a small degree of astigmatism and proportionately reduced vision, while another who is highly organized and suffers from the same disability may attain normal or supernormal vision and pay for it. Optical efficiency is important, but the treatment should be executed considering the patient as a whole, including his environment, physical ability, nature, and amount of work, as well as his psychological reaction to life as a whole, to ensure visual comfort.

It must be remembered that gross visual error does not give rise to discomfort; it simply results in failure of visual function and hence complete rejection. Small errors, on the contrary, tend to give rise to greater discomfort. Unless these small errors are corrected with punctilious care, they may be perpetuated in some other form, and the symptoms may be unrelieved. Good vision with comfort has been found to be significantly associated with optimally prescribed correction.

Comfort is not only associated with correction; it is also affected by the right solution proposed in the form of the right lens and the right frame, together with a good fit. Fitting a spectacle frame snugly is an art, and this is where optometry goes beyond the paradigm of science and merges with art. An optometrist should have a fine sense of observation and a sound understanding of a well-fitted spectacle frame. He also needs to remember that every patient has different anomalies, and he should fit the spectacle frame to ensure comfort for the patient, not a flat surface for a square or pretty look only. However, the fact remains that it is not possible to predict beforehand how comfortable he will find his new glasses in everyday life.

Since "comfort" is a subjective and psychological concept, determining whether a prescribed correction will be comfortable is a nuanced task for clinicians. The decision relies on the clinician's judgment, interpreting both objective and subjective findings in consideration of patient symptoms, habitual correction, and immediate feedback. The clinician presumes that the tailored prescription will provide comfort. He faces similar challenges when the patient feels discomfort after using the prescribed correction. The patient cannot pinpoint the precise reason for his discomfort. The clinician has to make an effort to discover the reason for the patient's discomfort by questioning him and making another judgement based upon his responses, again using his experience and evidence.

Adaptation

Adaptation is a crucial consideration in prescribing refractive correction. When an individual receives a new prescription, a brief period of adjustment is often necessary before using it comfortably. The adaptation duration varies based on factors such as age, the magnitude of correction, changes from habitual correction, and the type of correction.

This adaptive process enables the visual system to acclimate gradually, ultimately enhancing visual comfort. Initially, visual acuity might decrease with the new correction, but over time, the visual system learns to optimize it. Changes in refractive correction may also impact binocular vision, leading to eye strain and alterations in visual perception.

Binocular vision, essential for depth perception and spatial localization, relies on the primary visual cortex in the brain's occipital cortex. While most individuals seamlessly adapt to new corrections, some may experience initial discomfort and hence difficulty in adjusting.

The neuromuscular mechanisms of the ocular system play a role when a new correction is worn. Plus correction relaxes accommodation, while minus correction induces accommodation. Accommodation is linked with convergence. The prismatic effects also come into play—plus correction introduces a base-in prismatic effect, easing muscle tension, while minus correction introduces a base-out prismatic effect, placing additional strain on muscles. The visual system continually adapts to diverse contexts, making transient adjustments in sensitivity or perception when exposed to new stimuli and exhibiting lingering after-effects upon stimulus removal. This adaptation is a matter of time, with some individuals adapting swiftly, others requiring more time, and those unable to adapt needing unique considerations. This is where refractive correction goes beyond the paradigm of science and merges with art.

Visual adaptation has the potential to affect almost every aspect of a person's life. The consequences may include a number of physical and mental unhealthy days and overall dissatisfaction. One of the ways the visual system adapts to new refractive correction is through the changes in accommodation function. Another way the visual system adapts to a new refractive correction is through changes in the activity of the neurons in the visual cortex of the brain. When a new correction is introduced, the neurons in the visual cortex need to adapt to the changes in the visual input to ensure that the visual image is perceived accurately. This process can take some time, but eventually, the visual system will adapt, and the person will be able to see clearly with the new correction.

Satisfaction

The visual satisfaction transpires when an individual develops a positive feeling for his correction and this happens when he is able to cope with his occupational needs unconsciously and he continues with it comfortably for a prolonged period of time. This is demonstrated in the **Figure 13.1.**

Occupation encompasses how individuals engage with their environment, whether at work, home, or in daily life, each having specific or general requirements. These interactions manifest as behavior. Visual satisfaction often results from behavioral ease, closely linked to vision. This satisfaction emerges when an individual can see clearly, comfortably, and swiftly adapts to their new correction.

Chapter 13: Prescribing and Counseling

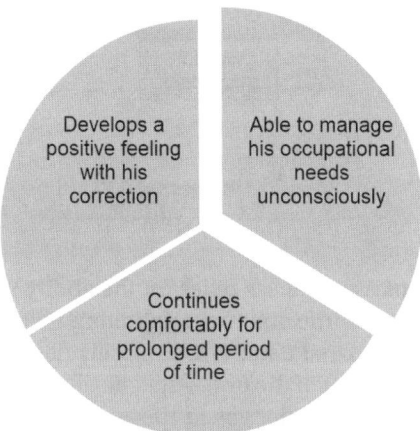

Fig. 13.1: Visual satisfaction triad.

The visual process is a complex process. Multiple factors influence the visual comfort which in turn contribute significantly to visual satisfaction. As a general rule visual acuity of 20/20 forms no true basis for visual satisfaction. An individual may be able to read 20/20 in the clinic and may still be complaining of dissatisfaction with his vision.

Visual satisfaction also fluctuates throughout the day and with different tasks. Most individuals challenge their own visual system with different visual tasks and challenging situations on a given day. Continuous near vision tasks for hours, high contrast demands in low light conditions, glare while driving, exposure to air-conditioned environment at workplace or demand for peripheral vision during sports are all very important considerations to assess someone's visual satisfaction.

In general, most studies agree that visual satisfaction of any individual with his refractive correction is driven by three factors as shown in **Flowchart 13.2**.

Spatial awareness involves the cognitive skill of understanding one's position in space. This knowledge allows individuals to anticipate the proximity of objects as they move. It is a crucial aspect of perception, and difficulties in spatial awareness can lead to perceptual issues, causing individuals to appear clumsy or have challenges in interpersonal interactions.

Chapter 13: Prescribing and Counseling

Flowchart 13.2: Factors that drive visual satisfaction.

```
        Spatial
       awareness
        ↙     ↘
  Visual  ←→  Visual
efficiency    comfort
```

Effective spatial awareness relies on the ability to automatically process task-specific information, facilitating efficient acquisition and processing of spatial data. This is closely tied to the quick and coordinated movement of the eyes—specifically, the ability to fixate, converge, and focus. Challenges in these eye muscle skills, rather than issues with the eyes themselves, can impact spatial awareness.

In summary, achieving visual satisfaction is a multifaceted process involving physical, physiological, and psychological factors. Practitioners must consider numerous elements influencing daily activities to ensure visual satisfaction. While it is challenging to predict satisfaction during refractive correction measurements, adherence to fundamental guidelines increases the likelihood. Patients visit optometrists not only for vision disturbances but also for symptoms like eye strain, pain, headaches, dizziness, and vertigo. In these cases, satisfaction results from addressing and treating these symptoms through proper correction.

FACTORS THAT INFLUENCE PRESCRIBING DECISION

The measurement of refractive error is not the conclusive treatment in itself; the examiner must take into account what he is using as well as his overall personality and intelligence before taking a decision on what he should use as his vision correction. The clinician should appreciate and recognize this and allow his treatment advice to be guided by his knowledge, experience and discovered information. The three factors that must be included in decision-making process are shown in **Flowchart 13.3**.

Habitual Correction

Habitual correction refers to the regular correction that the patient is using either as spectacles or contact lenses. When determining a new

Chapter 13: Prescribing and Counseling

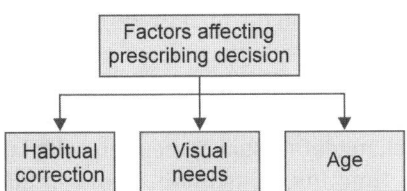

Flowchart 13.3: Factors that affect decision while prescribing refractive correction.

prescription, it is crucial for the examiner to take into account the patient's habitual correction. This consideration is essential because the patient's visual system has adapted to a specific way of perceiving the world with their habitual correction.

Visual perception is the complicated cognitive process of receiving, interpreting, and responding to visual stimuli. It takes place within the brain. While the retinal image forms the basis, visual perception integrates various aspects such as light sense, form sense, contrast sense, and color sense. Crucially, what individuals see is not merely a direct translation of retinal stimuli. Extensive cerebral editing occurs, involving the suppression or interpretation of information to align with past experiences. Visual perception is heavily influenced by previous encounters and stored information. Sensory receptors gather environmental information, which is then combined with pre-existing knowledge, enabling the brain to form conclusions about the external world based on stored information.

Therefore, careful consideration of the patient's habitual correction is crucial when prescribing new refractive correction to ensure a smooth adaptation process and optimal visual experience.

The brain plays a pivotal role in processing information received through the eyes, where visual perception and the interpretation of the environment are influenced by inputs from other sensory systems and an individual's past experiences. The brain's ability to process visual information can be compromised if there is a disruption in the contributions of each component. A sudden change in prescription has the potential to significantly alter the perception of the world, potentially causing discomfort, visual disturbances, and, in some cases, non-adaptation. Therefore, careful consideration of the patient's habitual correction is crucial when prescribing new refractive correction to ensure a smooth adaptation process and optimal visual experience.

A modification in spherical correction shifts the focal point within the eye, directly influencing visual acuity. The impact on a person's vision depends on the magnitude of the correction change. Additionally, it influences depth perception and spatial awareness since alterations in how light is refracted and focused can affect the perception of distance and spatial relationships. Generally, the brain adapts to changes in visual perception, with larger corrections requiring more time for adjustment, while smaller changes are accommodated relatively quickly.

Cylinder correction is prescribed when the cornea has an irregular shape, leading to different light refractions in various eye meridians. This correction compensates for the irregularity, improving vision. Unlike improving acuity on a Snellen's chart, cylinder corrections enhance the quality of distorted images and create a contrast-enhancing effect. Therefore, it is advisable to exercise caution and avoid unnecessary adjustments to the entire cylinder correction, as the primary goal is to maintain optimal vision quality rather than making wholesale corrections.

The cylinder axis indicates the location of astigmatism in the eye. The impact of changing the cylinder axis depends on the amount of the cylinder. Smaller corrections may not significantly affect visual performance, while larger corrections notably impact image quality. Care is exercised when adjusting the cylinder axis, especially in asymptomatic patients. it is often best to maintain the accustomed axis to avoid issues like spatial disorientation or eye strain, even if visual acuity could be slightly improved at a different axis.

An unintended alteration in binocular balance can lead to incongruity between the eyes, causing abnormal spatial perception. Likewise, a modification in near addition affects the depth of focus and the habitual near viewing distance. These changes impact the accommodation function and the convergence function. Some individuals may find this experience uncomfortable, experiencing unusual sensations and struggling to adapt to the new correction.

To prevent potential issues, it is essential for the examiner to consider the habitual correction as a benchmark when prescribing a new correction. There are three key areas as shown in **Flowchart 13.4** where the clinician can use the habitual correction as a reference.

- ❖ If the patient is not experiencing any symptoms with their current correction, the clinician may choose to avoid making unnecessary changes to the prescription.

Flowchart 13.4: Use of habitual correction.

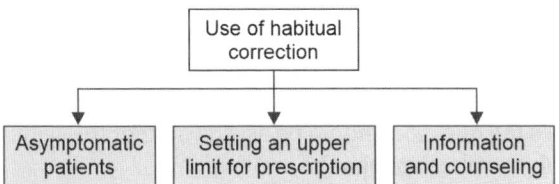

- ❖ The habitual correction can be utilized to establish an upper limit for changes in the new prescription. This ensures that adjustments remain within a range that the patient is accustomed to.
- ❖ The information from the habitual correction serves as a benchmark to explain the new prescription to the patient. This aids in counseling the patient on what changes to expect and facilitates a smoother adaptation process.

A change in spherical correction not only alters the focus but also changes the magnification of the image. Plus lenses magnify the image, creating a false sense of proximity, while minus lenses result in minification. This magnification effect can distort the perception of distance and spatial relationships. In the case of cylinder lenses, the impact is more pronounced. These lenses elongate the image in one direction, leading to significant degradation and distortion of image quality. It is crucial to consider these effects when prescribing corrective lenses, as they directly influence how individuals perceive and interact with their surroundings.

It is generally agreed upon that spherical correction should not be altered by more than 0.75 D to 1.00 D, cylinder by 0.50 D to 0.75 D, and axis by 10 degrees. In cases where larger changes are deemed necessary, it is imperative for the clinician to thoroughly explain and counsel the patient about potential difficulties and the need for adaptation. Clear communication helps manage patient expectations and ensures a smoother transition to the new prescription.

Further, it is always suggested that the examiner must also be chary of invariably altering the corrections at the routine eye examination if he finds a little change in refraction in the following scenarios:
- ❖ Minor changes in refraction in the absence of symptoms
- ❖ Small introduction of cylinder correction where none was present previously.
- ❖ Small alteration in the cylinder axis

The change may result in the development of symptoms which were not present previously.

Also, even in a scenario where the patient reports symptoms, the finding that his present correction is in some marginal degree incorrect should not always be taken as an indication to alter them. In all cases the question should be asked whether the symptoms can reasonably be related to change in refraction.

Understanding the patient's current correction is crucial, not only for evaluating the need for any alterations but also to reduce the likelihood of developing symptoms that may lead to visual discomfort and dissatisfaction. It is essential to acknowledge that reasons for non-adaptation are diverse and unique to each individual. Therefore, prescribing a new refractive correction requires careful consideration.

Visual Needs

Visual needs play a crucial role in determining the appropriate refractive correction for an individual. Visual needs refer to the specific requirements of an individual with regard to their occupational and lifestyle needs. Occupations are everything we do in our lives. In other words, occupations explain how we relate to our environment. The hypothesis is that occupational and lifestyle needs generate the visual needs that form the basis for vision correction. Visual and occupational performances are directly linked, and this relationship is intuitively obvious. But the problem is that the science is weak. As professionals, we are able to measure vision in many different ways and very accurately, but we cannot connect the resulting improvement in vision with its effect on occupational performance.

Understanding visual needs requires the examiner to do a visual task analysis to estimate the overall visual demand, and this would include consideration of the following information:

- ❖ Target size
- ❖ Target distance
- ❖ Static and dynamic states of the target
- ❖ Contrast of the target against its background
- ❖ Color of the target and background
- ❖ Illumination and position of luminaires
- ❖ Environmental distractors
- ❖ Surface reflectivity of the surroundings
- ❖ Duration of the demand
- ❖ Patient's position and posture

There are three most important characteristics of occupational activities. These are:
1. The activities involve the individual completely.
2. The activities are meaningful to the individual.
3. The activities include processes that are repetitive in nature.

All occupational interactions may be summarized as behaviors. Vision and visual responses are one such behavior. 90% of the interaction is through vision. Any deficiency in vision and the visual system may influence the interaction adversely and thereby affect occupational performance, which is the main reason for visual dissatisfaction.

In order to understand the visual needs, the examiner has to understand the patient and his occupational environment and then discover the visual needs, considering the interaction that might happen between him and his environment.

Age

Patient's age is the foundation of visual needs as age determines the occupational and lifestyle needs. Aging has a huge impact on the vision and visual needs of the patients. It is important that the clinician understands changes in eyes, visual system and visual needs that happen with age and prescribe the correction accordingly. Among all the factors, age remains the most important guiding factor for prescribing the refractive correction. Other factors such as the patient's visual needs, occupation, and lifestyle are all the function of age. It is, therefore, prudent to have an age-specific approach for understanding the fundamental guidelines for prescribing refractive correction.

FUNDAMENTAL RULE FOR PRESCRIBING CORRECTION

The prescription for refractive correction should be considered in conjunction with the symptoms and age of the patient. Where there is an obvious refractive error associated with a visual defect, the indication to prescribe correction is clear; apart from such an obvious indication, however, there are other factors that may lead to a decision in the realization that the ametropia discovered is a kind or degree that is unlikely to be the sole cause of trouble. For example, in children, a small degree of hypermetropia or astigmatism is natural. Many subjects between the ages of 20 and 40 have static refraction. It has been observed that there is a slight but steady increase in hypermetropia during middle age, between the ages of 40 and 60. A subject who was emmetropic at 30 years of age may show 0.25 D of hyperopia at around 45–50 years and 0.75 D at around 60 years. At extreme old age, after around 60 years of age, a trend towards myopia may develop. Recognizing these age-specific trends, it becomes evident that prescribing refractive correction requires an approach tailored to each age-group. Establishing fundamental guidelines based on age-specific considerations appears to be the most appropriate method for determining when and how to prescribe refractive correction.

In light of these age-specific nuances, we can discuss the prescribing of refractive correction to align with distinct age groups as shown in **Figure 13.2**. This approach acknowledges the dynamic nature of visual changes across the lifespan, providing a more effective and targeted strategy for prescribing refractive correction.

In children emmetropization is essentially completed by the age of 6 years. As a result, the prescription of a small amount of hypermetropia is generally avoided in routine clinical practice. The decision to prescribe corrective lenses in children is multifaceted and involves careful consideration of factors such as strabismus and amblyopia. In cases where strabismus or amblyopia is present, the decision to prescribe corrective lenses becomes crucial. Corrective lenses can play a significant role in addressing these visual abnormalities and promoting normal visual development. The details of this decision-making process are thoroughly explained in Chapter 20.

18–40 Years (Adult Population)

In the age group of 18–40 years, adults typically enjoy stable and healthy eyesight, with the most common vision-related issues arising from visual stress. Symptoms such as eye strain, accommodative spasm, asthenopia, headaches, and nonvisual acuity-related pain are prevalent in this demography. These problems may manifest with

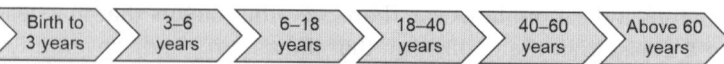

Fig. 13.2: Age grouping.

or without specific symptoms, making the alleviation of symptoms a primary objective in prescribing corrective measures.

Addressing the specific visual needs of individuals within this age range is crucial, given the variations in occupational demands. Prescribing correction should not only aim to enhance visual acuity but also consider the unique visual requirements associated with specific professions or activities. Recognizing and accommodating these needs can significantly improve visual comfort and overall satisfaction with corrective measures.

In-depth counseling plays a pivotal role in the management of visual stress among adults. Many individuals in this age group develop suboptimal habits, such as incorrect viewing angles, poor posture, inadequate illumination, and uncomfortable seating. These habits can contribute to visual stress and discomfort over the course of the day. Therefore, along with prescribing correction, addressing and correcting these habits through counseling is essential for long-term visual well-being.

While static refraction is common in this age group, caution is advised when considering changes in prescription during routine re-examinations. When a patient seeks a new pair of spectacles due to the physical deterioration of their existing pair, it is prudent to confirm that the refraction is indeed static. In cases where minor changes in refraction are detected without accompanying symptoms, it may be reasonable to exercise restraint in altering the correction. Minor adjustments, especially in cylinder axis or the introduction of a small cylinder where none was previously present in the habitual correction, should be carefully evaluated, considering the overall impact on visual comfort and well-being. This approach ensures that changes in prescription are made judiciously, prioritizing the patient's comfort and minimizing unnecessary modifications.

Correction in Case of Adult Hyperopia

- ❖ Adult hyperopia may present with a range of complications, necessitating regular assessments.
- ❖ Refractive correction decisions should be tailored to individual cases, with asymptomatic patients potentially left uncorrected.
- ❖ Symptomatic patients, experiencing issues like eye strain, dizziness, asthenopia, and headaches, should be corrected to alleviate their specific symptoms, apart from addressing reduced visual acuity.

Habitual Undercorrected Patients

- Patients accustomed to undercorrection should not receive full hypermetropic correction.
- The ciliary muscles are habituated to maintaining a significant accommodative tone, making it challenging to adjust to full correction.
- Full correction may induce myopia in such cases, leading to indistinct distance vision and potential intolerance.
- It is advisable to continue undercorrecting hypermetropia in these individuals, even if symptoms like headache or eye strain persist.

Eye Strain and Accommodative Spasm

- In the presence of marked eye strain symptoms, it is beneficial to alleviate accommodation by correcting as much of the total hypermetropia as possible.
- Addressing the entire error is essential in cases of accommodation spasm to ease ciliary muscles and indirectly relieve convergence by reducing accommodation.
- Conversely, in latent divergent squint cases, undercorrection, by stimulating accommodation, may inadvertently stimulate convergence.

Simple Myopia

- Simple myopia primarily requires refractive correction.
- Overcorrection should be avoided, but a comfortable full correction is recommended.
- In low myopia, prescription usually seldom requires change but in high myopia, full correction can rarely be tolerated. This is because the images formed by strong concave lenses are diminished in size, bright and clear. The patient, who is accustomed to interpret hazy diffusion circles, is intolerant of them. In such cases correction is prescribed with which greatest visual acuity is obtained without distress.

Astigmatic Correction

- Small astigmatic error does not require correction provided there is no symptoms of eye strain and asthenopia. Since the end objective clinical refraction is to prescribe a correction that the individual can use comfortably for sustained period

of time, undercorrection of astigmatic in most situations is recommended.
- ❖ Extreme care must be taken to alter the cylinder axis. It is a good practice to avoid altering cylinder axis even if the visual acuity improves at a slight different axis from that to which the patient is used to. The theoretically correct axis may lead to a complaint of spatial disorientation.

Management of Uncorrected Anisometropia

Adults, detected with uncorrected anisometropia should be encouraged to wear full refractive correction especially when symptoms of asthenopia or muscle imbalance are present. The correction may be increased periodically to reach to full correction.

40–60 Years (Middle-aged Population)

Prescribing refraction correction for individuals aged 40–60 years requires a nuanced approach considering natural aging processes. The prominent factor in this age range is the onset of presbyopia, stemming from a gradual decline in the ability to accommodate for near vision. Consequently, the primary goal is not only to enhance visual performance for distance vision but also to address near vision by prescribing an additional plus correction, known as near addition, to support accommodation.

Alongside the onset of presbyopia, individuals aged 40–60 years may experience an increased incidence of ocular diseases and systemic health conditions. Fluctuating vision in this middle-aged population can be attributed to systemic issues such as diabetes, high blood pressure, and medication regimens for conditions like high cholesterol, thyroid disorders, anxiety, depression, and arthritis. These medications may induce temporary changes in refraction. Additionally, early symptoms of cataracts, glaucoma, and macular degeneration can contribute to alterations in refractive correction during this period.

Near Addition Prescription

It is common practice to initiate near vision correction by adding +0.75 D to the distance correction. The following guidelines should be followed while prescribing the near addition power:
- ❖ Near addition prescription is need based.
- ❖ Near addition prescription varies based upon reading distance.

- Typically, the same near addition is prescribed for both eyes. Notably, unequal near addition may signal the presence of medical issues.
- When prescribing near addition, it is advisable to undercorrect rather than overcorrect to minimize challenges related to accommodation and convergence functions.
- A practical tip is to ensure that the patients can comfortably read not only at their habitual reading distance but also about 12-15 cm further away. This precaution helps guard against overcorrection.
- If a correction brings the near point closer than 28 cm, adding convergence with prism and accommodation with a sphere may be necessary.

Temporary Corrections

Temporary changes in refractive correction between the ages of 40-60 years can be influenced by various factors, including both physiological and external elements. The following considerations are critical:

- Sudden increases in blood glucose levels can alter refractive error. In such cases, a temporary minus correction might be prescribed to ensure clear vision for distance objects.
- Fluctuations in blood pressure levels may impact the flexibility of the eye's lens and alter its shape, leading to temporary changes in vision. Individuals experiencing a sudden increase or decrease in blood pressure might notice shifts in their ability to focus clearly.
- Dehydration can influence the thickness and shape of the cornea, leading to temporary changes in refractive correction.
- Stress and anxiety may contribute to changes in accommodation, affecting the ability of the eyes to focus properly.
- Hormonal fluctuations, especially in women experiencing menopause, can influence tear production and ocular surface changes, contributing to temporary changes in vision.
- Individuals prone to migraines or headaches may experience temporary changes in vision associated with these episodes.

In individuals aged above 60 years, the emphasis shifts towards enhancing patient satisfaction. The visual satisfaction transpires when an individual develops a positive feeling with his correction, he is able to cope with his most visual needs unconsciously and comfortably for a sustained period of time. This is discussed in detail in Chapter 21.

Chapter 13: Prescribing and Counseling

COUNSELING

In the contemporary landscape, the pervasive influence of Darwin's theory of survival of the fittest necessitates a re-evaluation of clinicians' roles. The practice philosophy is changing from the old paradigm of diagnosing and prescribing to taking care of the patient as a whole and keeping them well. Clinicians are now expected to go beyond clinical procedures, incorporating psychotherapeutic techniques into their practice.

Psychotherapy, viewed as the art of utilizing words and establishing a strong therapeutic relationship with patients, is now an integral part of the overall medical procedure. Its purpose is to shape patients' perceptions of reality and assist them in embracing themselves as they are. Recognizing the psychosocial dimensions of a patient's situation holds profound implications for their well-being. This paradigm shift requires clinicians to perceive the patient as a whole, considering the context of the visit.

When integrated into the practice protocol, this approach yields extraordinary results, leading to positive consequences. The clinician's ability to acknowledge the psychosocial aspects of a patient's condition allows for a more meaningful connection and a more effective therapeutic process. This, in turn, empowers patients to handle various aspects of their lives in a more constructive manner.

Figure 13.3 outlines the three fundamental pillars of patient counseling in optometry practice, elucidating the core principles that clinicians should refine and master to achieve optimal results.

This is where the counseling gets into the vision care practice. Patient counseling is the process of providing information, guidance, and support to patients regarding their eye health, visual conditions, refractive correction, options available for solutions and other related associated factors. The main goal of patient counseling is to empower patients to make informed decisions about their vision care, improve their understanding of their ocular and visual conditions, and help them manage their vision effectively. Counseling aims at helping the patient understand and accept themselves "as they are" so that they can help themselves.

Counseling is an important part of the eye care process and it should be done after the measurement of refractive error together with discussion for prescribing correction. It covers a discussion on a range of topics, which includes:

Chapter 13: Prescribing and Counseling

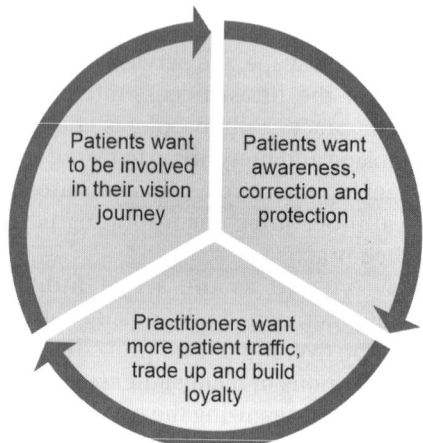

Fig. 13.3: Fundamentals of patient and practitioner interaction.

- Explain prescription
- Address the patient's concern
- Explain different options for vision correction
- Cost involvement
- Professional recommendation
- Educate patient on adaptation factor

Explain Prescription

When explaining the prescription for refractive correction, effective communication is paramount to ensure the patient gains a comprehensive understanding of their refractive error. Initiate the explanation by breaking down the patient's refractive error into simple terms, clarifying concepts such as nearsightedness, farsightedness, or astigmatism, and elucidate how each condition impacts their vision. Proceed to delve into the prescription details, providing a clear explanation of the terms involved. Outline the significance of the sphere, cylinder, and axis values in the prescription. Help the patient understand how these elements contribute to addressing their specific visual needs. Emphasize the importance of measuring the interpupillary distance, as this measurement ensures the lenses are precisely aligned with the patient's eyes, optimizing visual clarity. If prism correction is included in the prescription, articulate its purpose and how it assists in addressing particular visual challenges. Ensure the patient comprehends the necessity and function of each component in their prescription. Additionally, take the time to communicate any specific instructions integral to the treatment plan. This may include details about when and how to wear corrective lenses, any adjustments to be made over time, and potential lifestyle considerations that can enhance the effectiveness of the prescription.

Address the Patient's Concern

Encouraging patients to voice their questions and concerns about their prescription is a crucial component of delivering quality care and fostering patient satisfaction. To address these concerns effectively, begin by actively listening to the patient without interruption or judgment. Demonstrate empathy to create a supportive environment that encourages the patient to freely share their thoughts.

When a patient expresses a concern, rephrase it in your own words to ensure a clear understanding and validate their perspective. This simple step helps acknowledge the patient's feelings and concerns. Subsequently, provide the patient with accurate and relevant information tailored to address their specific worries.

Several common concerns may arise during clinic visits, including:
- "Is my prescription too strong?"
- "Do I need glasses for such a small correction?"
- "Why is my lens power increasing so rapidly?"
- "Will I go blind eventually?"
- "Why can't I read the smallest letters in the test chart?"
- "How frequently should I get my eyes examined?"
- "What is better for me—spectacles or contact lenses?"
- "Can I use sunglasses?"
- "Do I need to take any medicines?"
- "What is the axis, and why do I need it?"

As a clinician, it is your professional duty to reassure patients and address their concerns, ensuring they feel at ease in seeking vision care from you. This process of effective communication not only improves clinical outcomes but also enhances patient value and builds long-term loyalty. By taking the time to understand and respond to each patient's unique worries, you contribute to a positive and collaborative patient-practitioner relationship.

Explain Different Options for Vision Correction

There are several options available for vision correction, including eyeglasses, contact lenses, and refractive surgery. Each option comes with its distinct advantages and limitations, making the optimal choice contingent upon the specific needs and preferences of the patient. Therefore, it is imperative for the practitioner to comprehensively explain the risks and benefits associated with each option, ensuring the patient is well-informed in making a decision aligned with their lifestyle and visual requirements.

While recommending the most suitable option, the practitioner should also provide insights into the diverse types of contact lenses and ophthalmic lenses available. A thorough discussion should cover the features, advantages, and benefits of each type, empowering the patient with knowledge about the latest advancements in vision correction. This is crucial because the continuous evolution of products introduces new options that patients may not be familiar with.

In detailing contact lenses, the practitioner may delve into various types such as daily disposables, extended wear, and toric lenses for astigmatism. Highlighting the unique attributes of each type helps the patient understand the potential benefits and considerations associated with their use.

Similarly, in discussing eyeglasses, the practitioner can explore different lens materials, coatings, and designs. This includes progressive lenses, anti-reflective coatings, and high-index materials, among others. Offering a clear overview of these options enables the patient to make an informed choice based on their lifestyle, visual preferences, and budget constraints.

By providing a comprehensive understanding of the array of vision correction options and their associated features, advantages, and benefits, the practitioner ensures that patients are equipped to make choices that align with their individual needs and preferences. This proactive approach not only facilitates informed decision-making but also underscores the practitioner's commitment to delivering personalized and up-to-date vision care.

Cost Involvement

When it comes to counseling patients about the cost involved in vision correction, it is essential to provide them with transparent and accurate information about the different options and their associated costs. He should also inform about the options for financing and insurance facilities, if any.

Chapter 13: Prescribing and Counseling

Professional Recommendation

Patients indeed rely on their practitioners for professional recommendations in the realm of vision care. As the expert in the field, patients seek guidance, consultation, and product recommendations from practitioners who base their suggestions on knowledge, experience, and expertise.

The practitioner's role involves a thorough consideration of the patient's medical history and relevant factors to recommend the most suitable solution for their visual needs. This recommendation should be made with the patient's best interest at heart, ensuring that it aligns with their lifestyle, preferences, and overall well-being.

While patients retain the autonomy to make decisions about their health, professional recommendations serve as invaluable tools, particularly in unforeseen incidents or complex situations. These recommendations are grounded in the practitioner's understanding of the patient's unique circumstances and are designed to optimize visual outcomes.

It is crucial for practitioners to effectively communicate these recommendations, explaining the rationale behind the suggested solution and addressing any concerns the patient may have. This dialogue fosters trust and confidence in the practitioner's expertise, encouraging patients to make informed decisions about their vision care.

Educate Patient on Adaptation Factor

In addition to providing recommendations and prescribing corrective measures, it is essential for practitioners to educate all patients about the potential adaptation process to their new correction. While not every patient may experience adaptation issues, offering a clear explanation helps prepare individuals for possible adjustments and fosters a more informed and comfortable experience.

By discussing the adaptation period, practitioners can address common concerns that patients may have, such as changes in visual perception or comfort. This proactive communication ensures that patients are aware of the potential for an adaptation phase and are better equipped to navigate it if it occurs.

Furthermore, practitioners should take the opportunity to educate patients about their prognosis. This includes discussing the likelihood of changes in their corrective prescription over time and the anticipated pace of such changes. Providing this information helps manage patient expectations and allows them to make more informed decisions about their eye care.

Additionally, practitioners can educate patients on proactive measures to potentially slow down or prevent the progression of certain eye conditions. This may include lifestyle adjustments, protective measures, or specific interventions that align with the patient's eye health needs. In summary, patient education regarding potential adaptation to new correction and understanding the prognosis is an integral part of comprehensive eye care.

Follow-up Schedule

The examiner must advise to follow up with him at regular intervals to monitor any changes in their vision and ensure that their eyeglass or contact lens prescription is up-to-date. The recommended follow-up schedule will depend on several factors, including the patient's age, the severity of their vision problems, and any underlying medical conditions. The common guidelines are:

Children should have their vision checked regularly, starting at around 6 months of age, and then again at 3 years of age and before they start school. After that, they should have their eyes checked every 1–2 years, or more frequently if needed.

Adults under 40 with no vision problems should have their eyes checked every 2–3 years. If they wear contact lenses or have a family history of eye disease, they may need more frequent eye exams.

Adults over 40 should have their eyes checked every 1–2 years to check for age-related vision problems, such as presbyopia, cataracts, and age-related macular degeneration.

MULTIPLE CHOICE QUESTIONS

1. **Overcorrection of refraction error is often prescribed in which of the following cases?**
   a. Intermittent exotropia or exophoria
   b. Defocused image
   c. Dry eyes
   d. Diabetes

2. **Which of the following factors contribute to non-adaptation to new refractive error?**
   a. Magnitude of refractive error
   b. Patient's age

Chapter 13: Prescribing and Counseling

   c. Patient's existing ocular condition
   d. All of the above
3. **Which of the following is not the symptom of light sensitivity?**
   a. Reduced blinking
   b. Poor concentration
   c. Narrowing of the palpebral aperture
   d. Epiphora
4. **Which of the following statements regarding overcorrection is not true?**
   a. Overcorrection pushes the focal point behind the retina.
   b. Overcorrection induces accommodation.
   c. Overcorrection creates stimulation for the posterior segment of the eye to elongate.
   d. Overcorrection completely rules out as an useful strategy to prescribe in the practice of clinical examination of eye for vision defect.
5. **Which of the following statements is not correct for astigmatic correction in infants and toddlers?**
   a. Astigmatism associated with spherical errors should always be corrected.
   b. Oblique astigmatism should always be corrected as it is amblyogenic.
   c. Younger children can accept high cylinder power far more easily than adults.
   d. Astigmatism more than 1.50 D should not be corrected.
6. **Which of the following is not the true objective of patient counseling during eye examination?**
   a. Help patients understand their ocular and visual condition.
   b. Empower patients to make informed decision about their vision care.
   c. Educate patients about the latest advancement in eye examination technologies.
   d. Prepare patients to accept themselves "as they are".
7. **Which of the following statements is not true while considering the habitual correction as benchmark to decide prescription for new refractive correction?**
   a. The clinician may avoid altering the prescription for refractive correction if the patient does not have any symptoms.
   b. The clinician may use the data pertaining to habitual correction to set the upper limit to make changes in spherical, cylinder and axis.

Chapter 13: Prescribing and Counseling

    c. The clinician may use the data pertaining to habitual correction to explain the new prescription of refractive correction to counsel the patient for adaptation.
    d. The clinician may use the data of habitual correction to ensure that the patient gets full satisfaction with his new correction.

ANSWER KEY

| 1. a | 2. d | 3. a | 4. d | 5. d | 6. c | 7. d |

SELF-PRACTICE QUESTIONS

1. Under what conditions does an optometrist thinks of prescribing overcorrection of refractive error? Explain.
2. What is measured as refractive error is not always prescribed as refractive correction? Explain with examples.
3. Why do some patients find it difficult to adapt to new refractive correction, while many can adapt quickly? Explain.
4. How can you try and avoid factors that may lead to non-adaptation with new refractive correction?
5. What causes dissatisfaction to a new refractive correction for a patient?
6. How would you explain your patient about the change in refractive correction?
7. 'The wholesale correction of refractive error is a more negative evil'. Explain.

14 CHAPTER

Refraction in Myopia

CHAPTER OUTLINE

- Classification of Myopia
- Treatment of Myopia

Myopia, a common refractive error, occurs when parallel rays of light focus in front of the retina when the eye is at rest. Traditionally, the primary concern associated with myopia has been blurred distant vision, a symptom often effectively addressed with appropriate minus power lenses. However, there has been a recent shift in perspective on myopia due to its potential long-term complications.

Beyond affecting the clarity of vision, myopia is now recognized for its broader impact. It can limit occupational choices and, more significantly, contribute to an increased risk of vision-threatening conditions. Blurred distance vision remains a major symptom, and while it can be improved with corrective lenses, the myopic eye poses significant challenges. The high prevalence of myopia underscores its importance as a public health concern.

Practitioners are increasingly recognizing the need for myopia control strategies. Addressing myopia goes beyond providing clear vision; it involves managing the potential risks associated with this refractive error. Myopia has been linked to conditions such as retinal breaks, detachment, and glaucoma, posing a threat to long-term visual health.

This paradigm shift in the understanding of myopia emphasizes the importance of proactive measures to control its progression and reduce associated risks, ultimately safeguarding the long-term visual health of individuals with myopia.

CLASSIFICATION OF MYOPIA

Myopia can be classified based on various factors. Based on degree of myopia it may be classified as shown in **Table 14.1**.

The classification of myopia into different degrees based on its magnitude helps in risk assessment, clinical management, patient education and research and epidemiology. It facilitates the collection of data for studies on the prevalence and progression of myopia in different populations. It also aids in understanding the impact of myopia on public health and in developing strategies for myopia control and prevention.

Myopia may further be classified into two categories:

Simple Myopia and Pathological Myopia

Simple myopia is characterized by variations within the normal limits of the optical system which may be an increase in curvature of the cornea and the lens surface, a shallow anterior chamber, a high refractive effectivity of the lens or a great axial length of the globe. Simple myopia may be congenital or it may first appear between the age of 5 years and puberty and then progress during the growing age until adolescence is passed when the eyes stabilize. All the time, however, whether or not progression occurs, in the majority of myopic cases, the eyes remain healthy and visual acuity can be corrected to expected standards with appropriate correction.

Pathological myopia is degenerative myopia which is accompanied by degenerative changes occurring particularly in the posterior segment of the eye. It is usually associated with lengthening of the anteroposterior axis of the eyeball and is by and large progressive in nature. Degenerative myopia occurs most commonly as an isolated developmental condition. It may also appear in association with other ocular disease or with general disease or it may also be present as a congenital anomaly.

There are two more classifications of myopia. They are:

Table 14.1: Different degrees of myopia.	
Magnitude of myopia	Grades of myopia
0.25 D to 3.00 D	Low myopia
3.00 D to 6.00 D	Moderate myopia
6.00 D to 10.00 D	High myopia
Above 10.00 D	Very high myopia

Night Myopia and Pseudomyopia

Night myopia is the result of increased spherical aberration in low illumination. Night myopia induces reduction in contrast. Patient's focus drifts toward a resting level of accommodation which is not zero, thus inducing some degree of myopia. Night myopia may be symptomatic, and patients may report blurred vision or halos around lights at night. Symptomatic night myopia requires correction, such as wearing nighttime driving glasses.

Younger patients who are engaged more in near vision task sometimes report pseudomyopia which results in blurring of distance vision brought about by spasm of the ciliary muscles. Patient appears to have myopia due to an inappropriate accommodative response. The diagnosis is done by cycloplegic refraction using a strong cycloplegic like atropine or homatropine eye drops. Delayed subjective refraction may also be applied to determine pseudomyopia. Progressive myopia requires relatively frequent alterations in the prescription. Refractive development can be ascertained through a history, previous patient record and referral information. They need more frequent consultations to monitor refractive changes.

Myopia can be the result from the secondary causes because of several reasons, some of the common among them are:
- Contact lens-induced corneal edema
- Trauma-induced corneal edema
- Changes because of cataract
- Blood sugar imbalance
- Drug induced
- Convergence-induced secondary myopia

In any of the above cases the onset of blur may be either sudden or insidious. The distance blur is affected in more than one ways as it may fluctuate with the time of the day, it may be temporary, or binocular vision may be affected more than the monocular vision. Care must be taken in altering the lens prescription. If spectacles are to be prescribed, they need to be considered only as an emergency and temporary measure.

▋ TREATMENT OF MYOPIA

The treatment of simple myopia primarily involves prescribing corrective lenses to achieve clear vision. The goal is to eliminate the symptoms associated with blurred distance vision. Achieving a clear retinal image of distant objects requires correcting the full extent of myopia. However, there are considerations before prescribing the correction.

Full correction may not be acceptable to an adolescent who has never worn glasses before. This is because of his habit of not using accommodation for near vision. So a little undercorrection is advisable which can be comfortably used.

In higher degree of myopia, the full correction is rarely tolerated largely because the image formed by strong concave lenses is diminished, very bright and clear. The patient accustomed to hazy diffusion of circles, is intolerant of them. Therefore, the correction is prescribed with highest possible acuity obtained without distress.

Low myopia is always fully prescribed. In low myopia a little change in correction is expected after the age of adolescence and therefore the patients may be confidently advised to return for checkup only when they notice deterioration in vision with corrected lenses. They may also be reassured that the change is unlikely before the age of 40 years.

Awareness of the patient's habitual prescription is of paramount importance in judging changes in myopic correction. Generally, once a patient is adapted to higher minus correction, it is difficult for them to readjust to a reduction in minus correction. This is due to perceived increase in contrast of the target produced by the concentration of the image. The patient subjectively interprets this apparent increase in intensity as an increase in clarity of vision.

Fogging method of subjective refraction is not very critical in case of high myopia as the insufficient spherical minus lens in front of uncorrected eye, is enough to blur the distant vision and does not allow the patient to bring the focus onto the retina by accommodation. However, in very low myopia, fogging method of subjective refraction can prove useful to prevent overcorrection. The duochrome test is very useful for myopic patients. It is advisable to correct the defect only up to the point where the objects on red background are slightly clearer than green objects.

Room length is very critical for appropriate correction in myopia. A room length shorter than 20 feet will be shorter than optical infinity which implies both vergence and accommodation are in play, resulting in undercorrection and fluctuating results.

Room light can have an impact on myopic refraction measurements, particularly during eye examinations. A dimly lit room will

Chapter 14: Refraction in Myopia

result in increase in spherical aberration, which can result in a false myopic refraction measurement. On the other hand, a brightly lit room may cause hyperopic shift, which can result in undercorrection in myopia.

Although myopia would appear to be the least troublesome of all refractive problems, the maximizing of visual potential with comfort and safety needs refracting skills, experience, and clinical judgment.

MULTIPLE CHOICE QUESTIONS

1. **What is myopia?**
   a. Myopia is a vision defect in which rays of light coming from infinity focus before retina.
   b. Myopia is a vision defect in which rays of light coming from infinity focus behind the retina.
   c. Myopia is a condition in which rays of light coming from infinity focus on the retina.
   d. None of the above

2. **A myope wearing -10.00 Dsph spectacle correction in his both eyes, says that he sees better if he pushes his glasses closer to his eyes. How is he changing his effective lens power?**
   a. He is making his correction stronger.
   b. He is making his correction weaker.
   c. He is creating telescopic effect with his glasses.
   d. He is adding base in effect.

3. **Which of the following variations in the optical components of eye is not considered to be responsible for myopia shift?**
   a. An increased curvature of corneal
   b. A shallow anterior chamber
   c. A greater axial length of the globe
   d. Low refractive index of the lens

4. **Accommodation can worsen far vision in:**
   a. Emmetropia
   b. Myopia
   c. Hyperopia
   d. Astigmatism

ANSWER KEY

| 1. a | 2. a | 3. d | 4. b |

Chapter 14: Refraction in Myopia

SELF-PRACTICE QUESTIONS

1. A 25-year-old myopic patient who is able to see reasonably well at distance without correction is in the clinic where the clinician is examining his eyes for refractive correction. The clinician feels that minus spherical lens is absorbing more during subjective refraction. Why is this happening, and what can be done to determine if it is needed?
2. A 70-year-old patient is found to have a -1.00 diopter change in refractive error in each eye from his prescription of one year ago. What are the possible etiologies of this myopic shift? What are the considerations before giving the patient a prescription for a new pair of glasses incorporating this myopic shift?

15 CHAPTER

Refraction in Hypermetropia

CHAPTER OUTLINE

- Correction of Hypermetropia
- Subjective Refraction in Hypermetropia

The optical condition of a hypermetropic eye necessitates an increase in converging power for a clear image, achievable either through the eye's natural mechanisms or artificial means, typically the use of convex lenses. The eye itself increases the converging power by the influence of accommodation. The artificial means of increasing converging power of the eye points to the use of convex lenses.

The accommodation is age dependent. So long as the accommodation is active, a certain amount of hypermetropia is corrected by the normal physiological tone of the ciliary muscles which is latent hypermetropia. The remaining portion that remains uncorrected in normal circumstances is termed as the manifest hypermetropia. Manifest hypermetropia is made up of facultative hypermetropia and absolute hypermetropia. Facultative hypermetropia is overcome by an effort of accommodation and absolute hypermetropia is not corrected by accommodation.

It would be good to understand the two terms—the tone of the ciliary muscles and the effort of accommodation. Though they are related but they are different concepts. The tone of the ciliary muscle refers to the level of contraction or relaxation of the muscle at rest, i.e., without any active effort of accommodation. In other words, it is the baseline level of tension in the muscle when the eye is not actively focusing on a particular object. On the other hand, the effort of accommodation refers to the active contraction of the ciliary muscles that occurs when the eye is actively trying to focus on a near object. The effort of accommodation is the amount of work required by the ciliary muscles to achieve this change in lens shape.

CORRECTION OF HYPERMETROPIA

The correction of hypermetropia is being decided in light of patient's ability to compensate for close work and other symptoms. Therefore, each case should be dealt with on its own merit and should be dealt with in terms of the factors as given by **Flowchart 15.1**.

Age

Age is an important criterion for prescribing correction in case of hypermetropia. Newborn babies are born with some degree of hypermetropia which is usually to the tune of 2.00 D to 3.00 D. Hypermetropia initially increases to reach at peak by 6 months and then reduces through the process of emmetropization by the age of 12 months. At around the age of 6 years the visual system centers around emmetropia with a deviation of ±1.00 D. So manifest hypermetropia up to the age of 6 years may not be corrected unless the patient shows the signs of poor binocularity, suppression, strabismus or poor school performance.

Between the age of 6 and 18 years, small amount of error may require correction especially when they are causing visual stress or when they report ocular fatigue. If the suspicion of strain is suggested by more definite signs like headache, dislike of work, early tiring, rubbing of the eyes, itching, twitching of the lids or combination of them, an examination should be made. Plus lens can be prescribed conservatively. Plus power, if prescribed, should be cut to aid adaptation. It should be remembered that in children above the age

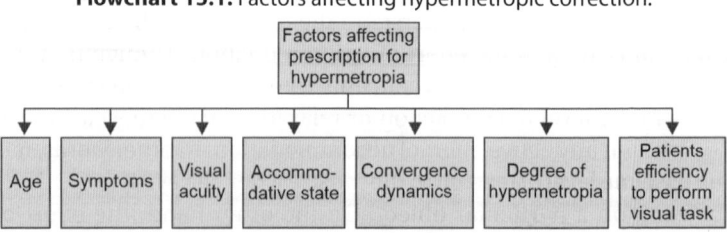

Flowchart 15.1: Factors affecting hypermetropic correction.

of 6 years, hypermetropia tends to decrease with growth. Therefore, they should be examined every year and their correction should be trimmed down, if necessary. The younger the patient and greater the latent hypermetropia, the greater is the legitimate undercorrection.

In adults between the age of 18 and 40 years, refractive state of eye is fairly stable. In such cases, hypermetropia is corrected to improve near vision. The need for re-examination depends upon several factors. If full correction is worn and the patient is not of presbyopic age, re-examination is hardly needed except when symptoms arise. After the age of 40, the increase in hyperopia may indicate added plus for distance acuity as well as for near acuity and for visual comfort. Even if the distance correction needs to be cut to assist adaptation, the full magnitude of hyperopia needs to be included for near correction. In later life around the age of 60 years when the accommodation has gone and all the hyperopia has become absolute, distance correction is always necessary. **Table 15.1** summarizes the age-related criteria for hypermetropia correction.

Symptoms

The fundamental principle of clinical refraction is to prescribe the refractive correction to treat symptoms. In a subject that is asymptomatic with no accommodative and convergence adverse relationship, small amount of hypermetropic refractive error may not be prescribed to him. However, if the subject is symptomatic, even with small amount of hypermetropic, correction needs to be prescribed.

Table 15.1: Age-related correction criteria for hypermetropia.	
Age range	Prescribing correction criteria
Birth to 3 years	Avoid correcting manifest hypermetropia
3–6 years	Avoid correcting manifest hypermetropia unless the patient shows the signs of poor binocularity, suppression, strabismus or poor school performance
6–18 years	Small amount of hypermetropia is corrected only in case of symptoms
18–40 years	Hypermetropia is corrected to improve near vision
40–60 years	Hypermetropia is corrected to improve visual acuity and visual comfort
Above 60 years	Prescribe full correction

In the lower degree of hypermetropia, particularly in young people in whom accommodation is active, symptoms of hypermetropia are usually entirely absent. The subject neither reports visual symptoms, nor any ocular or referred symptoms. In higher degree the symptoms are marked and the subject may report all types of visual, ocular and referred symptoms.

When the error is large the accommodative power falls short to attain clear vision for distance vision. Most patients with hyperopia in their youth are usually able to compensate for poor near vision through the accommodative ability. However, when their accommodative ability is substantially reduced, the correction for near vision is inevitable. In case of old population poor distance vision is the major complaint as entire hypermetropia turns into absolute. Therefore, correction should be prescribed to improve visual acuity.

If hyperopia remains untreated especially in case of children it can lead to strabismus and/or amblyopia. It is, therefore, important that the examiner should also look at the clinical signs together with symptoms before taking a decision on prescribing correction in hypermetropia. **Table 15.2** shows the several symptoms and clinical signs that are critical for clinical decisions.

The following guideline is helpful in making clinical decision:

- ❖ Optimal correction of hypermetropia is prescribed, with consideration for possible near addition to enhance the patient's binocularity, particularly in cases of esophoria or esotropia.
- ❖ Plus correction needs to be minimized in case of exophoria or exotropia so that the accommodative-convergence induced by over-accommodation can cause a secondary turning in of the eyes and lessen the amount of manifest exophoria.

Table 15.2: Signs and symptoms.

Symptoms	Signs
Blur vision	Rubbing of eyes
Headache	Forehead wrinkling
Eye strain	Squinting of eyes
Eye fatigue	Reduced accommodative ability
Asthenopia	Increased near point of convergence
Ocular pain	Muscle imbalance
Vertigo	Reduced stereopsis

❖ In cases of excessive convergence, every endeavor should be made to influence the patient to wear the spectacle even at the cost of some discomfort. When there is a tendency for latent convergent squint, the whole of the error requires correction and the correction should be constantly worn. This is to relieve convergence indirectly by relieving accommodation.

❖ In cases of latent divergent squint, deliberately under-correcting the hypermetropic error is employed to stimulate accommodation, ultimately encouraging convergence.

Visual Acuity

Unlike myope, most hyperope usually does not complain of blur vision at distance. However, some of them may complain of difficulties in seeing at close distance in which case the required correction should be prescribed. Distance blur is ordinarily not indicated until age reduces the accommodation amplitude too greatly even for distance acuity demands. Temporary failure of ciliary muscles may result in obscuration of vision in which case plus correction may be prescribed. The uncorrected visual acuity in hypermetropia varies with the degree of optical error and the proportion which cannot be overcome by accommodation. Visual symptoms in the higher degree of the error are marked, for nothing is seen clearly, but in low degree, when the accommodation is active and is able to overcome the error, as usually seen in youth, they may be entirely absent. Facultative hypermetropia does not by itself involve any decrease in visual acuity, but absolute hypermetropia affects distant vision much in the same proportion as myopia as given in **Table 15.3**.

The corrected visual acuity frequently does not come up to the standard, particularly in the higher degree of error. The visual

Table 15.3: Expected reduction in visual acuity in different degrees of hypermetropia.		
Degree of hypermetropia	*V/a based on feet*	*V/a based on meter*
+0.50 D	20/25	6/7.5
+0.75 D	20/40	6/12
+1.00 D	20/80	6/24
+2.00 D	20/160	6/48
+3.00 D	20/250	6/75
+4.00 D	20/400	6/120

deficiency may be due to lack of retinal development to some degree particularly in the case of high errors. Perceptual factors probably play a considerable part in its etiology. When the subnormal vision is bilateral, as is the case when the refractive error was not corrected in early childhood, the acuity improves to some extent after wearing correcting spectacle for some months. However, when there is inequality of vision in two eyes, unilateral amblyopia is common even in the absence of squint. The same difficulties favor the development of a convergent accommodative squint.

Accommodative State

The influence of accommodation in hypermetropia is of considerably significant. So long as accommodation is active, a certain amount of the optical error is corrected by the normal physiological tone of the ciliary muscle. It thus appears that a high hypermetrope or a low hypermetrope with no accommodation power, can see nothing distinctly unless the accommodation is active and the error lies within his facultative limits. On the other hand, the constant accommodative effort which is made automatically in instinctive attempt to obtain distinct vision frequently leads to fatigue and distress, to disorientation between accommodation and convergence and to other troubles. All these symptoms are of course; considerably more marked when close work is undertaken.

Because of the added accommodation required by the uncorrected hyperope, the complaint that the patient is most likely to present is blur vision at near point and/or asthenopia. If presented by a pre-presbyopic hyperope, such blur is manifested mainly during reading or prolonged closeup work. The relative magnitude of near-point difficulty is probably directly proportional to the patient's amplitude of accommodation.

Often subjects who have extensive near vision task complaint that they find their distance vision is blurred for an initial short duration before it becomes clear. This happens because of accommodative spasm. When there is a spasm of accommodation the whole of the error requires correction and the correction should be constantly worn. Every effort has to be made to induce the patient to wear the spectacle even at the cost of some discomfort.

Convergence Dynamics

While the accommodation provides retina with a clear and sharp retinal image, vergence functions are critical for fixation and stabilizing the retinal image. The efficient performance of a task depends a lot on the efficient functioning of these two elements of vision. If an individual is incapable of performing his visual tasks efficiently, it is quite likely that his visual system is compromised in some respect in one of these two functions directly or indirectly. If there are any disturbances in vergence function, the individual develops discomfort or becomes fatigued quickly, reducing his visual performance. Symptoms commonly associated with accommodative and vergence disfunctions are blurred vision, headache, ocular discomfort, ocular or bodily fatigue, diplopia, motion sickness and loss of concentration during a task performance. These symptoms can effectively be treated with proper lens correction and vision therapy.

Adequate correction is needed in case of excessive convergence as in accommodative spasm and the patient is influenced to wear correction even at the cost of some discomfort. Conversely, in the presence of a latent divergent squint, undercorrection works that may stimulate convergence by stimulating accommodation.

Degree of Hypermetropia

If a subject is using full correction and he has not yet reached the presbyopic age, change of correction is hardly necessary except when fresh symptoms arise. However, there may be situations when the patient may be able to adapt to full correction of hypermetropia. This may be because the ciliary muscles have been accustomed to maintain a considerable amount of accommodative tone, which can be renounced only with difficulty, thus rendering them effectively myopia. The patient may complain of indistinct distance vision with some strange symptoms to which he may not be able to adapt. It is, therefore, advisable to undercorrect the total hypermetropia. On the other hand, the headaches and symptoms of asthenopia may persist if a part of the hypermetropia remains uncorrected. We are thus, faced with a dilemma the solution of which frequently calls for clinical judgment. Therefore, the most practical method is to consider each case on its merits, to determine the manifest hypermetropia. Correcting the patient as nearly to his total hypermetropia as possible while remaining within the limits consistent with comfort and good vision, at the same time paying regard to his age, to the state of his accommodation, his symptoms, his muscle balance, his general physical and nervous state, and his vocation. The younger the patient, the greater is the latent hypermetropia and greater the legitimate undercorrection.

Patient's Efficiency to Perform Visual Task

Finally, the capacity of the ocular muscles to perform work serves as an index of the general constitutional state and the onset of fatigue here should be considered suggesting its imminence elsewhere. Eye strain is a symptom of general strain. The treatment should not be confined to the optical correction alone, but should include an inquiry into the general physical and nervous state and if necessary, should involve a reorganization of the habits and activities of the individual so that he lives within the limits of his capabilities.

■ SUBJECTIVE REFRACTION IN HYPERMETROPIA

Fluctuating accommodation can confuse the retinal focus presented by each change of lens combination before the eyes; accommodation must be maintained at the relaxed state. Therefore, fogging method of subjective procedure is preferred for determining the refractive error, especially for the older children or younger adult patients.

A common case for hypermetropic patient who reduces his accommodation during retinoscopy but on subjective testing will accept only a much reduced convex sphere. In this circumstance it may be advantageous to keep the fellow eye fogged by a high plus lens, rather than being screened out by an opaque disc during subjective testing in any event, hypermetropia will often accept somewhat higher spherical correction binocularly.

In a high hypermetropia and originally healthy eyes, may fail to attain 6/6 vision, a situation particularly common when the use of spectacle has been unduly delayed.

Some avid computer users most often complain that their distance vision does not clear immediately. It takes a little more time. This may be because of accommodative spasm, i.e., their accommodation locks at near and takes little more time to relax. Delayed subjective method of refraction may be more useful in such cases.

MULTIPLE CHOICE QUESTIONS

1. **What optical condition characterizes hypermetropia?**
    a. Increased axial length
    b. Excessive corneal curvature

Chapter 15: Refraction in Hypermetropia

c. Inadequate converging power
d. Retinal detachment

2. Which of the following is not true about hypermetropia?
   a. Manifest hypermetropia is the strongest plus lens which the patient can accept for clear distant vision.
   b. Latent hypermetropia is the residual hypermetropia masked by ciliary tone and involuntary accommodation.
   c. Latent hypermetropia can be unmasked by cycloplegic refraction.
   d. Facultative hypermetropia refers to hypermetropia that cannot be overcome by accommodation.

ANSWER KEY

| 1. c | 2. d | | | | | |

SELF-PRACTICE QUESTION

1. A 26-year-old patient, who was diagnosed with latent hyperopia and received a glasses prescription following cycloplegic refraction, is now reporting intolerance to the new glasses. How should this issue be addressed or managed?

CHAPTER 16

Refraction in Astigmatism

CHAPTER OUTLINE

- Symptoms
- Treatment
- Tests for Astigmatic Correction

Simple astigmatic error usually degrades and deforms the retinal image. They do not create defocus of retinal image. The image is distorted having an elongation in the meridian of greatest power together with rotating displacements of the image of all lines in space, not parallel with or perpendicular to the axis of the lens. Two types of distortions are produced:
1. Meridional aniseikonic error.
2. Declination error, objects may appear tilted or rotated due to unequal refraction in different meridians.

SYMPTOMS

Astigmatism is a common refractive error that can result in visual defects, but beyond the visual aspects, it can contribute to eyestrain. The constant effort to achieve clear vision, especially in hypermetropic (farsighted) and mixed astigmatism, places a significant strain on the eyes due to accommodative stress, particularly in cases of small astigmatic errors.

Notably, small astigmatic errors often do not manifest noticeable symptoms and may be considered physiological, requiring no specific treatment. However, when symptoms of eyestrain are present, they can be diverse.

Chapter 16: Refraction in Astigmatism

In instances of oblique astigmatism, individuals may unconsciously tilt their head to one side, a habit that, particularly in children, could potentially lead to the development of scoliosis. Additionally, there may be a tendency to partially close the eyelids, creating a stenopeic slit effect. This is done in an attempt to enhance clarity by blocking out rays from one meridian, making the viewed object appear more distinct.

Understanding these nuances in astigmatism and its associated symptoms is crucial for addressing eyestrain effectively and considering appropriate interventions when necessary.

TREATMENT

Smaller amounts of simple astigmatism often do not significantly impact visual acuity but may cause symptoms like eye strain. If no symptoms are present, correcting minor astigmatism may be unnecessary. However, if symptoms arise, correction becomes essential.

Correction for larger astigmatic errors is necessary due to the potential for multiple symptoms. Caution is crucial in such cases, as any disparity in correcting the two eyes can induce artificial heterophoria, especially when not looking through the optical centers of the lenses. Incorrect positioning of the spectacle frame can further disrupt binocular vision. Monocular vision may be tolerable in extreme cases.

Prescribing astigmatic correction for individuals with high errors who have not used correction before requires careful consideration. The patient may find the unaccustomed cylinder power intolerable. One strategy is to undercorrect the cylinder and add half of the uncorrected portion algebraically to the spherical correction.

Changing the cylinder axis should be avoided whenever possible, even if it leads to improved visual acuity. Such alterations may cause spatial disorientation and asthenopic symptoms. If a decision is made to change the axis, patients must be informed about potential symptoms during the initial adjustment period.

Regular re-examination is advisable for patients with significant astigmatism, especially in children. Pure astigmatism in adults tends to change minimally until later in life. Understanding these considerations is crucial in ensuring effective correction and addressing potential complications associated with astigmatism.

TESTS FOR ASTIGMATIC CORRECTION

A number tests types and charts can be used to test astigmatism, common among them are:

Clock Chart

Clock chart **(Fig. 16.1)** is used to determine the cylinder component using subjective technique of refraction.

Jackson Cross Cylinder Test

Jackson cross cylinder **(Fig. 16.2)** is one of the most popular tests used for determining astigmatic correction today. The technique does not require fogging of eye and can be used to determine both the amount of cylinder correction as well as axis of cylinder.

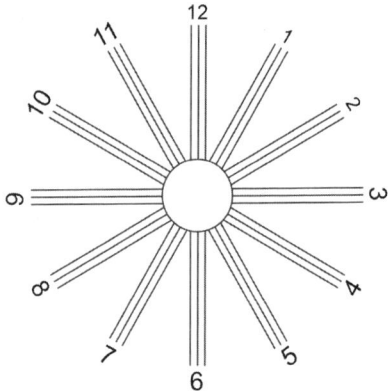

Fig. 16.1: Clock chart.

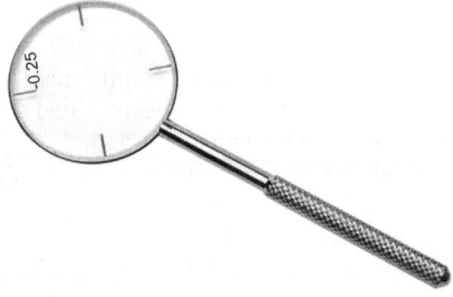

Fig. 16.2: Jackson cross cylinder.

Fan and Block Test

Fan and block test **(Fig. 16.3)** is used to determine the cylinder component using fogging method of subjective refraction.

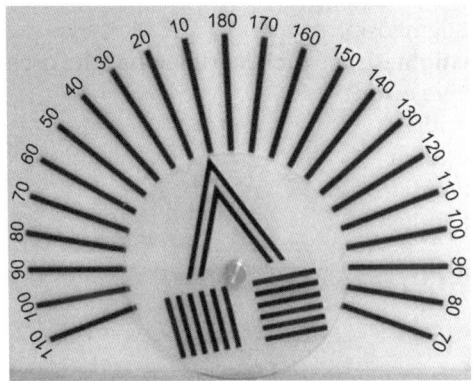

Fig. 16.3: Fan and block chart.

Stenopeic Slit

Stenopeic slit can be very effectively used to determine the power required to correct each principal meridian subjectively.

Astigmatic Letter Chart

Dr Pray's astigmatic letters' **(Fig. 16.4)** has been designed to measure the power and axis of astigmatism with the orientations of the stripes in degrees 180, 165, 150, 135, 120, 105, 90, 75, 60, 45, 30 and 15.

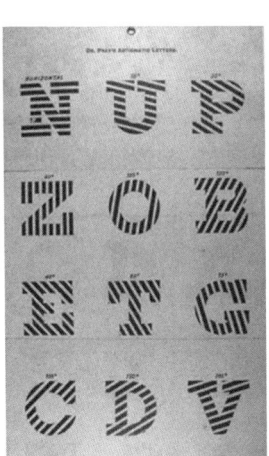

Fig. 16.4: Dr Pray's astigmatic letter.

MULTIPLE CHOICE QUESTIONS

1. In which type of astigmatism both focal lines are located in front of the retina in an unaccommodated eye?
   a. Simple hypermetropic eye
   b. Mixed astigmatism
   c. Compound hypermetropic eye
   d. Compound myopic eye

Chapter 16: Refraction in Astigmatism

2. Which type of astigmatism shows an increasing trend with increasing age?
   a. Oblique astigmatism
   b. Irregular astigmatism
   c. WTR astigmatism
   d. ATR astigmatism

3. In WTR astigmatism which meridian has the greatest amount of refractive error?
   a. 45° meridian
   b. 90° meridian
   c. 135° meridian
   d. 180° meridian

ANSWER KEY

1. d	2. d	3. b			

SELF-PRACTICE QUESTIONS

1. A 30-year-old patient having just begun wearing the new correction complains of difficulties. He says that with their new glasses, the top of his desk looks slanted, and when walking he has some nausea and the floor seems to be coming up at him. His previous prescription is BE -1.75 + 1.00 × 90 and new prescription is RE -2.00 + 1.25 × 75, LE -1.75 + 1.50 × 105. What is the most likely cause of these symptoms and what can be possible management?

2. In the fan and block test chart, under fog, how would you proceed to determine the amount of cylinder and the cylinder axis when the patient reports that the 3–9 O'clock spoke is more distinct than 12–6 O'clock spoke?

CHAPTER 17

Refraction in Presbyopia

CHAPTER OUTLINE

- Symptoms
- Correction of Presbyopia
- Test for Near Addition
- Premature Onset of Presbyopia

Presbyopia **(Fig. 17.1)** is a common age-related condition affecting individuals in their 40s and beyond, resulting in the loss of the ability to focus on close-up objects. This occurs due to the failure of accommodation, the eye's mechanism for adjusting focus to see near objects clearly at a normal reading distance.

The failure of accommodation in presbyopia can be attributed to two key factors as shown in **Flowchart 17.1**.

Physical Changes in the Crystalline Lens

The crystalline lens undergoes gradual changes, becoming harder and less elastic with age or in conditions such as cataracts. This

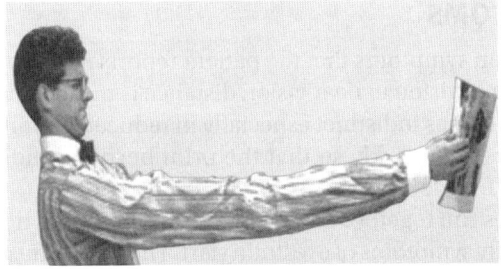

Fig. 17.1: Presbyopic patient.

Flowchart 17.1: Failure of accommodation in presbyopia.

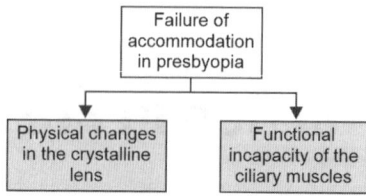

reduced elasticity prevents the lens from deforming adequately, making accommodation challenging. When the lens becomes too rigid, the contraction of the ciliary muscles is insufficient to induce the necessary changes in lens shape.

Functional Incapacity of the Ciliary Muscles

The ciliary muscles play a crucial role in accommodating the lens by altering its shape. However, muscular weakness or debility may arise at any age. This aspect of accommodation failure is termed physiological accommodation.

The distinction between physical and physiological accommodation is significant, highlighting the dual nature of the presbyopic challenge. Physical accommodation falters when the lens loses elasticity, while physiological accommodation diminishes due to the weakened capability of the ciliary muscles.

The changes in the crystalline lens occur gradually and persist throughout life without sudden alterations. Initially, individuals may not experience difficulty, but over time, the near point at which clear vision is possible moves farther away. When this distance extends beyond the typical reading distance, reading becomes challenging, marking the onset of presbyopia.

SYMPTOMS

The common symptoms that the patient reports in presbyopia are:
- Blurring of vision at near vision distance is most common. Small print becomes indistinct especially in reduced illumination.
- The eyes tire quickly so that the print becomes indistinct after reading for a few minutes.
- The lines run together and overlap and sometimes double.
- Gradually symptoms of eyestrain start. The ciliary muscle working near its limit tire and accommodative effort strained to its limit

and acting in excess of convergence, gives rise to distress—the eyes feel tire and ache, headache comes on.
- Some patient complains of glare while reading books.

The patient may complain in different ways. Some of the examples that are commonLY seen in practice are:
- I have to stretch my hands to read as shown in **Figure 17.1**.
- I have difficulties in threading a needle.
- Myopes report removing of their spectacles for near vision task.

A hyperope starts life with his near point considerably farther away, the decline in accommodative power is noted sooner. The opposite holds true in case of myopes. In case of low myopia, presbyopia will be delayed. Emmetrope in most situation, behaves in the same way as hyperopes behave. Thus, presbyopia is a relative term. It varies with individual and also with his habit. A person with a habit of reading complains of discomfort sooner than a person who does not have reading habit.

CORRECTION OF PRESBYOPIA

The primary goal of treating presbyopia is not necessarily to restore accommodation but to provide additional correction for near vision for individuals who have experienced a physiological decline in their ability to accommodate.

Presbyopia necessitates the use of different prescriptions for various distances. Typically, a presbyopic patient requires at least two prescriptions: one for distance vision and another for close-up tasks. An additional near addition is prescribed, and its strength is determined by factors such as age, preferred working distance, and the best-corrected distance visual acuity. The strength of the near "add" generally increases with age.

Preferred working distance varies among individuals, influenced by factors like height and arm length. Knowing the patient's habitual reading distance is crucial for prescribing the appropriate near addition. While the average is considered to be around 40 cm, individual variations exist. When inquiring about reading distance, it is essential to ask where the patient feels comfortable holding the near task.

Presbyopia correction can be achieved through either separate spectacles for distance and near vision or multifocal lenses. Another option is to use distance-correcting contact lenses along with reading spectacles containing the necessary near addition. Multifocal contact lenses have proven effective in correcting presbyopia. Surgical interventions are also available, including monovision correction, where the dominant eye is corrected for distance, and the nondominant eye is corrected for near vision. However, monovision may impact depth perception, and some individuals may find it uncomfortable, especially for activities like driving or extended periods of reading. Careful consideration and discussion with the patient are essential in determining the most suitable correction method for their specific needs.

TEST FOR NEAR ADDITION

In general, lowest plus spherical correction that gives clearest vision at habitual near distant is prescribed, the strength of which depends upon the age of an individual, preferred reading distance and the best corrected distance visual acuity. Once the distance refraction is completed, any of the methods as detailed below may be applied to determine near lens addition for an individual:

- ❖ Amplitude of accommodation
- ❖ Balanced range of accommodation
- ❖ Cross grid test
- ❖ Near duochrome test
- ❖ Trial and error method

Amplitude of Accommodation

The first step is to measure the amplitude of accommodation. You may use either push-up method or minus lens to blur method or any other method that you are comfortable with. It serves as a starting point for determining the near addition for the patient using following formula:

$$\text{Add power} = \frac{1}{\text{Working distance (meters)} - \frac{1}{2}(\text{amplitude of accommodation})}$$

The near addition is prescribed that allows him to use one-half to two-thirds of the total amplitude of accommodation.

Balanced Range of Accommodation

Negative relative accommodation (NRA) is the measure of maximum ability to relax accommodation while maintaining clear, single binocular vision at a specified distance. Positive relative accommodation (PRA) is the measure of the maximum ability to accommodate while maintaining clear, single binocular vision at a specified viewing distance. NRA is determined by adding plus power lens binocularly until the patient is no longer able to read the fine prints on the test card. The PRA is determined by adding minus power lenses until the patient is no longer able to read the fine prints. The difference between the NRA and the PRA is called the relative accommodative amplitude. Using these data the clinician may achieve the indicated addition as under:

Example:
- PRA –0.50 D
- NRA +2.00 D
- Range 2.50

Therefore, indicated required addition is +2.00 – (2.50 / 2) = +0.75 D.

Cross Grid Test

The cross grid test is usually used when the clinician uses phoropter for subjective refraction.
- Place the cross grid **(Fig. 17.2)** at a near point distance
- Reduce room illumination
- Put ±0.50D cross cylinder with minus axis vertically in front of both eyes with distance correction in place.
- Now ask the patient which set of lines are clear and sharper—horizontal or vertical
- Expected answer: Horizontal lines
- Add plus lens binocularly until vertical lines are clear and sharper
- Then reduce plus to achieve equal clarity and sharpness
- That's the end point

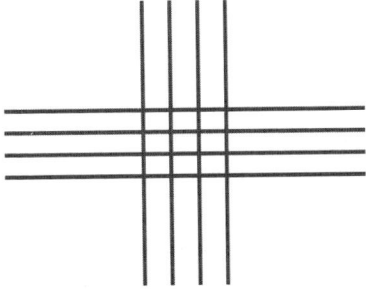

Fig. 17.2: Cross grid chart.

Near Duochrome Test

The near duochrome test can be done using phoropter and also with trial frame refraction using handheld duochrome test designed for the purpose. If done with trial frame follow the following procedure:
- Ask the patient to hold the near duochrome test in his hand with distance correction in place in the trial frame at a distance as decided.
- Duochrome with black rings or letters may be used. Keep both eyes open and ask the patient which black rings are clearer or darker. Three possible responses can be expected:
  1. Either black rings on green background is clearer and darker which indicates the need for plus lens.
  2. Or, black rings on the red background is clearer and darker which indicates the need for reduction of plus power.
  3. Rings on both sides—red and green background appear similar.

In a young patient with active accommodation the preference for red and green will be alternate indicating that there is no need for any near "add". Uncorrected or undercorrected presbyopes will have marked green preference. The most important thing to note is that this test applies only for a particular fixation distance used during the test. If the test distance is moved towards the eyes about 5 cm, the green preference will again be dominant and if the test distance is taken away by 3 cm from the fixation point, the red preference will become dominant.

Once the near addition is determined by any of the above methods, put the proposed near addition lens in the trial frame in front of the distance correction, ask the patient to hold the reading text chart and make sure that he has fairly good visual performance at a range of distance of his normal near working distance.

Subjective Refraction at Near

In general practice subjective refraction at near is mostly used to determine the near addition using following approach:
- Put the patient's distance refractive correction into a trial frame.
- Keep the room lights on and use a reading lamp.
- Determine by history the near visual tasks the patient would like to perform and the relevant working distances and ask the patient to hold the reading test chart at the habitual reading distance **(Fig. 17.3)**.

Chapter 17: Refraction in Presbyopia

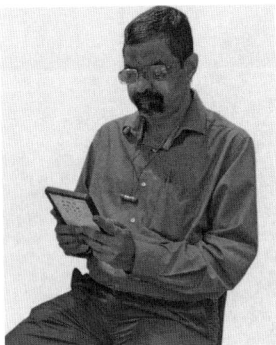

Fig. 17.3: Patient demonstrating his habitual reading distance.

- Explain the procedure: "I am now going to determine the power you need for your reading glasses."
- Ask the patient to hold the near vision test chart at the distance the patient would like to read/work.
- Determine a tentative addition. This is most easily obtained from the patient's age and working distance. **Table 17.1** shows tentative additions for different ages which can be used to select the first trial lens.
- Introduce the tentative addition to the trial frame and ask the patient to read the smallest print possible at their preferred distance.
- Measure the acuity in both eyes.
- Make necessary changes in the trial lens to improve the visual acuity. Add +0.25 Dsph and check the visual acuity. If visual acuity improves replace −0.25 Dsph by +0.50 Dsph. If the best visual acuity is achieved, do not change further. Instead of adding +0.25

Table 17.1: Shows tentative additions for different ages.	
Age	Near addition
40 years	0.75 D
42 years	1.00 D
44 years	1.50 D
46 years	1.75 D
48 years	2.00 D
50 years	2.25 D

Chapter 17: Refraction in Presbyopia

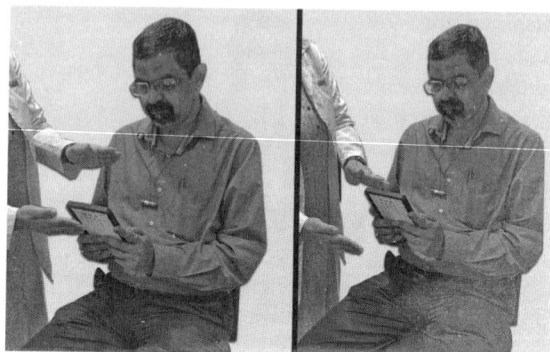

Fig. 17.4: Checking the range of clear vision.

Dsph, you may add –0.25 Dsph and then go back to +0.25 Dsph based upon the patient's response. However, before adding any lens you may alter the distance of reading test chart. If the visual acuity improves by taking the reading test chart a little farther away, you may add plus or vice versa.

* Stop adding lenses when best visual acuity at the habitual distance is achieved.
* Determine the range of clear vision **(Fig. 17. 4)** with the reading add, by asking the patient to bring the chart as close to them while still in focus and as far away while still in focus. This is very important to ensure sufficient depth of field.
* Record the final additions, the visual acuity and range of clearest vision obtained with the additions.

Always remember that near power should always be prescribed based upon patient's need. It is good to undercorrect than to overcorrect as too strong near addition tends to create difficulties that the patient may experience with accommodation, convergence and depth of field which will be inconveniently limited.

Many practitioners decide the prescription for near vision additions, leaving a percentage of amplitude of accommodation in reserve. The question is how much percentage of amplitude of accommodation is to be left in reserve? There is no norm. The most commonly adopted figure has been one-half or one-third of available amplitude. The rationale for this assumption seems logical because using all of the available accommodation is not sustainable without discomfort. In order to focus an object at a distance of 25 cm, an emmetrope needs to use 4.00 D of accommodation. For comfortable reading one-third of accommodation should be kept in reserve. If the person has 6.00 D of amplitude of accommodation, he can use 4.00 D of accommodation for his near vision task comfortably, keep the 2.00 D in reserve. However, if the patient is myope, the amount of accommodation required will be less and if he is hyperope, the amount of accommodation required will be greater than 4.00 D and a plus lens will be added.

PREMATURE ONSET OF PRESBYOPIA

Usually onset of presbyopia is expected to be around the age of 40 years. The premature onset of presbyopia should always excite suspicion factor that there are factors other than physiological involved. In the following cases premature onset of presbyopia is commonly observed:

- ❖ The failure of accommodation may be due to sclerosis of lens or development of cataract.
- ❖ Presbyopia is said to appear early after suppression of ovarian function.
- ❖ Glaucoma is said to the reason for early presbyopia.
- ❖ The general health is also frequently associated with ciliary weaknesses. It has been noted that conditions like anemia, diabetes, lactation, tuberculosis are all associated with early presbyopia.

The final prescription for presbyopic correction can be specified in two formats; either as the distance refraction plus the reading addition required for close work tasks, or as the final distance and reading prescription whereby the final near vision prescription is the sum total of the distance correction plus the near vision addition. The practitioner should select one format or the other and be consistent, so the prescription is not misinterpreted. Where an intermediate or occupational specific addition has been found, this should also be specified separately on the final prescription.

MULTIPLE CHOICE QUESTIONS

1. **Near addition should be prescribed....**
    a. Based upon patient's age
    b. Based upon monocular test of near addition
    c. Based upon subjective examination and patient's visual needs
    d. All of the above

2. **The onset of presbyopia does not depend on which of the following?**
   a. Near vision task
   b. Sex of the patients
   c. Refractive state of the patients
   d. Amplitude of accommodation
3. **Which of the following is not correct for the occurrence of presbyopia?**
   a. Loss of elasticity of the sclera
   b. Sclerosis the lens fibers
   c. Reduced elasticity of the lens capsule
   d. Reduced contraction of the ciliary muscle
4. **What is the expected value of amplitude of accommodation for a 40-year-old individual?**
   a. 1.00 D
   b. 3.00 D
   c. 5.00 D
   d. 8.00 D

ANSWER KEY

| 1. c | 2. b | 3. a | 4. c |

SELF-PRACTICE QUESTIONS

1. What is presbyopia? What causes presbyopia?
2. A patient complains that when he tries to read, he feels his arms are not long enough, how would you like to deal with him?
3. A 45-year-old emmetropic presbyope who uses only reading glasses says, "I can read clearly without my reading glasses when I am at sea beach, but I cannot read at my home". Write how would you like to handle?

18 CHAPTER

Refraction in Anisometropia

CHAPTER OUTLINE

- Symptoms
- Vision in Anisometropia
- Correction in Anisometropia

Anisometropia represents the condition in which a patient's refractive error significantly differs between the two eyes. To what degree the term significant implies is unclear, as the threshold of inequality resulting in adverse symptoms is unique to an individual. Most commonly, a refractive difference of 2.00 D is considered significant in defining the presence of anisometropia. Anisometropia causes aniseikonia which is unequal size of retinal image formed on two retinae. The development of anisometropia is often thought to have genetic component, the mechanisms are not clear. Factors associated with the development of binocular anomalies, such as amblyopia and strabismus have also been shown to be associated with anisometropia. Amblyopia resulting from hypermetropic anisometropia is mostly refractive amblyopia. As little as +1.00 D of hypermetropic anisometropia can cause a breakdown of central fusion and result in amblyopia. However, in myopia the anisometropia amblyopia is avoided. Mild to moderate myopic anisometropia does not result to amblyopia. Strabismus occurs when both the eyes are not aligned. The lack of coordination between two eyes because of difference in refractive error keeps us from being able to focus both eyes on the same point in space. Diplopia occurs because two eyes send different images in terms of size to our brain, causing double vision and confusion.

SYMPTOMS

Most patients with anisometropia may not show any symptoms, however there may be cases of symptomatic patients. The common symptoms that are observed in anisometropic patients are as under:
- Headache
- Eyeache
- Patients may also experience vertigo and spatial distortions, sometimes so severe that ambulation may be hazardous, as steps and curbs may appear tilted.
- Decreased reading stamina
- Adaptation difficulties with new correction

VISION IN ANISOMETROPIA

Binocular vision in anisometropia is rarely perfect and attempts for fusion frequently brings in the symptoms of accommodative asthenopia. With higher degree of anisometropia, fusion is usually impossible and may turn to be alternating or uniocular. Alternating vision occurs when the patient starts using one eye for distance and other for near. This occurs most commonly in case when one eye is emmetropic or moderately hypermetropic and the other is myopic. On the other hand, if the error in one eye is higher and visual acuity is also not good, it may be excluded all together from the vision process.

The unequal refractive error prescribed in optical correction most often result in aniseikonia which may create significant adaptation difficulties. It is difficult to measure aniseikonia and this is where the difficulty in solving the aniseikonic problem starts. The Space Eikonometer, an instrument that was designed to measure small amounts of aniseikonia, is no more available, though there has been some report of development of computer software for the purpose. In general, it has been estimated that each 0.25 D difference between the refraction of two eyes causes 0.50% difference in the size of retinal images. A difference of 5% has been considered to be the limit that can be tolerated by an individual.

Very often the patient faces difficulties when his eyes move from the primary gaze. This is because of the artificial heterophoria created because of side gaze vision. With 2.00 D difference in optical correction, 1D prism of deviation is incurred if the gaze deviates 5 mm from the optic axis. The effect is manifested in hypermetropia because of the narrowing of effective visual field of binocular vision.

The worst side is patient tends to suppress the image in one eye if the refractive error is great which may lead to amblyopia in suppressed eye. This is very critical in case of children.

CORRECTION IN ANISOMETROPIA

Each case must be dealt individually with attention being paid to the amount of discomfort and the disability from which the patient is suffering without correction and the amount of discomfort he experiences with the correction. Spectacle correction does not work for the individual in most cases. However, several efforts have been made to correct anisometropia with spectacle by prescribing smallest frame size and unequal base curves in two eyes. Patients have been advised to turn the head for side gaze, instead of eye to minimize the effect of induced prism. For a presbyope progressive addition lens with shorter corridor length has been seemed to be easier to adapt. Spectacle frame fitting must be stable and well maintained all through. It is important that vertex distances are minimum and consistent. Pantascopic angle used while refraction may also affect visual performance. Prism may be used to treat secondary muscular imbalance. Contact lenses are successful modality of treatment. Contact lens minimizes the difference in image sizes and also eliminate the resultant prism.

In children under the age of 12 years, every attempts should be made to induce the full correction to be worn. In adults an attempt should be made to wear full correction and the spectacle should be used constantly. The initial difficulties may disappear after a few week's difficulties. Most of such patient will unable to tolerate it. If the optical correction fails to give comfortable vision, binocular vision may be abandoned.

MULTIPLE CHOICE QUESTIONS

1. **Which of the following is true for anisometropia?**
   a. It occurs when the two eyes have different refractive errors
   b. Both the eyes are not oriented in the same parallel axis
   c. Difference in image sizes
   d. Subluxation of one of the eye
2. **Anisometropia amblyopia is:**
   a. Unilateral
   b. Bilateral

c. Unilateral and bilateral both
d. Detected in patient with dyslexia
3. **In hypermetropic anisometropia, aniseikonia can be reduced by which one of the following methods?**
   a. Decreasing the distance between the spectacle lens and cornea
   b. Increasing the front curvature of the spectacle lens without changing the lens power
   c. Reducing the thickness of the spectacle lens without changing the lens power
   d. Using high refractive index glass

ANSWER KEY

1. a   2. a   3. a

SELF-PRACTICE QUESTIONS

1. How can you minimize a patient's symptoms of altered space perception, when prescribing new correction?
2. How would you deal with the factors related to lens design in order to alter the lens magnification?

19 CHAPTER

Refraction in Aphakia

CHAPTER OUTLINE

- Vision in Aphakia
- Correction in Aphakia

Aphakia is a condition characterized by absence of lens from the pupillary area of the eye. Usually, the lens is removed surgically. Occasionally, it may be because of perforating wound or ulcer. Rarely, it could be absent because of congenital defect. The parallel rays of lights are brought to focus approximately 6-7 mm behind retina when the anteroposterior diameter of the eye is between 23-24 mm. The dioptric system of the eye must be supplemented by strong converging lenses of about +10.00 D or +11.00 D, if the eyes were originally emmetropic.

The condition has following characteristics in general:
- The aphakic eye is strongly hypermetropic
- Presence of against the rule astigmatism
- Absence of accommodation mechanism
- Absence of clear vision which hinders fixation also
- The posterior focal point lies behind the eyeball

VISION IN APHAKIA

The high plus spectacle lens correction produces enlargement of image in aphakia as correcting lens moves forward from the position of natural crystalline lens. Theoretically, it has been said to have an effect on visual acuity. A visual acuity of 6/9 corrected with spectacle lens corresponds to acuity of 6/9P or 6/12 in an eye with its optical system unaltered. Each diopter of plus power leads to nearly 2-3%

magnification of image. When the objects appear larger they appear falsely closer than reality, and this leads to physical in-coordination. The brain also takes some time to adapt to this.

Another disadvantage is the restrictions of visual field. The higher magnifications produced by high plus lenses reduces the field of view through the high plus lenses. It produces a blind area or scotoma in the patient's periphery. It means the object disappears in between the field of view through the lens and the object field immediately visible outside the lens edge where the object reappears again. The presence of above scotoma leads to another unique phenomenon called "Jack-in-the-box". The object lying in the periphery of the patient's visual field is not clear as the light arising from the objects lying immediately near the lens edge does not pass through the lens. The patient only perceives the presence of object. The patient tends to move his head towards the object to see it clearly; the object comes to the area of scotoma and thus disappears. The patient turns his head further so that the object comes in front of the spectacle lenses in the visible area and thus it reappears. This sudden disappearance and reappearance of the objects is called Jack-in-the-box phenomenon.

The edge of a convex lens acts as a prism. The higher the power of the convex lens the greater is the prism angle. The light falling on the prism bends towards its base; therefore, greater the angle more will be the bending. In aphakic lenses, the light falling at the edge of the lens bends towards the center of the lens and does not reach the pupil and therefore they are not seen, resulting in a scotomatic area in the visual field. Since the edge of the lens is present all around the lens, it gives rise to a ring-shaped scotoma. The position of ring scotoma moves with the movement of eyes. It is, therefore, called "roving ring scotoma".

The effect of plus lens is noticed as light scattering and thus reducing the light intensity. The person notices the effect as reduction in contrast.

CORRECTION IN APHAKIA

Aphakia is most commonly characterized by high degree of against the rule astigmatism immediately after the surgery which diminishes rapidly to about 2.00 D to 2.50 D in 6 weeks of time and further to smaller values in next 3 months. It is, therefore, safer to prescribe the correction after 6 weeks of the surgery. However, if the spectacle is desired before this, a temporary spherical equivalent is a practicable approach. However, the new small incision sutureless cataract

Chapter 19: Refraction in Aphakia

surgery produces less corneal toricity than those of larger wounds. The prescribing of postoperative correction has been reported as early as 3 weeks after the operation. Postoperative astigmatism is likely to be similar to that seen preoperatively.

Since accommodation is absent, the patient needs a separate correction for distance, near as well as for intermediate distances.

Retinoscopy does not work as an objective mode of refraction because of the poor fixational ability of the patient. Keratometer and autorefractometer both provide good starting point. Fogging method of subjective correction is of no use. Stenopeic slit can be used very effectively for quick and accurate subjective correction.

MULTIPLE CHOICE QUESTIONS

1. **Each diopter of plus lens power leads to how much amount of image magnification?**
   a. 3%
   b. 4%
   c. 2%
   d. 2.5%
2. **Which of the following is not correct regarding aphakia?**
   a. Reduction of visual field is common
   b. There is increasing magnifications
   c. Ring scotoma of aphakia is created by the prismatic effect of the lens
   d. None of the above
3. **Regarding aphakia which of the following is not true.**
   a. The aphakic eye is strongly hypermetropic
   b. Presence of with the rule astigmatism
   c. Absence of accommodation mechanism
   d. The posterior focal point lies behind the eyeball

ANSWER KEY

1. a	2. d	3. b				

SELF-PRACTICE QUESTIONS

1. What is aphakia? What causes aphakia?
2. Explain how different does the world look around an aphakic individual?

20 CHAPTER

Pediatric Refraction

CHAPTER OUTLINE

- Development of Vision
- Emmetropization
- Amblyopia and Strabismus
- Retinopathy of Prematurity
- Measuring Refractive Error in Children
- Prescribing Refractive Correction in Children

The American Academy of Pediatrics defines "pediatrics" as the medical specialty focused on the physical, mental, and social well-being of children from birth to young adulthood. Pediatric clinical care is a specialized discipline that enables clinicians to identify developmental issues early, address specific health concerns in children, and facilitate their transition into adulthood. It necessitates an understanding of developmental challenges, proficiency in specialized tests, effective communication skills, and patience. The field is particularly challenging, as improperly executed refractive correction can potentially be more detrimental than beneficial.

Children acquire visual abilities over time, similar to how they learn to walk and talk. At birth, a child's vision is stimulated by various visual inputs, though they may not distinguish between two targets or shift their gaze between objects. Their primary focus is on objects approximately 8-10 inches from their eyes. As they grow, children learn to:

- ❖ Focus their eyes
- ❖ Move their eyes accurately
- ❖ Coordinate the use of both eyes
- ❖ Utilize visual information to understand and interact with the world

Chapter 20: Pediatric Refraction

Any issues with a child's eyes and vision during infancy can lead to developmental delays in these abilities. When examining a child's eyes, clinicians must possess comprehensive knowledge of normal eye development and the process of emmetropization. Prescribing refractive correction requires careful consideration of several factors:

- ❖ Understanding how a child's vision and visual system develop over time is crucial for appropriate interventions.
- ❖ Recognizing the natural process of emmetropization, which involves the eyes adjusting to achieve optimal focus, is essential for prescribing accurate refractive corrections.
- ❖ Knowledge of the development of visual disorders, such as strabismus and amblyopia, is vital for early detection and intervention.
- ❖ Considering the impact of premature birth on visual development is crucial, as premature infants may face additional challenges related to their eyes and vision.

DEVELOPMENT OF VISION

Understanding the age-related development of visual functions is crucial for practitioners involved in pediatric eye care. The early years of a child's life are particularly significant as anatomical and physiological changes in the cortical system reflect the maturation of visual function.

Visual acuity is notably poor at birth, but there is rapid maturation during the first year, with adult-level visual acuity reached by the age of 3 years. The approximate Snellen's equivalent visual acuity at birth is considered as 6/300, improving to 6/6 by the time the child is 5 years or older. Normal eye movement is essential for the proper development of the visual system, and abnormal eye movement is often the first sign of developmental abnormalities.

Accurate focus over short distances is achieved by newborns, and adult-like accommodation function develops by 3-4 months. While accommodative convergence to a near target is present in the first month, precision in convergence takes time to develop, with accurate convergence typically not achieved until 6 weeks of age. Stereopsis, the ability to perceive depth, is not present at birth but emerges suddenly around 2-3 months and is largely complete by 6 months. Fusion and stereopsis develop concurrently.

Structural development of the eye continues postnatally. The macula develops later than the rest of the retina, and the fundus lacks pigmentation, taking nearly 6 months to resemble an adult-like picture. The pupil is small during infancy, increases to an average size of 7 mm by the age of 12 years, and then gradually decreases throughout life. The cornea, initially flat at birth, gradually acquires curvature, reaching an adult-like diameter by 2 years of age.

Additionally, color vision undergoes development with trichromacy typically achieved by 3 months and dichromacy by 2 months.

EMMETROPIZATION

Emmetropization is indeed the process by which the eye adjusts its refractive properties along with the growth of axial length to achieve clear vision at a distance without the need for corrective glasses or surgery. This natural process is particularly active during the early years of a child's life, helping the eyes to reach a state of emmetropia, where light focuses precisely on the retina for clear vision without the aid of corrective measures.

Refractive Error

Refractive error in newborn babies indeed varies, and most full-term newborns are born with some degree of hypermetropia, which tends to reduce with age. The average hypermetropia at birth is typically in the range of +2.00 D to +4.00 D, and it is often symmetric. Additionally, astigmatism in the range of 1.00 D to 1.50 D is commonly present, with a higher prevalence of against-the-rule astigmatism in newborns. Anisometropia of around 1.00 D may also be observed at birth.

While most infants exhibit hypermetropia initially, a small percentage may show myopia at birth. However, this myopia often tends to resolve and reach emmetropia by toddler age, unless there are complicating factors such as a history of premature birth, neurodevelopmental delay, or a family history of degenerative myopia. Premature babies, especially those with low birth weights, may have a higher risk of developing myopia.

Axial Length

The axial length of the full-term newborn eye is indeed in the range of 16–18 mm. After birth, there is extensive growth, and by the age of 3 years, a child's eye typically grows to around 22–23 mm. The mean adult axial length values are indeed in the range of 22–25 mm.

The relationship between axial length and refractive error is well-established. A change of 1 mm in axial length is often associated with a change in prescription of approximately 2.00 D to 2.50 D. Moreover, a change of 1.00 D in myopia is roughly equivalent to a 0.30 mm increase in axial length.

It is also accurate that the child's eyes reach their maximum size, typically in the range of 24-26 mm, during puberty. This period of growth and development is critical in understanding and managing refractive errors and visual health in pediatric patients.

Emmetropization Mechanism

The process involves coordinated changes in different refractive components of the eye along with alterations in axial length. Changes in childhood include an increase in axial length, vitreous depth, corneal curvature, and anterior chamber depth, coupled with a decrease in crystalline lens power and thickness. These changes occur together, leading to a small net change in refractive error. Both hypermetropia and astigmatism tend to reduce with age, with hypermetropia initially increasing and then decreasing through the process of emmetropization. The prevalence of astigmatism drops by the age of 4-5 years. Around the age of 6 years, the visual system tends to center around emmetropia with a deviation of ±0.75 D.

The first year of life is marked by rapid changes in refraction and growth. Hypermetropia increases initially, reaching its peak by 6 months, and then decreases through emmetropization. The most rapid decline in hypermetropia occurs between 6 months and 2 years of age in normally developing eyes. By 12 months, average infants typically have hypermetropia of not more than 2.00 D. After the age of 3 years, the rate of emmetropization slows down. Genetic predisposition, environmental factors (such as visual experience), and external influences (like refractive error or disease) can affect emmetropization. When emmetropization does not occur properly, refractive errors like myopia, hyperopia, or astigmatism may result.

The process of emmetropization needs to be respected when correcting refractive errors in children. Inappropriate correction during the developmental period may adversely affect the natural process. Critical considerations for prescription include recognizing that refractive errors characteristic of a child's age may decrease without intervention. Partial correction of hyperopic error from around the first year of life allows emmetropization to proceed.

Infants with hyperopia not reducing without intervention may be at a higher risk of developing strabismus or amblyopia. Refractive corrections that completely remove blurs may halt emmetropization and lead to higher final refractive errors. Full hyperopic correction may be reserved for infants and young children with esodeviation. Strabismic children should be monitored for increasing amounts of anisometropia.

AMBLYOPIA AND STRABISMUS

Amblyopia and strabismus are significant developmental disorders often observed in early childhood, resulting from factors that disrupt normal visual development. Patients with amblyopia may report poor vision or diplopia and may adopt compensatory postures like head tilting. There are three fundamental types of amblyopia:

1. **Strabismic amblyopia:** Resulting from misalignment of the visual axes.
2. **Anisometropia amblyopia:** Arising from unequal refractive errors between the eyes.
3. **Refractive amblyopia:** Caused by significant refractive errors, usually in both eyes.

Strabismus is defined as a misalignment of the visual axes and is not typically present at birth. Most neonates initially have transient divergence misalignment. Constant exotropia and intermittent exotropia are more common, while esotropia is rare. Normal eye alignment is the result of an active visual process during early life. The understanding is that most forms of strabismus are not congenital, but is the problem in visually guided motor learning. When eyes do not line up together, the straight or straighter eye becomes dominant. The visual acuity of this eye stays normal because the eye and its connection to the brain are working as they should. The misaligned or weaker eye, though, does not focus as it should and its connection to the brain does not form correctly.

Strabismus usually can be treated effectively when found and treated early. If it is not treated, the brain eventually will ignore the visual images of the weaker eye. This change is called amblyopia, or "lazy eye" which can make vision blurry, cause double vision, and harm a child's depth perception. Experts do not completely understand the cause of strabismus, but it results from the failure of the eye muscles to work together. Idiopathic strabismus is the most common type. Other conditions that can also cause strabismus are duane syndrome, moebius syndrome, thyroid eye disease, nerve damage, cerebral injuries, fracture of the orbital wall.

RETINOPATHY OF PREMATURITY

Retinopathy of prematurity (ROP) is an eye disorder that primarily affects premature infants. It is a potentially blinding condition that can occur when a premature infant's retina does not develop properly. The underdeveloped blood vessels can cause abnormal growth of blood vessels or bleeding in the retina. The premature cornea lacks luster and clarity. The other characteristics traits are shallow anterior chambers, miotic pupils, and bluish irides.

To prevent ROP, premature infants are monitored closely, and their oxygen levels are carefully regulated to avoid fluctuations that could contribute to the development of the condition. In the case of retinopathy of prematurity, clinical refraction may be more challenging due to the potential for abnormal eye growth and development.

In some cases of ROP, the retina may develop abnormally, causing the eye to grow in a different shape than normal. This can lead to refractive errors such as nearsightedness, farsightedness, or astigmatism. Additionally, infants with ROP may have reduced visual acuity, which can make it difficult to obtain an accurate refraction. Prescribing refractive correction in ROP can be challenging due to the potential for abnormal eye growth and development.

It is important to note that refractive correction may need to be adjusted over time as the infant's eyes continue to develop. Close monitoring and follow-up visits with the ophthalmologist are essential to ensure that the prescription remains appropriate and that any changes are detected and addressed promptly.

The other complications in relation to child's birth that can disrupt normal eye development are low birth weight, oxygen deprivation, infections and trauma. Infants with low birth weight may be at increased risk particularly if they are associated factors like prematurity or oxygen deprivation at birth. Oxygen deprivation at birth can cause damage to the developing retina. Infections that occur during pregnancy or delivery can also increase the risk of refractive error in infants. Trauma during delivery, such as head injury or trauma to the eye can also increase the risk of refractive error in infants.

MEASURING REFRACTIVE ERROR IN CHILDREN

Measuring refractive error in children, especially in preverbal ones, poses significant challenges due to their age and the dynamic nature of their refractive conditions. Clinicians must tailor their techniques to align with the age-specific status of the visual system and the child's response capabilities. Infants, lacking verbal responsiveness and behavior control, necessitate objective methods like retinoscopy and autorefraction. As toddlers and preschoolers develop communication skills, a combination of objective and subjective techniques becomes feasible, including preferential looking tests and engagement strategies. For preschoolers and beyond, subjective refraction with age-appropriate charts and binocular vision assessments becomes more applicable. The evolving milestones of development and variations in visual functions and ocular structures underscore the need for an age-specific approach. Recognizing that critical milestones are achieved at different ages, a refractive error measurement program can be designed in three broad categories to accommodate the evolving needs of children.

- Birth to 3 years
- 3–6 years
- 6–18 years

Birth to 3 Years (Infants and Toddlers)

Infants are nonresponding and their behavior cannot be controlled. It is, therefore, best to examine their eyes when they are alert and on the lap of their mother. The clinician needs to rely more on objective method of examination that can be executed quickly. The procedure starts with history taking and followed with visual acuity assessment to be completed with the assessment of refractive error.

History Taking

Since children of this age group do not complain most of the history is obtained from the parents of the children as observed by them. Therefore, parents are asked questions. A good case history should include questions related to child's birth, behavioral abnormalities as well as general health. **Table 20.1** shows some of the simple questions that are useful in such cases.

Chapter 20: Pediatric Refraction

Table 20.1: Questions for history taking in infants and toddlers.

Questions in relation to	Questions
Pregnancy and birth history	• How was mother's health during pregnancy? • Any infectious disease during pregnancy? • Alcohol intake and/or smoking? • Was the delivery normal or cesarean delivery? • Were forceps used at the time of delivery? • Was the delivery difficult? • Was his birth premature? • What was the birth weight? • If so, was oxygen given?
Developmental history	• Does your child have any developmental delays? • Age when milestones achieved rolling, sitting, crawling, walking, etc.
Family history	• Family history of strabismus and amblyopia • Family history of congenital cataracts, retinoblastoma • Family history of neurological disorder • Family history of poor vision
Behavioral history	• Parental observation of crossed eye • Does your child show abnormal eye movements?
Child's eye and general health	• Is there any concern regarding child's hearing ability? • Has your child had any injuries to the eyes or head? • Does your child have any neurological disorders? • Does your child seem to have trouble focusing on objects?

Measuring Visual Acuity

Visual acuity serves as a precise indicator of macular function, yet in newborns, its development is incomplete, progressing rapidly within the initial year. Subjective evaluation in preverbal children is nearly impossible, necessitating qualitative measurement through behavioral and electrophysiological techniques distinct from those used in adults.

The electrophysiological approach, utilizing visually evoked potentials (VEP), objectively measures visual acuity by assessing brain activity through scalp electrodes. Conversely, the preferential looking (PL) technique, widely applied for behavioral estimation, relies on the observation that infants prefer patterned stimuli over blank ones.

Notably, VEP methods indicate quicker acuity maturation, contrasting with PL acuity, which reaches adult levels only by 36 months, exhibiting a gradual increase with age. VEP acuity is constrained by structural and neural changes in ocular media and the visual pathway, while PL acuity is influenced by attention, oculomotor development, and examiner proficiency.

Clinicians must be cognizant of age-appropriate threshold limits when measuring visual acuity. The clinician should measure the binocular acuity first and then move to measure monocular acuity. While measuring monocular acuity eye patch should be used to cover an eye in place of trial frame or occluder. Estimation of visual acuity in infants and toddlers can provide direction for remainder of the examination. The recommended tests to measure visual acuity in this age group are fixation preference test and preferential looking test.

Refraction

Refraction is essential for assessing the normal development of a child's visual system and identifying any issues with binocular vision. Investigating the refractive state of the eyes and comparing it with age-related norms is crucial.

Unlike adults, subjective refraction is impractical for infants and toddlers due to poor fixation, zero response, and limited attention span. Objective refraction, particularly retinoscopy, proves more reliable. Traditional autorefractometers are unsuitable due to their size and inadequate accommodation control.

Two effective methods for infants and toddlers are cycloplegic retinoscopy and near retinoscopy. Cycloplegic refraction involves using eye drops to relax eye muscles, preventing over-focusing during the examination. This method is most effective when the baby is well-cyclopleged and quietly fixates on the retinoscope light.

Near retinoscopy, or the Mohindra technique, is conducted in complete darkness with the nontested eye occluded. It is useful for screening higher refractive errors, especially when cycloplegic methods are unavailable or refused. The retinoscopy is performed from a distance of 50 cm and a working compensation of -1.25 D is used to arrive at the results.

The average refractive error in babies from birth to one year is approximately $+2.00$ D of hyperopia with a deviation of 2.00 D. Astigmatism up to 2.00 D is common in children under 3 years old. These information help clinicians in understanding and addressing refractive errors in young children, ensuring timely interventions for optimal visual development.

3–6 Years (Preschool Children)

Preschool development spans the crucial ages of 3–5 years, marking a significant period where many large and transient refractive errors from infancy typically resolve by around 3 years of age. Several key developmental considerations should be taken into account during refraction assessments in this age group:

- Most preschoolers can communicate verbally, enabling the use of subjective techniques with some limitations. However, it is essential that these techniques are quick and nonthreatening to ensure cooperation.
- The axial length of the eye in this age group generally falls between 21.50–22.50 mm, but there exists a wide range of normal variation. Some children may have axial lengths that deviate from the average.
- There is a notable range of developmental hypermetropia between ages 3 and 6. Initially around +2.00 D, hypermetropia decreases, and by approximately age 6, the visual system tends towards emmetropia with a deviation of ±1.00.
- The prevalence of astigmatism decreases by ages 4–5, with a shift towards with-the-rule astigmatism.
- Anisometropia detected during the preschool years may remain stable.
- Myopia is rare in this age group, and its presence should prompt suspicion of another neurodevelopmental or ocular anomaly, especially in the absence of a positive family history of degenerative myopia.
- Almost half of children with amblyopia are identified during the preschool years, highlighting the importance of early detection and intervention during this critical developmental stage.

History Taking

A good case history in case of preschool children should include questions related as mentioned in **Table 20.1**. Additionally, following questions may be added on case to case basis:
- Does the child rub his eyes frequently?
- Does the child avoid coloring activities, puzzles, and other detailed activities?

- Does the child sit close to the television or hold a book too close?
- Does the child squint or tilt his head?

Measuring Visual Acuity

Measuring visual acuity at this age group is a little less challenging as most children develop the necessary response skills to allow subjective acuity testing. However, it is still useful to limit the amount of verbal interaction especially in case of younger preschool children.

Age-specified test charts are recommended. The 3 years old child can respond to well to match simple forms and shapes though demonstration and imitation. Broken wheel acuity cards that uses Landolt C target is appropriate for this age group. The chart requires very little verbal interaction.

The LEA symbol chart which consists of four optotypes—circle, square, apple, and house can also be used with great success. The child simply has to find a matching block or point to the shape that matches the target presented.

The HOTV test can also be completed by many preschoolers. HOTV chart is a vision screening test chart that determines relative visual acuity for distance vision using the four letters H, O, T and V.

Refraction

Retinoscopy is the most ideal technique for the younger children in this age group for measuring refractive error. Static retinoscopy and cycloplegic retinoscopy are the two recommended test. Cycloplegic retinoscopy is the valuable technique for first evaluation of preschool children. It should also be used in cases of strabismus and high refractive error. A quick and less threatening subjective refraction can also be tried in preschoolers.

6–18 Years (School Age Children)

Children in this age group demonstrate increased capabilities and independence, enjoying an active lifestyle with peers and displaying enhanced motor skills. While eye examination techniques align closely with those used for adults, age-appropriate adjustments to instructions and targets are often necessary. Some techniques applicable to infants, toddlers, and preschoolers may also be relevant, especially for children under 8 years old. Key developmental considerations for this age group include:

- Following preschool age, the majority of children are typically emmetropic, although a small percentage may develop myopia before starting school.
- Instances of new astigmatism or anisometropia are commonly associated with the onset of myopia.
- Hyperopia, hyperopic astigmatism, and hyperopic anisometropia usually do not emerge anew during this developmental stage.
- Smaller refractive errors can be addressed at this age, particularly since they are linked to symptoms such as asthenopia, focusing problems, and visual fatigue, especially with increasing visual demands.
- During this stage, children with amblyopiagenic levels of hyperopia may be identified. Their vision problems often go undetected and unsuspected, potentially contributing to poor school performance.

History Taking

Children in this age group should actively participate in the comprehensive history-taking process, given the significant link between vision and learning. It is crucial to incorporate inquiries about their school performance to uncover the specific vision-related issues affecting their learning. Additionally, tailored questions can be posed to discern the child's symptoms more precisely.

Strategically crafted questions can also aid in identifying signs and symptoms of vision problems that may be associated with attention deficit hyperactivity disorder (ADHD). A common visual condition linked to ADHD is convergence insufficiency, manifesting as reduced ability to focus during near work, poor fixation, loss of place while reading, word skipping or repetition, compromised visual memory, and impaired reading comprehension.

Moreover, symptoms such as excessive talking, heightened physical movement, impatience, impulsive actions, and interrupting conversations may also be explored, providing valuable insights into potential visual or attention-related challenges.

Refraction

The refraction techniques should undergo a major shift in older children. Cycloplegia refraction takes the back seat and plays complementary role. The reasons for this shift are:

- ❖ Attention and accommodation can be controlled to distant target at this age.
- ❖ The accuracy of retinoscopy is improved.
- ❖ Myopia is more common refractive error and is more accurately determined by skillful static refraction.
- ❖ Habitual and preferred amount of accommodation are revealed by skillful static refraction. Adaptation problems occur if the habitual or preferred amounts of accommodation are ignored in older children.

Objective refraction can be performed using following techniques:
- ❖ Static retinoscopy
- ❖ Cycloplegic retinoscopy
- ❖ Autorefractometry

Cycloplegic refraction may be performed in case of children below the age of 8 years and/or in conditions like strabismus, amblyopia or significant hyperopia. Autorefractometry is a very quick way for objective measurement of refractive error and is very useful for older children. Objective refraction can be followed by the comprehensive subjective refraction especially with children above the age of 8 years. Subjective refraction allows the clinician to fine tune the prescription based on the patient's subjective experience. It takes into account factors such as the patient's age, occupation, and visual needs, as well as any complaints the patient may have about their vision. Thus it allows for a more personalized prescription that is tailored to the patient's individual needs and preferences. There are three techniques of subjective refraction that can be used on case to case basis. These are:

- ❖ Monocular subjective refraction
- ❖ Binocular subjective refraction
- ❖ Fogging method of subjective refraction

Binocular subjective refraction is recommended in cases involving nystagmus, significant phoria, latent hyperopia, pseudomyopia, anti-metropia, hyperopic anisometropia, and unilateral amblyopia. Monocular subjective refraction can be conducted using fogging techniques or without fogging, employing the manifest monocular subjective refraction technique. While all methods offer accurate measurements of refractive error, the selection of a specific method may hinge on factors like age, individual characteristics, and practitioner preference.

PRESCRIBING REFRACTIVE CORRECTION IN CHILDREN

The developing visual system of the children is considered most susceptible to the interference especially in the first few years of development. A prescription for refractive correction for a child can do more harm than any good, if an inappropriate refractive correction is prescribed as it may affect the ongoing optical and neurological development in infants and toddlers. It can also affect developing brain because of abnormal sensory input as can occur in amblyopia. The clinician must consider several critical factors before prescribing the refractive correction. Some of the common factors to consider are:

- Age of the child
- Normal developmental visual milestones
- Type and magnitude of the refractive error
- Presence of amblyopia
- Presence of anisometropia and associated strabismus

Birth to 3 Years

At birth, infants generally exhibit hyperopia along with some degree of astigmatism, and their eyes undergo rapid changes. Emmetropization occurs swiftly during the first year of life and continues up to 5 years, requiring a normal visual system and environment. Timely and age-appropriate correction of refractive errors is crucial for proper visual development, encompassing visual acuity, binocularity, and overall growth.

Hypermetropia

Uncorrected hypermetropia can lead to amblyopia and esotropia. Amblyopia may arise if hypermetropia persists, especially during near vision tasks. Full correction is recommended if strabismus is present. Even low amounts of hypermetropia can result in refractive accommodative esotropia, increasing the risk of amblyopia. Prescription of hypermetropia should involve full cycloplegic correction, with the degree of correction dependent on the age. Partial correction may be considered for larger refractive errors, leaving room for emmetropization, provided amblyopia and strabismus are ruled out. In the absence of esotropia, it is not necessary to correct low hyperopia. As a rule hypermetropia is corrected earlier than myopia.

Myopia

Correction of myopia is suggested for high values exceeding 5.00 D in children below the age of two, as they primarily engage in near vision activities. Low myopia up to 3.50 D may not necessitate immediate correction, especially as it does not pose a high risk of amblyopia due to unaffected near vision. Prescription of glasses in low myopes is ideally done at ages three to four when children start showing interest in distant viewing. Over-correction should be avoided, aiming for the lowest power needed for optimal visual acuity. Intermittent exotropes should be prescribed even with the smallest myopic correction with the aim of inducing convergence, to overcome exotropia. A little over correction may also be considered in such case.

Astigmatism

Astigmatism, not overcome by accommodation, can be amblyogenic if cylindrical power exceeds 1.5–2 D. Correction is advised, particularly for astigmatism associated with spherical error or exceeding 1.5 D. Oblique astigmatism should always be corrected as it is amblyogenic. High cylindrical powers are generally well-accepted by children, and under-correction is discouraged. Smaller cylindrical powers (<1.5 D) may be prescribed in older children with mildly reduced visual acuity.

Anisometropia

Anisometropia is a common cause of amblyopia, with hypermetropic anisometropia being more amblyogenic than myopic anisometropia. A difference of >1.5 D in hypermetropia is considered amblyogenic and should be corrected early. Myopic anisometropia up to 3.00 D poses a low risk of amblyopia. Beyond 3.00 D, early correction is recommended. Aniso-astigmatism, with a difference of >1.50 D, should also be corrected early.

Anisometropia also has the potential to impair binocular vision. In cases of anisometropia, the best correction for each eye is assessed first. Then the binocular correction is assessed, noting the following:
- ❖ Binocular visual acuity for distance and near should be noted.
- ❖ The presence of diplopia and whether this is due to aniseikonia or a manifest strabismus, with the correction.

3–6 Years (Preschool Period)

Clinically, the preschool period signals the end of the critical period of development. During this period, a child's sensitivity to amblyopia development rapidly declines. There is less concern that a full correction will interfere with any beneficial process. The effect of refractive interventions is more readily demonstrable because newly acquired refractive problems do not cause regression of visual functions that have already developed. Nonstrabismic binocular vision may begin to be seen in the school years. This is the age when full correction of refractive error determined with or without cycloplegia could be given. Refractive errors that remain by this age, when the vast majority of children have achieved emmetropia, are not likely to go away naturally. Adaptation to full correction of any refractive error, including astigmatism or anisometropia, is rarely problematic at this age. The objective of prescribing refractive correction between the ages of 3 and 6 years is to address any vision problems that may be affecting their development and academic performance. Uncorrected refractive error, such as nearsightedness, farsightedness, or astigmatism, can lead to difficulties with reading, writing, and other activities that require visual acuity. More frequent eye examinations are recommended during this period to monitor any changes in their refractive error and ensure that any visual problems are detected and addressed as early as possible. This is the period when parents can be told that there is little likelihood that the child will outgrow an abnormal refractive error. Prescribe for refractive errors when stable for age.

The most common reason children are first prescribed correction at this age is for an 'old' problem that is first determined at this age, such as hypermetropia, astigmatism, or anisometropia that have been present for some time.

Hypermetropia

In children below the age of 6 years, some degree of hypermetropia is physiological and therefore the correction is given only when the error is high, binocular vision is disturbed or if strabismus is present.

Myopia

Myopia is rare at this time frame and should raise suspicion of some other anomaly in the absence of family history of degenerative myopia. Degenerative myopia presents before school age with high refractive error. Reduced vision and staphyloma formation may be apparent immediately or may develop later in the life.

Astigmatism

Astigmatism of 1.50 D or greater should be usually corrected and lesser amount may be considered for correction based on the child's function and any accompanying refractive error.

Anisometropia

Stable anisometropia of 1.00 D or more should be corrected, unless equal, normal corrected acuity can be demonstrated in the clinic. The most common problem that initiates a prescription for spectacle around age 3 is accommodative esotropia. It is ironic that this age of peak refractive development is the age at which most amblyopiagenic refractive errors are first detected.

6–18 Years (School Age)

Under correcting for the purpose of maintaining emmetropization mechanism is no longer indicated. However, a new problem of adapting to spectacle prescription arises.

Myopia

Children typically develop myopia during their early stages of school years and retain good corrected vision throughout the life. Non-pathologic or simple myopia may have been characterized by normal corrected acuity, onset during the school age, progression that self-limits around 6.00 D and the absence of staphyloma formation. The standard of care for myopic children of school age children is full correction of the myopic error. Care should be taken to avoid prescribing excess amount of myopia in children who are insensitive to blur produced by minus lenses. Undercorrection enhances the possibility of myopia progression.

Hypermetropia

Older hyperopic children without esodeviation rarely require prescription of full hyperopic error as determined using cycloplegia. The clinician can rely on static refraction and prescribe the maximum plus that allows best distance acuity. If an esodeviation is present, the correction is determined as the amount that provides optimal binocular performance at distance and near. This may require a bifocal prescription. In case of amblyopia, prescribe best sensory correction because precise optical correction provides the basis of any possible acuity improvement.

Astigmatism

Refractive correction of astigmatic blur must be obtained optically. The first issue is to manage amblyopia, if the child has. In such case the clinician has a little choice but to prescribe the best sensory correction because precise correction provides the basis for any possible acuity improvement. Unfortunately, meridional amblyopes are generally without complaints until they are told to wear glasses. They may not perceive much visual benefit from the correction and full correction may cause complaints of asthenopia, vestibular symptoms or headache in a precisely asymptomatic child. Ideally, the clinician can obtain compliance by forewarning the parents and the child about the possible difficulties with adaptation, reassuring both that the vision will be comfortable in a few days. This can be difficult because difficulties are apparent immediately but benefits are not. The children who cannot fare better, their correction may be tapered down to reach to full correction eventually in amblyopic children. In children who do not have amblyopia, there is no harm in using under correction. The full astigmatic correction may cause complaints of asthenopia, vestibular symptoms or headache in a previously asymptomatic child. The correction may have to be reduced to obtain compliance. The goal should be eventual wear of full correction in amblyopic child.

MULTIPLE CHOICE QUESTIONS

1. **Which of the following functions is present at birth?**
   a. Streopsis
   b. Vertical Saccades
   c. Vestibulo-ocular reflex
   d. Accommodation

2. **Which of the following is found matured to adult levels at 6 months of age in the normal infant?**
   a. Visual acuity measured by preferential looking
   b. Astigmatism
   c. Smooth pursuit movements
   d. Contrast sensitivity measured by VEP

3. **Which of the following is correct for a 2 months baby?**
   a. Has no color perception
   b. Has gross fusion
   c. Can discriminate between red and green

d. Can accurately follow a fast-moving targets with smooth movements
4. **Most children are born with:**
   a. 1.00 D of ATR astigmatism that shifts to WTR after 5 years
   b. 1.00 D of WTR astigmatism that shifts to ATR after 5 years
   c. No astigmatism
   d. 1.00 D of ATR astigmatism that remains unchanged
5. **Full-term babies are born with hyperopia to the tune of:**
   a. +2.00 D to +4.00 D
   b. +1.00 D to +2.00 D
   c. +4.00 D to +6.00 D
   d. +5.00 D to +7.00 D
6. **Adult like accommodation function develops by:**
   a. 3–4 months
   b. 2–3 months
   c. 5–6 months
   d. 8–10 months
7. **Which of the following function cannot be measured by VEP technique?**
   a. Visual acuity
   b. Color vision
   c. Convergence
   d. Contrast sensitivity
8. **Which of the following statement is not correct for child's eye development?**
   a. Macula develops earlier than the rest of the retina
   b. Pupil is miotic during infancy
   c. Cornea is almost flat at birth
   d. Fundus lacks pigmentation at birth
9. **The natural process of emmetropization is a complicated process that does not include:**
   a. An increase in axial length
   b. An increase in vitreous chamber depth
   c. A decrease in the power of crystalline lens
   d. A decrease in corneal curvature
10. **Which of the following statement is not correct with respect of development of vision in children?**
    a. Refractive errors that are characteristics of child's age are not likely to be decreased without any intervention in most situations

Chapter 20: Pediatric Refraction

    b. Partial correction of hyperopic error beginning around the first year of life allows emmetropization to proceed
    c. Infants whose hyperopia does not reduce without intervention are more likely to develop strabismus, amblyopia or both
    d. Refractive corrections that remove blurs entirely may stop emmetropization and result in higher final refractive errors

11. **Which of the following test for visual acuity assessment is not based upon the principle of preferential looking?**
    a. Keeler acuity system
    b. Cardiff acuity test
    c. Teller acuity card
    d. LH symbols

12. **In children from birth to 3 years of age, which of the following factors should be considered before prescribing the refractive correction?**
    a. Prescribe for refractive errors when stable for age
    b. Prescribe for refractive errors when they are amblyogenic
    c. Prescribe for refractive errors when they affect vision development and behavior
    d. All of the above

ANSWER KEY

1. c	2. c	3. c	4. a	5. a	6. a	7. c	8. a
9. d	10. a	11. d	12. d				

SELF-PRACTICE QUESTIONS

1. Why it is important to think differently when it comes to examining and prescribing children below the age of 12 years for refractive error assessment?
2. Why it is necessary to be aware of the normal developmental visual milestone for a child before prescribing the correction for refractive error? Explain with reference to the normal developmental of various visual milestones.
3. A 6-year-old child shows the refractive error of +1.25 in each eye. Would you prescribe correction or not? Explain.
4. What do you think are the key challenges associated with the management of vision correction in pediatric population?

CHAPTER 21

The Geriatric Refraction

CHAPTER OUTLINE

- Aging Changes in Eyes
- Aging Changes in Visual Functions
- Measuring Refractive Error
- Prescribing Correction

The term "geriatrics" refers to medical care for older adults. However, it is difficult to define the age group precisely in terms of years. The common consensus is population aged 65 years and over belongs to the geriatric category.

Aging brings in lot of changes. While some of the changes are physiological, there are other changes that include biological changes, behavioral changes, psychological changes, and functional changes. These changes exert their effects in the lifestyle of the geriatric population.

Aging produces physiological changes in all the structures of the eye causing not only varied functional changes but also makes the eyes more susceptible to ocular diseases. The impact is seen as decline in task performance and reduction of visual function in the elderly population. The degree of functional losses varies from individual to individual, depending upon the optical and neuronal alteration and/or damage.

There may be pathological changes also in ocular structures that may lead to visual impairment. Visual impairment reduces the quality of life and increases the risk of falls, depression, and cognitive impairment. Visual impairment is a leading cause of disability. The most notable among them are listed below:

- Uncorrected refractive error
- Maculopathy
- Cataracts
- Glaucoma
- Retinopathy

These pathological conditions may affect the central vision, peripheral vision, contrast sensitivity and color perception of the elderly population.

Aging is also associated with several systemic diseases that can also affect vision. High blood pressure can damage the blood vessels in the eye and lead to a condition called hypertensive retinopathy that can cause vision changes or even loss of vision. Diabetes is another condition that can cause vision loss. High levels of blood sugar can damage the blood vessels in the retina, leading to diabetic retinopathy. It can also increase the risk of cataracts and glaucoma which also have potential for vision loss. Aging is the number one risk factor for the development of Parkinson's disease. Besides, elderly population may also suffer from cardiovascular disease, rheumatoid arthritis, etc., which can affect the vision in more than one way.

Many elderly individuals take varieties of medicines and often have complicated medical picture. Some of those medicines may have significant effect on vision and the visual system. Though nothing much can be done to minimize their effect, communication and full discloser of information is useful to provide most appropriate and individualized care.

AGING CHANGES IN EYES

The following is a brief overview of what happens to various ocular structures with aging:

Eyelids

Aging affects the elasticity of eyelids. The eyelid skin gets increasingly loose and thin. Lid laxity is further affected by reduction in orbital fat which causes eyes to 'sink in'. In some case the muscles that control eyelid movement may also weaken, leading to drooping or sagging eyelids. These changes can affect both the functions and the appearance of the eyelids.

Lacrimal System

The lacrimal system starts producing reduced tears, leading to dry eyes. The tear drainage channel is blocked or become less efficient, leading excessive tearing in the eyes. The tear film quality is also adversely affected. The changes cause a range of symptoms that include dry eyes, tearing eyes, irritation and discomfort.

Extraocular Muscles

The tonicity of the extraocular muscles diminishes with aging. The effect is seen as decrease ability to converge, maintain convergence and decrease smooth visual tracking.

Cornea

Corneal aging generates structural and functional changes including steepening of keratometry values, and a rotation of the axis of corneal astigmatism resulting in a shift from with-the-rule to against-the-rule astigmatism. Changes in corneal hydration alter change in corneal thickness, which in turn can affect refractive error. Corneal swelling produces increase in myopia or decrease in hypermetropia. Other corneal changes include increase in corneal fragility, decrease in corneal luster and corneal sensitivity.

Anterior Chamber

Anterior chamber is about 3 mm deep in the center in normal adults which becomes a little shallower in elderly population. The angle of the anterior chamber also gradually narrows with age and there is age-related reduction in aqueous outflow which may lead to elevation of intraocular pressure.

Ciliary Body

Ciliary body is the site of aqueous production. There are changes in the shape and tone of ciliary body with aging, which along with decrease elasticity of the lens capsule causes a decrease in the amplitude of accommodation resulting in presbyopia.

Iris

Iris becomes less reactive with age and more difficult to dilate pharmacologically. Aging is also associated with decrease in the amount of iris pigments.

Pupil

The pupil becomes smaller and less responsive to changes in light. That is why people in their 60s need more light for comfortable reading especially during night. It also serves to increase the depth of focus. As a result, during subjective refraction the just noticeable differences for older population may somewhat be larger than for younger adults.

Crystalline Lens

Aging leads to major changes within the crystalline lens, leading to several changes in the lens:
- ❖ Yellowing of crystalline lens age, causes more absorption of blue light and thus increases selective light transmission.
- ❖ The loss of the UV ray filter function increases phototoxic lesions of the retina which in turn may lead to increase in the incidence of age-related macular degeneration.
- ❖ Hardening of the crystalline lens caused by various biochemical and photochemical changes gradually restricts accommodation.
- ❖ Opacification of lens causes the appearance of senile cataract. Nuclear portion of the lens becomes denser with age and that this is accompanied by an increase in the index of refraction.

Vitreous

Vitreous undergoes the irreversible process of aging that are important in the pathogenesis of vitreous liquefaction, vitreous detachment and retinal disease. The changes are characterized by changes in the collagen fibrils, hyaluronic acid components, condensation of the vitreous gel and formation of optically empty spaces called lacunae. The elderly person may note spider like floater in front of eye which moves in the direction of gaze. Vitreous liquefaction is often followed by vitreous shrinkage leading to posterior vitreous detachment. In some case the elderly person may show symptoms of having curtain-like shadow in the field of vision which may point to a retinal detachment.

Retina

Retina shows several aging changes that affect almost every aspect of vision. There is a change in the integrity of photoreceptor cells with rods and cones, showing increased pleomorphism, decrease in number of cells in the posterior pole, decreased melanin content, increased lipofuscin content, and decreased volume of cytoplasm.

Choroid

The choroid is a layer of tissue in the eye that lies between the retina and the sclera. It contains blood vessels that supply oxygen and nutrients to the retina. As we age, there are several changes that can occur in the choroid, including thinning, degeneration and reduced blood flow to the retina. The changes in choroid lead to a reduction in the supply of oxygen and nutrients to the retina.

Sclera

Older population have sclera that is more dark, red, and yellow. In fact sclera coloration is a cue for the perception of age, and health. Sclera also thins with aging that increases visibility of blood vessels and also increases the risk of ocular diseases.

Clinical fundus examination that includes the examination of the inside back surface of the eye, made up of the retina, macula, optic disc, fovea and blood vessels shows gradual fading of fundus color, greater visibility of larger choroidal vessels and peripheral retinal degenerations. **Table 21.1** shows the aging changes in eyes.

■ AGING CHANGES IN VISUAL FUNCTIONS

Aging affects the vision in more than one ways. However, the degree of functional loss may vary from individual to individual depending upon optical and neuronal changes which can further intensify with environmental changes. The following is a brief overview of what happens to various visual functions as we grow:

Visual Acuity

Visual acuity in geriatric population is reduced. In most geriatric individual the best corrected visual acuity of 6/6 is not achieved during clinical refraction. The author has noticed in his private practice that the number of people who can be corrected to 6/6 visual acuity is significantly less after the age of 70 years. He also observed that the visual acuity improvement is more at lower level than at higher levels. However, near visual acuity improves significantly in most cases. The reason of loss of visual acuity in the absence of ocular pathology can be attributed to the neuronal loss in the brain.

Table 21.1: Aging changes in eyes.	
Aging changes in ocular structure	Impact
The fat pads supporting the eyes decrease	The eyes sink into their sockets
Reduction in goblet cell number and lacrimal gland mass	Progressive reduction in tear production
Reduction in extraocular muscle tonicity	Decreases ability to converge, maintain convergence, smooth visual tracking
Cornea becomes less sensitive	Subject may not notice eye injuries
Pupil size reduces	Makes it more difficult to see at night, poor dark adaptation
Pupil reaction slows down	Increases glare recovery time
Crystalline lens becomes yellowed	Loss of the UV ray filter function
Crystalline lens becomes less flexible	Restricts accommodation
Crystalline lens becomes cloudy	Causes the appearance of senile cataract
Vitreous inside the eye may shrink	Dark specks, floaters or flashing lights
Vitreous liquefaction	Retinal tears, retinal detachment, vitreo-macular traction, macular hole
Structural and functional alteration in lacrimal glands	Decrease in the lacrimal gland secretory function, dry eyes
Decrease in retinal cells sensitivity	Diminishes color vision
Decrease oxygen supply to rod-dense peripheral retina	Reduces visual field

Accommodation

Accommodation, which is the ability to focus at varying distances, reduces significantly with aging. The maximum amplitude of accommodation is at the age of 5 years. Thereafter, the amplitude of accommodation progressively decreases at a rate of approximately 0.30 D/years. The loss of accommodation is nearly complete by the age of 60 years. The sclerosing of the crystalline lens within the eye contributes to the loss of accommodation.

Vergence

It has also been documented that elderly people tends to be exophoric at near. This stresses the fusional convergence function that may result in discomfort, asthenopia, diplopia and overall difficulties in performing near viewing tasks. The effect is observed as changes in binocular vision and the elderly individual finds it difficult to converge and maintain convergence.

Eye Motility

The normal upward gaze rotation in young children is 40 degree but substantially reduces in elderly patients to 16 degree. There is a progressive symmetrical limitation that begins around the middle age. No specific reference has been accorded except for neurological disorder of aging and reduced use of the eyes in the upper field. Reduced tonicity of extraocular muscles restricts overall eye movement with significant reduction in smooth visual tracking.

Visual Field

Visual sensitivity is reduced with age which has corresponding impact on visual field with also shrinks in older population. The reasons attributed are the decreased oxygen supply to rod dense peripheral retina and reduced pupil size. The loss of visual field is the primary reason that increases the risk of falls, decrements in mobility and increased risk of bumping.

Contrast Sensitivity

Contrast sensitivity is relatively stable during the middle age, but it begins to show a mild but definite loss of high and middle frequency contrast detection. There may be several reasons like changes in crystalline lens and pupil but most researcher believe it is because of neuronal loss within the visual pathway. It is because of reduction in contrast sensitivity the elderly population requires three times more contrast to perform certain everyday tasks than younger population.

Light Sensitivity

The amount of light that reaches to retina is significantly reduced in aging eyes. It is because of reduced pupil size and increased media opacities. The elderly individual needs three times more illumination than younger individual to perform tasks.

Color Sensitivity

The ability to distinguish the entire color spectrum starts decreasing with age which is more demonstrated after the age of 70 years. Most noticeable changes occur at blue-yellow spectrum. It is usually because of yellowing of the crystalline lens that tend to absorb and scatter blue light, making it difficult to differentiate in shades of blue, green and violet. They can perceive bright colors at the warm end of the spectrum, such as red and oranges. However, the loss of color vision in general does not seem to affect day-to-day life.

Dark Adaptation

Older adults have serious difficulty seeing under low illumination and at night, even in the absence of ocular disease. They show dysfunction in dark adaptation and conversely to light adapt. This could be because of changes in retinal metabolism, miotic pupil and a decrease in function of the central nervous system.

Glare Recovery Time

Glare is very common in elderly population. They also find it difficult to recover from the effect of glare quickly. They take longer time. This may be because of irregular corneal surface, media opacities coupled with slowed pupil reaction time.

It is important to know the changes in visual functions that are common in aging population while assessing refractive error. These are normal changes and have a great toll on functional vision loss. However, these changes have varying degree of impact depending upon the amount of optical and neuronal alteration and also because of environmental factor. **Table 21.2** shows the aging changes in visual function.

Table 21.2: Aging changes in visual function.	
Visual functions	*Aging changes in visual functions*
Visual acuity	Difficult to increase BCVA to 6/6 in most cases
Accommodation	No role of accommodation post 60 years
Vergence	Exophoria is common
Eye motility	Restricted upward gaze
Visual field	Restricted visual field
Contrast sensitivity	Reduced contrast sensitivity
Light sensitivity	Need of more illumination to perform task
Dark adaptation	Dark adaptation slows down
Glare recovery time	Increased time to recover from glare
Color sensitivity	Reduced color sensitivity more at blue-yellow spectrum

MEASURING REFRACTIVE ERROR

All older people are not alike. The differences among older population are great. For majority of older adults the effect of aging changes is subtle to which they adapt. However, the speed with which information is encoded, stored, and retrieved slows down significantly. But on intelligence test many older adults outperform their younger counterparts. This has been attributed to their accumulated knowledge and experience.

Refractive error changes throughout the lifespan. Hyperopic shifts in refraction have been consistently reported in adults over 40 years of age, followed by myopic shifts after the age of 70 years. Majority of them also show changes in astigmatism with a shift from with the rule astigmatism in youth to against the rule astigmatism in old age population. Anisometropia, which is defined as the difference of 1.00D of refractive error between the two eyes, also appears to increase with aging.

The physiological changes in the ocular structure and their corresponding impact on visual functions affect the refractive error in elderly population. Pathological changes impair visual acuity and add to functional loss. In addition, there are influences of environmental and lifestyle factors also. Therefore, it is crucial to understand the normal aging process and changes that happen when caring for the geriatric population. This knowledge is essential for accurate assessment, diagnosis, and treatment. Caring for the geriatric population requires a precise understanding of aging versus illness. This can be extremely challenging. An important aspect of caring for aging population is to look at the aging care holistically.

While dealing with elderly population, the practitioner must use more imagination and flexibility in structuring the examination and management to suit these diverse individual needs. Even in the absence of established pathology, elderly people should be advised to have an eye examination at least once a year so that eye disease, which is often asymptomatic, may be detected and treated at the early stage, thereby preventing further vision loss and the associated negative impact on quality of life.

Refraction process in elderly population is by and large the same as the normal process of subjective refraction. However, the approach to refractive error assessment should be adopted with respect to their visual needs, ocular condition and reported symptoms of the individual. Based upon this philosophy the discussion with regard

to the approach to refraction procedure for older population may be grouped into two categories:
1. Routine geriatric refraction
2. Refraction in Visually impaired patients

Routine Geriatric Refraction

The opportunity to improve the day-to-day functional abilities of the elderly population through updating their lens prescription is very important as many of them may be asymptomatic or using the outdated lenses. In general the common reason why they seek eye examination is they want to read and watch television. The distance vision per se is not very significant for them. There are some who tests as because they need a change of spectacle either because the existing glasses have broken or for social reason. Accordingly, the battery of tests applied can be modified. In general, the following considerations are important while examining them for refractive error assessment:

- History taking is very important to understand their ocular and visual conditions, visual needs and expectations, general health, environment and social requirements.
- Measuring uncorrected visual acuity, acuity with existing correction and pinhole acuity is critical to set the goal together with the knowledge of existing correction and findings of objective measurement of refractive error.
- Trial and error method or manifest monocular subjective refraction is more appropriate than fogging method or cycloplegic refraction. This is because the effects of accommodation on refractive error measurement are minimal.
- The physiological changes in the eye suggest that just noticeable difference of the purpose of trial lens selection during subjective refraction should be slightly larger. The general assumption that is made during the course of subjective refraction for youths is that 0.50D of change produces an incremental change in acuity by one line. This may not be true in case of elderly population.
- Reaction time to stimulus changes is markedly increased among the elderly population. So it is important to allow a little extra time to elicit patient's response during subjective refraction.
- The duochrome test for spherical end point may not yield reliable results. This is because yellowing of crystalline lens in aging eyes tends to reduce transmission of shorter wavelength, which

may alter the subject's preference for one color. It may also be because of the fact that the visual acuity is not adequate to discern a difference. Yellowing of the lens causes a red shift, leading to under-plussing. Over 55 years of age, the chromatic aberration of the eye drops significantly because of which the dioptric interval of the red and green stimulus reduces, especially with a small pupil. Therefore, the test may be ineffective.

- ❖ Binocular balancing may not be fruitful for elderly population because of the no role of accommodation process after the age 60 years.
- ❖ A transient change in refraction may be noted due to changes in local or systemic causes, if any. Diabetes, hypertension and other systemic condition affects the eyes in more than one way.

Refraction in Visually Impaired Patients

Visual impaired population has been defined as the best corrected visual acuity worse than 20/40 but better than 20/200. Impaired visual acuity in elderly population is characterized by decreased clarity or sharpness of vision that may include reduced central visual acuity, reduced field of vision, poor contrast sensitivity and reduced color perception. **Table 21.3** shows the common aging ocular diseases. These impairments are coupled with the general visual loss seen due to simple aging in the form of loss of accommodation, poor binocular vision, poor low light vision, muscle weakness and increased glare recovery time. In many case the effect of one or more systemic diseases also adds to the reduced visual functioning.

Impaired visual acuity is consistently associated with decreased quality of life in older persons, including reduced ability to perform activities of daily living and work, reduced mobility that increases the risk of falls and other unintentional injuries. Since visual impaired

Table 21.3: Ocular diseases that are common because of aging.	
Common aging eye diseases	Impact
Maculopathy	Disease in the macular functioning that causes central vision loss
Cataracts	Clouding of the crystalline lens of the eye
Glaucoma	Rise in fluid pressure in the eye
Retinopathy	Disease in the retina often caused by diabetes or high blood pressure

patient tend to have high prevalence of uncorrected refractive error, a good refraction is likely to yield a substantial improvement in visual acuity and improve the quality of life.

Objective refraction either by retinoscopy or by autorefractometer may not be possible in many cases of media opacity, optical irregularities, and small pupil size. Therefore, subjective refraction is more important in such cases. Use of hand-held trial frame and trial lenses rather than phoropter is recommended as it allows eccentric head and eye position, most patient would like to acquire.

Significant refractive error in the form of high myopia, high hyperopia and high astigmatism may be associated with certain ocular condition which must be carefully measured. High astigmatism greater than 5.00 Dcyl is mostly a form of irregular astigmatism. The practitioner must be alert for these deviations from the routine norms in order to diagnose and manage the high ametropic patient.

Refraction in visually impaired patient is although a time taking procedure, but yields enormous satisfaction for both patient and practitioner. The patient gets what he could not get from many and the practitioner gets a job satisfaction of doing something great for someone which in turn is followed by lots of blessings for him. In this way a good refraction is in the best interest of the practitioner to look at the opportunity to differentiate his practice. He must approach every case of vision impairment as if the patient needs either +20.00D or –20.00D of spherical with 8.00D of cylinder lens and apply more dynamic methods. Repeated presentation to certain patient may be necessary to yield satisfactory results. It is quite likely that the practitioner would need to look at options beyond theoretical methods of general refraction procedure.

Though objective method of refraction does not provide satisfactory results, it can be used as a good starting point for the subjective refraction. Keratometer gives the insights of corneal irregularities and indication of the presence of a large amount of astigmatism that may be missed otherwise. This can be used even if the patient has nystagmus. The clinician should attempt to elicit a viewing posture that reduces or eliminates the nystagmoid eye movements and then measure corneal curvatures. Radical retinoscopy can be performed in situations where reflex cannot be observed due to media opacity. Autorefractometer may not work in many cases because of several reasons. Small pupils, inadequate fixation, opacities of ocular medias, corneal irregularities, and ametropia beyond the range of the equipment. The clinician should consider subjective refraction as the primary method for assessing refractive error. He has to be more dynamic and ready to try all usual and unusual processes. The idea is not to apply the methods of refraction but to elicit some clues on which a meaningful refraction can be performed.

Some of the unusual processes that can be undertaken effectively are:

Flexible Test Distance

Usually the refraction in case of patients with sub-normal vision is started with the fact that substantial vision cannot be improved even with correction. The approach needs to be changed and objective should be modified to measure the residual visual acuity so that it can be effectively used to ensure functional independence of the patient. All attempts are aimed to achieve even the slightest improvement in the acuity so that necessary way forward can be suggested. Standard test distance may not be very critical. The test charts may be kept at 3 meters distance, instead of 6 meters that provides relative distance magnification and enables the patient appreciate more lines on the chart. In case the patient is insensitive to lens changes at 3 meter distance, the test chart may be placed at 2 meters or even at 1 meter.

Changing Illumination

Proper illumination is necessary for visually impaired patients. Light should be adjusted on the printed charts and should not shine on the subject's eyes. Entire test chart should be uniformly illuminated to minimize the effect of glare. Besides room light should have rheostat to allow changing room illumination that is comfortable to the patient. Reducing room illumination often improves the comfort and response of achromats and other light sensitive patients during refraction and provides better visual acuity.

Use of Halberg Trial Clip

Halberg clip (**Fig. 21.1**) is a very useful monocular trial frame. It can be used for over refraction in conjunction with the patient's own spectacle frame. Halberg clips are either two cell or three cell trial lens holder that can be attached to the patient's spectacle. With the Halberg clip, the clinician perform an over refraction to determine the amount of lens power that needs to be added to the existing

Chapter 21: The Geriatric Refraction

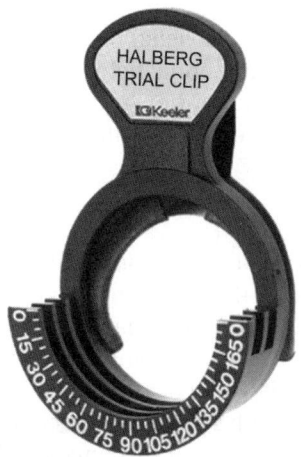

Fig. 21.1: Halberg trial clip.

correction to decide the actual full refractive correction. When the Halberg clip refraction is completed, it often happens that the axis of cylinder in the over refraction does not coincide with the cylinder axis in the existing correction. All that is needed is to take the spectacle with the over refraction lenses and place on the lensmeter, where back vertex power of the combination can be measured. The measurement gives the full refractive correction. Halberg refraction is very valuable especially in case of high lens prescription and also in cases where only subtle improvement in acuity is recorded with substantial change in refractive error.

Stenopeic Slit

Stenopaic slit determines the refractive error in each of the meridians individually. The care must be taken to decide the axis of cylinder correction as the patient's choice of the slit position may not always identify the axis of astigmatic correction especially in visually impaired patients. In some patient it may represent an area of unobstructed vision. It should be clearly understood that the slit is helpful only as a guide to the subjective refraction.

Application of Contact Lenses

Contact lenses are often of great value in improving the acuity of the people with distorted corneas, and high refractive errors.

Contact lenses are particularly important for people with high refractive error and reduced visual fields. Such people must scan to realize a meaningful functional field; if they have to scan behind a thick corrective lens, they either suffer from the lens aberrations or scan by moving their head to maintain their visual fields in clear part.

Use of Prism Lenses

The average subject's accommodation declines so that in the late 50's an addition of more than +2.50 D often becomes necessary. It is to be remembered that near point closer than 28 cm is rarely acceptable for regular wear. Therefore, when demand for fine work requires higher addition than +3.00 D, it would be prudent to add convergence with base in prism together with spherical correction. Prism will help the subject maintain convergence for sustained period of time and make reading easy.

During subjective refraction procedure in geriatric patients the clinician often frustrates when they notice that in spite their hard effort, the visual acuity does not improve. In such situation they can take the help of some screening test using simple tools and without having the need to refer to understand the possibility of improvement in visual acuity and adjust their expectations with regard to end result of the refraction procedure and make necessary recommendations to the patients. Some of the tests that they can use for the purpose are listed below:

Use of Maddox Rod

Maddox rod can be used as a simple test of macular function in patients who do not have totally opaque ocular media. Maddox rod is held in front of the eye to be tested and the light source is held approximately 14 inches or 35 cm away. If the patient observes an unbroken red line, the clinician may assume the macular integrity. On the other hand if the patient observes a discontinuity in red line, it may represent the presence of large scotoma and raise the possibility of macular disease.

Use of Photostress Test

The test can be used during routine examination to differentiate between macular or optic nerve pathology by shining light on pupil using ophthalmoscope. Photostress test is a gross test of dark adaptation in which the visual pigments are bleached by light. This causes a temporary state of retinal insensitivity perceived as scotoma by the patient. The recovery of vision is dependent on the ability of photoreceptors to re-synthesize visual pigments. In normal patients the recovery time is 15–30 seconds. Increased recovery time beyond 30 seconds is indicative of macular disease.

Use of Pinhole Test

The pinhole occluder works by reducing the amount of light that enters the eye and increasing the depth of focus. The subject looks through the hole at the distance object and the clarity of the image is noted which can help the clinician to continue trying for improvement or abandoning the further effort. Pinhole also be used as two point discrimination test to assess the macular functioning using two pinholes. The patient is asked to look through two pinholes (2 mm diameter) behind which a light is held. The holes are held two inches apart at a distance of 2 feet from the eye. If the patient can perceive two lights, it implies macular functioning is normal.

PRESCRIBING CORRECTION

While in younger and adult population the correction is prescribed to treat the symptoms, the geriatric vision correction is more driven by patient satisfaction. The visual satisfaction transpires when an individual develops a positive feeling with his correction, he is able to cope with his most visual needs unconsciously and comfortably for a sustained period of time. This may have specific requirements at home or at work or have general requirements in terms of navigating through the life.

Symptoms presented are varied and nothing much can be done for many of them by refractive correction. In great majority of cases refractive correction is prescribed to improve the functional vision, rather than visual acuity. This is because some patients over the age of 60 years lose sight beyond normal because of the cumulative effect of age-related changes and changes because of aging ocular disease. And it becomes impossible to improve visual acuity in such cases. Therefore, counseling together with prescription plays an important role for visual satisfaction of the elderly population.

In general the decision for prescribing refractive correction is driven by multiple considerations; some of them are listed below:

❖ The results of the objective correction may be prescribed in some cases.
❖ Trial framing may be done and the patient may be asked to choose the best correction for him.
❖ The refractive correction may be altered even if the visual acuity does not improve as measured on test chart but yield increased satisfaction in terms of functional vision.
❖ While prescribing near vision correction convergence may be added with plus spherical to improve reading stamina.
❖ Often in the practice it is possible that the patient is over misused, the clinician may keep the prescription same, because of the fear of blur experience if the minus correction is reduced if the patient is not symptomatic. However, if the patient reports symptoms of asthenopia or headache, the clinician may reduce minus with sufficient explanation to the patient for such decision.
❖ Sometimes the clinician prescribes a correction simply using his intuitions because he feels it right. It is true that intuitions can be fallible; it prompts further thinking and action. Pairing gut feeling with analytical thinking helps in better decision making. However, only an experienced practitioner can do it with great grit.

MULTIPLE CHOICE QUESTIONS

1. **Which of the following is not a normal physiological change that is being observed in the aging eyes?**
   a. Loss of accommodation
   b. Reduced transmittance of ocular media
   c. Pupillary miosis
   d. Rise in fluid pressure in the eye
2. **Accommodation is maximum at the age _____ and is nearly over at the age _____.**
   a. 5 years, 60 years
   b. 18 years, 65 years
   c. 10 years, 70 years
   d. 21 years, 75 years
3. **Which of the following is not correct with regard to duochrome test for elderly population?**
   a. Yellowing of crystalline lens causes a red shift, may lead to under-plusing

Chapter 21: The Geriatric Refraction

    b. Over 55 years of age, the chromatic aberration of the eye drops markedly, so the dioptric interval of the red and green reduces, especially with a small pupil

    c. Duochrome test for spherical end point yields reliable results in all cases of elderly population

    d. The duochrome test is not used with patients whose visual acuity is worse than 6/9, because the 0.50 D difference between the two sides is too small to distinguish

4. **Which of the following statement about geriatric vision is not correct?**
   a. Hyperopic shifts in refraction have been consistently reported in adults over 40, followed by myopic shifts after age 70
   b. A shift occurs from with the rule astigmatism in youth to against the rule astigmatism in old age population
   c. Anisometropia appears to increase with aging
   d. A poor vision in any of the eyes is always the result of amblyopia

5. **Which of the following statement is not correct about aging changes in the human eyes?**
   a. Arcus senilis appears as a gray-white ring at the edge of the cornea. It is common among people older than 60. Arcus senilis does not affect vision
   b. The muscles that work to regulate the size of the pupils weaken with age. The pupils become smaller, react more sluggishly to light, and dilate more slowly in the dark
   c. Thinning of the conjunctiva
   d. Thickening of the conjunctiva

6. **With aging the visual efficiency of the individual reduces, which of the following statement is incorrect in this regard?**
   a. Older people take more time to recognize objects and focus on object at different distances
   b. Moving objects are harder to see
   c. Smooth visual tracking improves
   f. Color sensitivity diminishes

7. **Photo stress test is performed to diagnose**
   a. Macular disease
   b. Optic nerve diseases
   c. Glaucoma
   d. Nerve conduction

8. **Why do we say that carrying out clinical refraction procedure in visually impaired patient is very challenging?**
    a. Objective refraction does not provide appropriate results
    b. Presence of media opacities, scotoma and optical irregularities
    c. Pupil size and location
    d. All of the above
9. **Which of the following statement is incorrect with respect to aging eyes?**
    a. Loss of cells in the ganglion layer and retinal pigment epithelial
    b. Meibomian gland dysfunction
    c. Increased blood flow in retina
    d. Loss of endothelial cell count
10. **Which of the following is the most common cause of cataracts?**
    a. Congenital
    b. Aging
    c. Trauma
    d. Uncontrolled blood glucose levels
11. **Which of the following condition is associated with the development of cataracts?**
    a. Loss of central vision
    b. Loss of peripheral vision
    c. Cloudy, hazy vision
    d. Black spots in vision

ANSWER KEY

1. d	2. a	3. c	4. d	5. d	6. c	7. a	8. d
9. c	10. b	11. c					

SELF-PRACTICE QUESTIONS

1. Describe the retinal changes that happen due to aging.
2. Why visual efficiency reduces in elderly population?
3. Explain the criticalities involved in the assessment of refractive error of visually impaired elderly population?
4. A 75-year-old male patient visits your clinic for visual disturbances produced by his spectacle. You examine and noticed that there is no change in refraction and you also noticed that his existing spectacle lenses are full of scratches and therefore you advise to change the spectacle lenses. But the patient says that whenever he changes

Chapter 21: The Geriatric Refraction

his spectacle lenses he has lots of difficulties and finds it difficult to adjust with the same. How would you like to manage?

5. A 70-year-old male patient is in your clinic for refraction. While doing subjective refraction you start feeling frustrations as because the visual acuity is not improving beyond 6/12 and the patient's inconsistent response is also confusing. How would you like to deal with the situation?
6. A 75-year-old patient who had been using only near vision glasses for many years finds that his near vision glasses are no more working for him and he can read without glasses better than with glasses? What could be the probable reasons?

CHAPTER 22

Refraction for Sports Athletes

CHAPTER OUTLINE

- Importance of Good Refraction in Sports
- Consideration for Prescribing Correction

Sports are highly visually demanding occupation. The significance of good vision cannot be overstated, as athletes rely on their eyes to swiftly fixate on targets, predict trajectories, make split-second decisions, and react promptly. Research underscores that even a minor uncorrected refractive error in one eye has the potential to profoundly impact an athlete's performance. Clear and accurate vision stands as the cornerstone of sporting excellence. In fact, nothing affects performance more than the ability to see clearly and correctly.

In the fiercely competitive world of sports, where the margin between success and failure is razor-thin, the eyes play a pivotal role in differentiating between a good player and a great one. Whether it is tracking a flying ball, returning a serve, making a crucial pass, or aiming to hit the ball, the eyes lead, and the body follows suit. In this high-stakes environment, where a single mistake or delayed reaction can jeopardize an entire sporting career, vision becomes the elusive factor that can elevate an athlete's prowess.

It takes the split second to sustain a potentially career ending injury. Athletes navigate dynamic and unpredictable environments, where hazards, opponents, or obstacles can emerge suddenly. Rapid visual processing enables athletes to perceive potential dangers, allowing them to take evasive action and make split-second decisions to avoid collisions. Any delay or impairment in visual perception during these critical moments can have severe consequences, including sustaining a career-ending injury.

While physical conditioning and mental toughness are acknowledged as vital components of athletic success, the importance of vision is often overlooked. Physical dominance makes an athlete good, mental toughness may make them great, but it is clear vision that can render them unstoppable. Despite the meticulous attention given to physical training and mental fortitude, the role of vision in sports is not always duly recognized. The truth is if you can not see it, you can hit it.

Hence, the goal of vision correction for sports athletes diverges from that of the general population. The primary focus is to evaluate players and athletes for their visual efficiency, establishing it as directly linked to their sporting performance. The objective is to discern the specific visual challenges impacting their abilities and determine the reasons for vision correction with the ultimate aim of enhancing their performance on the field.

IMPORTANCE OF GOOD REFRACTION IN SPORTS

Good refraction is indeed the cornerstone of optimal visual performance. Unless visual acuity is maximized during the refraction process, the subsequent steps in dispensing corrective measures lose their significance. This becomes especially critical when there is an intensified pressure of excessive visual demands on the visual system, such as those encountered in sports or other visually demanding activities. As a general rule, it is advisable to first prescribe for any significant refractive error because improper correction of refractive error:

- ❖ Result in either under or over-accommodation, resulting in disorders of accommodative functions. Such disorders can hinder an athlete's ability to focus on dynamic and rapidly changing visual stimuli, affecting their overall performance.
- ❖ Results in a high phoria and demands unusual negative or positive fusional vergence. This may affect an athlete's ability to maintain binocular vision and coordinate eye movements effectively, which is essential for activities requiring precision and accuracy.

- Creates an imbalance between the two eyes, leading to sensory fusion disturbances. Maintaining proper alignment and coordination is crucial for optimal visual performance, and disruptions can hinder an athlete's ability to perform at their best.
- Creates decreased fusional ability as a result of blurred retinal images. Reduced ability to fuse images can compromise an athlete's overall visual function, affecting their ability to process visual information accurately.

Even the small degree of refractive error may become a significant for someone. Therefore, the practitioner must take this decision based on additional testing and analysis of accommodative and binocular vision function so that he can answer whether the refractive error is the cause of the poor visual performance. This involves a more nuanced and holistic approach to vision care.

Two scenarios generally exist:
1. First, the athlete may present with significant accommodative and binocular vision problems. In such a situation, the low refractive error becomes significant as it will improve fusion and assist in management.
2. Another possible situation may be a patient with low refractive error, and all the accommodative and binocular testing results are within expected values. In this case, the practitioner may be left with no other possible visual basis for the patient's discomfort and must make a decision about prescribing the low refractive error. Experience shows that there is often an accommodative, ocular motor, or binocular vision disorder present in addition to low refractive error. It is very unusual to find a low refractive error in isolation that accounts for significant symptoms.

All myopic refractive errors, even 0.50D should be considered for correction in sports. Correction of 0.50D or more of anisometropia should be contemplated, especially if it requires accurate depth perception. In addition the effect of meridional anisometropia should be considered in athletes with asymmetric astigmatism. Correction of hypermetropia over 1.00D can alleviate fatigue, particularly in sports requiring sustained visual attention at the middle of the target. Astigmatism of more than 0.50D may reduce contrast and therefore should be considered. A young sport person with a little over minus correction will provide maximum distance visual acuity, albeit at the expense of having to exert a minor accommodative effort.

Chapter 22: Refraction for Sports Athletes

Once the full refraction is known, then refinements can be made, depending upon the visual need of the sport. A task analysis of the sport will assist in determining the specific visual demands and a careful refractive analysis can establish the best refractive compensation for use in that sport. For example, a myopic baseball player may be benefitted from an additional 0.25D of minus to improve contrast when playing in twilight conditions. Billiards has specific viewing distances that should be considered, especially for presbyopic athletes. Billiard's players often use single vision intermediate distance prescription for use during play. In sports like tennis where near visual acuity has minimal impact on performance, prescription of near addition may be avoided. In Golf also near visual acuity does not affect performance, however, clear vision is desirable for seeing the score card and identifying one's ball during the play. Such prescription becomes sports specific and is not prescribed for general use.

The toughest challenge for refractive error correction is created by shooters. Rifle shooters requires that the shooters clearly focus the target at far distance while carefully aligning the front and rear sights of the rifle with the target. There are four things in this equation—the aiming eye, the rear sight, front sight, and the target. The participant peeps through the sights, and sees three circles. He has to align these circles concentrically with the target in the middle. It is very important to have a clear picture of the sights than the target in rifle shooting. Once the sights have stabilized, pressure must be applied to the trigger to release the shot.

Pistol shooters are particularly affected by presbyopia because the front and rear sights must be aligned with the target with extreme precision. Front sight is positioned at an intermediate distance from the eyes and the difference in accommodative demand between sights and the far target creates significant blur for one distance when focusing at the other. The pistol shooters often want solution that provides image clarity at both the distances. Pistol shooters need a clear picture of sight. They require more additional plus power than rifle shooters. Younger shooter should be given little less near additional plus power so that they can also use the accommodation while keeping enough in reserve to avoid eye fatigue. The correction should be prescribed with an executive bifocal which will not induce image jump.

CONSIDERATION FOR PRESCRIBING CORRECTION

The following important consideration must be kept in mind while doing refraction for athletes and players:

- Even the smallest amount of refractive error must be corrected. In visually demanding occupation like sports, small amount of uncorrected myopia affects the visual performance. The visual system detects the blur and is left with no other option but to accommodate which effectively make them more myopic.
- In case of uncorrected low astigmatism, the visual system is in flux looking for a point focus and potentially causing a degree of accommodative spasm which ultimately makes it more difficult to relax accommodation sufficiently.
- Care must be taken while doing refraction in amblyopic eye. Peripheral awareness in this eye can be as good as other eye and uncorrected hypermetropia may have effect on the other eye and muscle balance between the two eyes.
- In squinting eyes, the abnormal retinal correspondence will contribute to a degree of depth perception which may be enhanced by same consideration as above.
- Refinement is very critical in sports vision refraction. Once the subjective refraction is determined, it is important to provide allowance for the required distance. For example, in shooting the athletes already have good acuity. Leaving them with correction at 6 meters will not give them sufficient flexibility and control at greater distance. It should also be remembered that in competitive situation, huge level of adrenaline will give them additional energy to accommodation that may not be seen during consulting room examination.
- The oculomotor balance may be affected by refraction. Uncorrected hyperopia can induce decompensated esophoria. Undercorrected myopia may force an athlete to go into overdrive searching for clear focus. The effect of overcorrection may be influenced by relationship between accommodation and vergence function which may vary from one person to another.

The mechanics of refraction applied is also extremely important, for example, binocular balancing and accurate testing of fixation disparity should be routinely practiced in sport-vision practice. Advice on refractive error cannot be given unless you know the dominant eye and which sport they particularly favor. This information is to be

Chapter 22: Refraction for Sports Athletes

kept in mind throughout the whole procedure. Peripheral awareness which is maximized by using high curve lenses and contact lenses can also be affected by residual uncorrected refractive error which will tend to diminish visual performance and eventually will make the athlete less peripherally aware.

MULTIPLE CHOICE QUESTIONS

1. **What is the main objective of sports vision assessment?**
   a. To examine the eyes and give them the appropriate lens prescription
   b. To elicit the ocular disorders and suggest a treatment plan
   c. To assess the visual system comprehensively, link the elements of the visual system to visual performance in the given sport and demonstrate how visual performance is affecting his sporting performance
   d. To examine the eye using most modern gadgets

2. **If refractive error is not fully corrected, it may lead to:**
   a. Either under or over accommodation
   b. Unusual demand of either negative or positive fusional vergence
   c. Decreased fusional ability as a result of blurred retinal images
   d. All of the above

3. **In which of the following sports near visual acuity does not affect sporting performance so much?**
   a. Golf
   b. Snooker
   c. Tennis
   d. Cricket

4. **A steady dominant eye is important:**
   a. To hold the visual system steady at the fixating target
   b. To enable the athlete to see the target more clearly
   c. To prevent the eyes from fatigue
   d. None of the above

ANSWER KEY

| 1. c | 2. d | 3. a | 4. a |

SELF-PRACTICE QUESTIONS

1. How can uncorrected refractive errors impact an athlete's ability to make split-second decisions in sports?
2. Do you believe that vision receives enough emphasis in sports training? Why or why not? How might awareness of the importance of vision be increased in the sports community?

23 CHAPTER

Refraction in Nonadaptation Cases

CHAPTER OUTLINE

- Importance of Effective Handling
- Psychological Condition of the Patient
- Goal of Re-evaluating Refraction in Cases of Nonadaptation
- Flow of Re-evaluating the Refraction

It is a truth that if you are a regular practitioner, you will occasional have unhappy patients who may need your help. Far-sighted practitioners have a well-defined plan to handle such cases that enables them not only to reduce the occurrence but also ameliorate their own pain as well as the pain of the patient.

IMPORTANCE OF EFFECTIVE HANDLING

Effectively managing cases of nonadaptation is crucial due to the unique challenges they present. These situations demand a distinctive approach since the patient not only faces difficulties but is also discontented, having lost trust in your practice. They are also under uncertainty about receiving good care and attention.

Addressing each such case may require 30–40 minutes of the clinical time, with some vehemently unhappy patients necessitating even more. This represents a loss for the practice. Moreover, navigating this colossal challenge often seems obscured, but an organized evaluation process may bring in good results. It assists the clinician in identifying the source of the problem and find appropriate solution, rebuilding trust, and working towards effective solutions.

Chapter 23: Refraction in Nonadaptation Cases

The significance lies not just in resolving the individual case but in preserving the reputation and overall success of the practice.

PSYCHOLOGICAL CONDITION OF PATIENT

The patient presenting with nonadaptation exhibits distinct behavioral patterns influenced by their emotional state. They express concerns about potential errors in their responses during the refraction process and harbor worries about the financial implications of having their glasses remade. These apprehensions contribute to a negative perception of both the practice and the practitioner, fostering emotions of anger and dissatisfaction that hinder rational behavior.

Effectively addressing these negative emotions is paramount, as mishandling can exacerbate the situation. The clinician's interaction becomes a pivotal factor in shaping the patient's perception—whether as an excellent, caring professional or as an insensitive practitioner undeserving of their trust.

Recognizing and understanding the patient's psychological condition is foundational in handling such cases successfully. Tailoring interactions and responses based on this understanding lays the groundwork for a positive resolution and the restoration of patient trust in the practitioner and the practice.

GOAL OF RE-EVALUATING REFRACTION IN CASES OF NONADAPTATION

The process of re-evaluating refraction in instances of non-adaptation encompasses a comprehensive examination aimed at uncovering the reasons behind the patient's struggles with the prescribed optical correction. Beyond addressing immediate concerns, the broader goals include rebuilding trust and collaboratively working towards a resolution.

It is essential to bear in mind that the purpose of refractive correction is to enhance vision, and its sustained use relies on the patient's comfort. A positive association with the correction develops when the individual can seamlessly integrate it into their daily activities, meeting occupational needs effortlessly and maintaining comfort over an extended period.

Success in this process lies in keeping the overarching goal in mind at every stage of re-evaluation, emphasizing a patient-centric approach and fostering an environment conducive to achieving lasting visual comfort and satisfaction.

FLOW OF RE-EVALUATING THE REFRACTION

Navigating the challenging task of re-evaluating refraction demands a structured approach for clinicians to pinpoint the root cause of the patient's struggles with the prescribed optical correction. A systematic evaluation becomes the cornerstone; empowering clinicians to unravel the complexities associated with nonadaptation cases and elevate the overall patient experience.

Commencing with patient counseling which includes assuring and reassuring the subject for utmost care, rather than traditional history-taking, becomes a prudent initial step. This form of counseling distinguishes itself from the typical clinical refraction process, requiring an abundance of patience. In this scenario, it is crucial to shed the authoritative demeanor, prioritize the patient's comfort, assure them of a resolution, allow them ample time to express themselves, and listen attentively. The cumulative impact of these initial actions is profound, often leading to a noticeable cooling down of the patient and a willingness to collaborate in finding solutions. Law 2 of clinical refraction says that the clinician must think beyond the paradigm of the routine process and drive all the tests and procedures to alleviate the patient's complaints and restore their lost confidence.

When considering the flow of re-evaluating refraction, particularly in cases of non-adaptation with spectacles, the approach may deviate slightly from the conventional clinical refraction flow, as illustrated in Graph 1. Our focus here will be specifically on cases related to non-adaptation with spectacles.

STEP 1: Entrance tests
- Counseling
- History taking
- Measuring visual acuity with spectacle
- Rechecking the spectacle lens
- Reassessing the spectacle frame fitting

STEP 2: Core tests
- Objective refraction
- Subjective refraction
- Near addition assessment

- Ruling out the impact of muscle imbalance
- Ruling out underlying condition

STEP 3: Refinement
- Trial framing

STOP: Represcribe and recounsel

Counseling

Counseling is the initial step in the re-evaluation process. Begin by creating a comfortable environment for the patient and encourage them to share their concerns. As the patient speaks, maintain active and attentive listening, interpreting their words to comprehend the underlying issues. Patients may struggle to articulate their problems precisely, so the clinician should work to discern the actual problem through careful interpretation. This step is pivotal in helping the patient regain a sense of assurance and establishes a foundation for collaborative efforts.

History-taking

History-taking for nonadaptation cases deviates from the routine clinical refraction process, requiring clinicians to ask pertinent questions to navigate the intricacies of the situation. The following set of questions is tailored to uncover crucial information:
- What specific challenges are you facing with your glasses?
- Is this the first instance of encountering such an issue, or have you experienced it before?
- How long have you been using the new spectacles up to today?
- Has the intensity of your difficulty remained consistent since you started using them?
- Have there been any changes in your lens or frame type? Was this a personal choice or a recommendation from someone?
- Do you notice any alterations in your difficulty when adjusting the position of your spectacles on your face or changing your posture?

These questions are designed to align with the goal of re-evaluating the prescribed refractive correction, aiming to gather information that helps identify the source of the patient's nonadaptation.

Measuring Visual Acuity with Spectacle

The subsequent step involves assessing visual acuity using Snellen's test chart with the prescribed spectacles. Examine visual acuity both monocularly and binocularly. Also change the vertex distance of the

Chapter 23: Refraction in Nonadaptation Cases

spectacle lens and carefully observe the changes in visual acuity. Extend the assessment beyond the clinical setting by evaluating vision in real-world environments outside the clinic. Encourage the patient to engage in various activities such as looking around, walking, and observing the floor, noting their perceptions of vision. Inquire about overall visual comfort during these activities. While rechecking visual acuity, it is crucial to keenly observe the visual postures the patient adopts to respond. This observation can provide valuable insights into how the patient is experiencing and adapting to their corrected vision.

Rechecking the Spectacle Lens

The next step involves a systematic recheck of the spectacle lens. Ensure the lens power aligns with the prescribed values using a lensmeter. Use a base measure watch to verify the base curve of the spectacle lenses. Examine the horizontal and vertical positioning of the optical center, confirming its alignment with the patient's interpupillary distance measurement and fitting height. Re-evaluate the lens material, design, and tints. Discomfort may also be linked to the lens prescribed. Additionally, compare these measurements with data from the patient's previous spectacles, if applicable, and make note of any deviations. This thorough re-evaluation ensures that the prescribed correction aligns with correctly with what was prescribed and measured as dispensing measurement.

Re-checking Spectacle Frame Fitting

The next step involves a meticulous re-check of the spectacle frame fitting. Place the frame on the wearer's face and carefully assess the overall fitting. It is essential to ensure that the spectacle frame sits squarely on the patient's face as it directly impacts the on-eye effectiveness of the prescribed correction as well as comfort. This evaluation should be conducted with attention to detail, following a sequential order to prevent any oversights. Refer **Figure 23.1** for the recommended sequential steps in assessing the spectacle fitting on the patient's face.

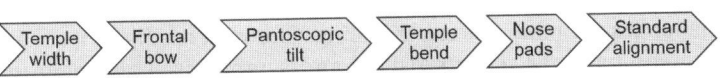

Fig. 23.1: Sequential steps of assessing fitting on patient's face.

Refining the fitting includes fine-tuning nose pads, considering the frontal angle, splay angle, and vertical angle of the nose pads. Additionally, compare the frame fitting with that of the patient's previous spectacle frame, if applicable, to identify any variations. This comprehensive assessment ensures that the spectacle frame not only provides the prescribed correction but also fits comfortably and effectively on the patient's face.

> It is crucial to bear in mind that a spectacle represents a symbiotic relationship between the lens and the frame. Viewing cases of nonadaptation should always involve considering the spectacle as a cohesive unit, rather than isolating the frame or lens individually. Whether the issue pertains to vision, comfort, or overall satisfaction, a holistic approach that encompasses both lens and frame is essential for a comprehensive understanding and resolution of nonadaptation challenges.

Observing the clinician at work instils a sense of confidence in the patient, encouraging active participation. Seizing this opportune moment, the clinician should actively engage the patient in the process, encouraging them to move forward and proceed with core tests.

Objective Refraction

Objective refraction involves performing retinoscopy over the patient's spectacles to gain insights into the correction. Furthermore, utilizing a keratometer can help estimate the approximate amount of cylinder correction, providing an opportunity for cross-check with the results obtained from an autorefractometer. This comprehensive approach ensures a thorough examination of the patient's refractive status, allowing for a more accurate assessment and refinement of the prescribed correction.

Subjective Refraction

Selecting the appropriate method for subjective refraction in non-adaptation cases is paramount to gather accurate and pertinent information. The choice should be tailored to address the specific challenges the patient is experiencing. Choose a method that aligns with the patient's reported signs and symptoms. This ensures a more targeted and effective subjective refraction process. In certain situations, binocular subjective refraction may be preferred over manifest monocular subjective refraction. This choice depends on the individual patient's needs and visual symptoms. The fogging method of subjective refraction proves effective in cases of latent hypermetropia, excessive accommodation in young patients, patients experiencing asthenopic symptoms, suspected over minus correction, cases of ocular deviation, and amblyopia. Consider delayed subjective refraction when accommodative spasm is suspected. Stenopeic slit is particularly useful in high astigmatic cases, providing a focused and precise evaluation of refractive errors. By aligning the choice of subjective refraction method with the patient's unique characteristics and reported issues, clinicians can enhance the accuracy of the refractive assessment, ultimately contributing to more effective vision correction. Lastly, the technique of over-refraction using a Halberg clip proves to be a valuable method for assessing the need for a change in correction. This approach involves placing the Halberg clip over the patient's existing correction to refine and fine-tune the prescription, ensuring optimal visual clarity and comfort.

> Spherical correction can be measured using multiple tests like Bichrome Tests, Subjective Method, Retinoscopy, Autorefractometer, Stenopeic slit.
> Astigmatic correction can be measured using Stenopeic slit, Jackson cross cylinder, Fan and block test chart, Dr Pray's Astigmatic Letters, Keratometer, Retinoscopy, Autorefractometer.

Near Addition Tests

Precision in prescribing near addition is paramount, and it should be based solely on the patient's needs rather than any other factor. Some practitioners may suggest higher additions for progressive addition lenses and slightly lower additions for other lenses, but this approach is not correct. Clinicians must always prioritize meeting the specific needs of the individual patient, irrespective of the lens type.

It is crucial to emphasize that prescribing a higher near addition not only deviates from the patient's specific needs but can also have repercussions on the design and efficacy of progressive lenses, potentially leading to adverse effects. As a result, clinicians should approach near addition tests with meticulous attention to the individual patient's visual needs only. Various tests can be employed to assess the appropriate near addition:

Subjective Refraction at Near

Utilizes subjective feedback to fine-tune the prescription for optimal near vision.

Near Duochrome Test

Evaluates near vision clarity and accommodative lag using a duochrome test.

Cross Grid Test

Assesses the patient's ability to maintain fusion and clear vision at near distances.

Amplitude of Accommodation

Measures the range of clear vision from distance to near, providing insights into accommodative capacity.

Balanced Range of Accommodation

Evaluates the patient's ability to maintain clear vision within a balanced range at various distances.

Additionally, conducting an over-refraction can further contribute to understanding the necessity for changes in the near addition. This comprehensive approach ensures that the near addition is precisely tailored to the patient's unique visual requirements, promoting optimal comfort and performance.

Ruling Out Muscle Imbalance

Finally, in cases of nonadaptation, re-examination should encompass a thorough assessment of muscle balance. If any imbalance is detected, the clinician may recommend the use of prism or prescribe orthoptic exercises as part of the intervention strategy.

Ruling Out Underlying Condition

Ruling out underlying conditions is imperative, and the examiner must be meticulous in ensuring that any potential diseases are thoroughly eliminated during routine examination. In cases where reading difficulties persist despite appropriate optical correction, it is essential to investigate whether the cause could be related to defects in the visual field or potential alexic or dyslexic anomalies. Excluding the presence of any underlying eye conditions is crucial for addressing nonadaptation. Conditions such as dry eye syndrome, ocular surface issues, or undetected pathology can significantly impact adaptation and must be considered in the diagnostic process.

Trial Framing

In cases of nonadaptation, the process of trial framing is essential for refining the correction in a real-world environment. The clinician should allocate ample time for the patient to wear the trial frame, observe, and provide feedback. This patient-centered approach ensures a thorough evaluation of the prescribed correction in the context of the patient's daily activities, enhancing the accuracy of the final prescription.

Represcribe and Recounsel

Finally, following a thorough examination and assessment, represcribe the correction based on the findings. The prescription may either remain the same or be adjusted as necessary. It is crucial to recounsel the patient, taking into consideration the challenges associated with correction, which are also influenced by the tasks the eyes are engaged in, and his visual environment. When diagnosing the reasons behind the condition, it is vital to acknowledge that comfort is a subjective experience that is not easily measured objectively. The patient's perception of comfort depends on the absence of bothersome factors and the presence of conditions conducive to smooth visual function.

Understanding the patient's psychology is paramount in the treatment of such cases. Individuals may adapt to new corrections in diverse ways, with some smoothly adjusting over time, while others may exhibit irrational behavior, expressing difficulties in using the new correction. Emphasizing the importance of adaptation and addressing any concerns or misconceptions is crucial. Patient understanding and cooperation play a pivotal role in successful adaptation. Clinical refraction serves as an opportunity for the practitioner to communicate effectively and address any psychological or emotional factors influencing nonadaptation.

This comprehensive approach ensures that the patient not only receives an accurate prescription but is also supported in the adaptation process, taking into account both optical and psychological aspects.

MULTIPLE CHOICE QUESTIONS

1. **What is the primary objective of re-evaluating refraction in cases of nonadaptation?**
   a. To prescribe higher additions
   b. To assess near vision only
   c. To identify reasons for difficulty in adapting
   d. To exclude subjective feedback
2. **What is crucial in ensuring successful adaptation in non-adaptation cases?**
   a. Ignoring patient concerns
   b. Rapidly changing prescriptions
   c. Patient understanding and cooperation
   d. Prescribing higher near additions
3. **What is the primary purpose of trial framing in nonadaptation cases?**
   a. To measure visual acuity
   b. To refine correction in real-world conditions
   c. To check eye muscle balance
   d. To assess ocular surface issues
4. **What test is useful in cases of high astigmatism for measuring astigmatic correction?**
   a. Stenopeic slit
   b. Cross grid test
   c. Near duochrome test
   d. Retinoscopy

ANSWER KEY

| 1. c | 2. c | 3. b | 4. a |

SELF-PRACTICE QUESTIONS

1. Provide a step-by-step guide on how a clinician should approach the re-evaluation of refraction in cases of nonadaptation.
2. Explain the importance of habitual correction while dealing with the cases of nonadaptation.

Bibliography

1. Akpek EK, Smith RA. Overview of age-related ocular conditions. Am J Manag Care. 2013;19(5 Suppl):S67-75.
2. Aronson JK. Ten principles of good prescribing. Available at https://www.cebm.ox.ac.uk/resources/top-tips/ten-principles-of-good-prescribing
3. Benjamin WJ. Borish's clinical refraction, 2nd edition, 2006.
4. Bennett CR, Bex PJ, Bauer CM, Merabet LB. The assessment of visual function and functional vision. Semin Pediatr Neurol. 2019 ;31:30-40.
5. Carlson NB, Kurtz D, Clinical procedures for ocular examination, 3rd edition, 2004.
6. Corboy JM, Norath DJ, Reffner R. The retinoscopy book: an introductory manual for eye care professionals, 4th edition, Jaypee Brothers Medical Publisher.
7. Fannin TE, Grosvenor T, Clinical optics, 1st edition, 1987.
8. Gittings NS, Fozard JL. Age related changes in visual acuity. Exp Gerontol. 1986;21(4-5):423-33.
9. Griffiths G. A strategy for sports vision assessment. Available at http://www.sportvision.co.uk/pdf/articlestrategy.pdf,
10. Griffiths G. Eye dominance in sport: a comparative. Available at https://www.sportvision.co.uk/assets/pdf/articleeyedominance.pdf
11. Griffiths G. The incidence of ametropia in elite sport. Available at https://www.sportvision.co.uk/assets/pdf/articleametropia.pdf
12. Harrington S. A protocol for the measurement of eye dominance in young children.
13. Jackson GR, Owsley C, McGwin G Jr. Aging and dark adaptation. Vision Res. 1999 ;39(23):3975-82.
14. Kerr DA. Trial lenses in vision correction. By Available at http://dougkerr.net/Pumpkin/articles/Trial_Lenses.pdf
15. Khurana AK, Khurana I. Anatomy and physiology of Eye, 1st Edition,1998.
16. Khurana AK. Theory and practice of optics and refraction, 2nd edition, 2008.

17. Lee L, Burnett AM, D'Esposito F, Fricke T, Nguyen LT, Vuong DA. Indicators for assessing the quality of refractive error care. Optom Vis Sci. 2021;98(1):24-31.
18. Lieberman JA 3rd, Stuart MR. The BATHE method: incorporating counseling and psychotherapy into the everyday management of patients. Prim Care Companion J Clin Psychiatry. 1999;1(2):35-38.
19. Lin G, Al Ani R, Niechwiej-Szwedo E. Age-related deficits in binocular vision are associated with poorer inhibitory control in healthy older adults. Front Neurosci. 2020;14:605267.
20. MacRae SM, Krueger RR, Applegate RA. Customized corneal ablation: the quest for supervision, 1st edition, 2001.
21. Michael R, Bron AJ. The ageing lens and cataract: a model of normal and pathological ageing. Philos Trans R Soc Lond B Biol Sci. 2011;366(1568):1278-92.
22. Musa MJ, Zeppieri M. Principles and Technique of Fogging During Subjective Refraction. [Updated 2023 Jul 19]. In: StatPearls [Internet]. Treasure Island (FL): StatPearls Publishing; 2024 Jan-. Available from: https://www.ncbi.nlm.nih.gov/books/NBK585051/
23. Pelletier AL, Rojas-Roldan L, Coffin J. Vision loss in older adults. Am Fam Physician. 2016;94(3):219-26.
24. Purves D, Augustine GJ, Fitzpatrick D, et al., (Eds.) Neuroscience. 2nd edition. Sunderland (MA): Sinauer Associates; 2001. Chapter 14, The Vestibular System. Available from: https://www.ncbi.nlm.nih.gov/books/NBK10819/
25. Purves D, Augustine GJ, Fitzpatrick D, et al., (Eds.). Neuroscience. 2nd edition. Sunderland (MA): Sinauer Associates; 2001. Types of Eye Movements and Their Functions. Available from: https://www.ncbi.nlm.nih.gov/books/NBK10991/
26. Rabbetts RB. Bannett & Rabbetts' clinical visual optics, 3rd edition, 1998.
27. Raharja A, Whitefield L. Clinical approach to vision loss: a review for general physicians. Clin Med (Lond). 2022;22(2):95-99.
28. Refraction and Prescribing, By Claire E. McDonnell, Available at https://arrow.tudublin.ie/cgi/viewcontent.cgi?article=1058&context=otpomart
29. Russell R, Sweda JR, Porcheron A, Mauger E. Sclera color changes with age and is a cue for perceiving age, health, and beauty. Psychol Aging. 2014 ;29(3):626-35.
30. Sachdev N, Cairns G, McGhee CNJ. An introduction to wavefront sensing in ophthalmology.2002; 6:50-53.
31. Salvi SM, Akhtar S, Currie Z. Ageing changes in the eye. Postgrad Med J. 2006;82(971):581-7.
32. Sebag J. Age-related changes in human vitreous structure. Graefes Arch Clin Exp Ophthalmol. 1987;225(2):89-93.
33. Sir Stewart Duke-Elder. System of ophthalmology, 1st edition,1970.
34. Stein HA, Stein RM, Freeman MI, The ophthalmic assistant, 8th edition, 2006.

35. The common sense of clinical refraction, By Gilbert Enechi, Available at https://www.researchgate.net/publication/348630716 NSE
36. The Three Dimensions of Vision Satisfaction, Available at https://www.opticianonline.net/cpd-archive/5059/#:~:text=Vision%20satisfaction%20is%20influenced%20by,discriminating%20efficiency%20and%20visual%20endurance.
37. Thibos LN. Principles of Hartmann-Shack Aberrometry, Available at http://www.carlomasci.it/biblio/aberrazioni_7.pdf
38. Ueta T, Makino S, Yamamoto Y, Fukushima H, Yashiro S. Pathologic myopia: an overview of the current understanding and interventions. Glob Health Med. 2020;2(3):151-55.
39. Webster MA. Visual adaptation. Annu Rev Vis Sci. 2015 ;1:547-67.
40. Williams D, Yoon GY, Porter J, Guirao A, Hofer H, Cox I. Visual benefit of correcting higher order aberrations of the eye. J Refract Surg. 2000;16(5):S554-9.

INDEX

Page numbers followed by *f* refer to figure, *fc* refer to flowchart, and *t* refer to table.

A

Aberration
 higher order 77*fc*, 80
 lower order 76
Accommodation 33, 337
 amplitude of 298, 366
 balanced range of 298, 366
 failure of 303
 in presbyopia, failure of 295
 mechanism, absence of 309
 positive relative 299
Accommodative
 disorder, implications of 34*t*
 esotropia 123
 spasm 264
 state 286
 stress 290
Acuity score 153
Adaptation 253
 problems 324
Airy disc, representation of 74*f*
Allen card test 146
Alternate occlusion test, procedure of 246
Amblyopia 159, 236, 316
Amblyopic eye 227
Ametropia 214
Anisometropia 236, 305, 321, 326, 328
 amblyopia 316
 correction in 307
 high 123
 management of uncorrected 265
 refraction in 305
 symptoms 306
Aniso-oxyopia 227
Antimetropia 227
Anxiety 265, 266
Aperture 73*f*
 size 73
Aphakia 309, 310
 correction in 310
 refraction in 309
Aphakic eye 309

Aplanatic curvature 80
Aqueous 1
 humor 5
Asthenopia 34, 63, 86, 263, 284
Astigmatic
 correction 124, 264, 365
  tests for 292
 errors, correction for larger 291
 eye 91*f*
 image 80
 letter chart 293
Astigmatism 92, 315, 326, 328, 329
 against-the-rule 91
 classification of 91
 degree of 124
 irregular 94
 presence of against rule 309
 prevalence of 321
 refraction in 290
 regular 90
 test 292
Athletes navigate dynamic 352
Attention deficit hyperactivity disorder 323
Auto lensmeter 179
 parts of 180*f*
Automated autorefractometer 211
Automated refractor's measurement system 213
Autorefractometer 120, 185, 210*f*, 210-214, 311, 324, 365
 advent of 210
 clinical use of 213
 components of 211, 211*f*

B

Back-lit chart 155*f*, 155
Badal optometer 212
Baseline data assimilation 172
Best corrected visual acuity 158
Billiard's players 355
Binocular balancing 342
 tests, two methods of 245, 246*f*

Binocular subjective refraction 227, 324
Binocular vision 39
    condition 228
    grades of 40*fc*
    in anisometropia 306
Binocular visual
    acuity 42
    field 51*f*
Blinking, increased 65
Blood sugar imbalance 277
Blur
    image, sources of 73*fc*
    vision 35, 60, 284, 287
        intermittent 60
Brain
    back of 41*f*
    occipital cortex 253
    via optic nerve 71
Break phenomena 203, 203*f*
Brow rests 209*f*
BWIS phenomena 203*fc*

C

Career-ending injury 353
Cataracts 236, 333, 342
    changes of 277
    posterior 158
        subcapsular 160
Chamber, anterior 334
Chart
    design 150
    types of 155
Cholesterol, high 265
Choroid 7, 7*f*, 336
Choroidal atrophy 94
Chromatic aberration 74
    causes of 75
Ciliary body 6, 334
Ciliary muscles 14, 14*f*, 95
    capability of 296
    contraction of 296
    functional incapacity of 296
Clear cornea 140
Clear crystalline lens 140
Clear ocular media 140
Clear vision
    checking range of 302*f*
    range of 302
Clinical refraction
    cardinal principle of 107

classification of tests used for
        purpose of 103*fc*
flow of 121*fc*
fundamental principle of 99, 283
goal of 106
intellectual process 111
laws of 100, 101*t*
methods of 117, 118*fc*
phases of 112*fc*
visit practice for 249*t*
Clock chart 292, 292*f*
Color
    perception 26
    sensitivity 338, 339
Coma 79*f*
Comatic aberration 78
Communication skills, effective 312
Condensing lens 189
Conjunctiva 7
Contact lenses 307
    application of 345
    induced corneal edema 277
    types of 270
Contrast
    detection 26
    perception 26
    sensitivity 27, 141, 338, 339
Convergence
    excess 35
    increased near point of 284
    induced secondary myopia 277
    insufficiency 123
Convex lens, power of 310
Cornea 1, 4, 4*f*, 229, 334
    anterior surface of 215
    surface curvature of 215
Corneal
    astigmatism 217
        estimation of 217
    curvature abnormalities 140
    radius, anterior 217
Corrected visual acuity 89
Counseling 116, 249, 267, 361, 362
    address patient's concern 269
    cost involvement 270
    educate patient on adaptation factor
        271
    explain prescription 268
    follow-up schedule 272
    professional recommendation 271

Index

Cross grid
  chart 299f
  test 298, 299, 366
Crystalline lens 1, 87, 335, 341
  changes in 296
  determine 229
Cycloplegic
  refraction 118
  retinoscopy 324
Cylinder
  axis 225
    changing 291
    estimating 203
    refine 237
  correction 258, 259, 232
  power 178, 182
    increases 213
    refine 237
Cylophoria 227

D

Dark adaptation 339
Darwin's theory 267
Data
  analysis 114
  assimilation 112
  synthesis 114
Decimal notation 142, 143, 143t
Defocused image 72
Defogging 230fc
Dehydration 266
Depression 265
Digital acuity system features 156
Digital test chart 156f, 156
Diplopia 35
Disorder, type of 34, 35
Distance
  angle of 1 minute of arc for 148f
  angle of 5 minutes of arc for 148f
  in meters 54
  increasing size in proportion to 149f
  test 150, 239, 244, 246
  vision 29
    clarity, delayed 34
    intermediate 29, 30
Divergence excess 35
Dominant eye 43
  tests for 47fc
Double vision 61
Dr Pray's astigmatic letter 293f

Dry eye syndrome 367
Duochrome test 341
  for spherical 243

E

Eccentric viewing 134, 154
Electromagnetic radiation 211
Emmetropization 314
  mechanism 315
Emotional state 360
Entrance tests 120, 361
Esophoria, basic 35
Exophoria 123
  amount of manifest 284
  basic 35
Exotropia, intermittent 123
Extraocular muscle 12, 12f, 13, 13fc, 62, 334
Eyeache 306
Eyeball, accessory organs of 9
Eyebrows 10
Eyelashes 10
Eyelids 10, 333
Eyes 1
  ability of 138
  accessory organs of 9f
  acuity 132
  aging changes in 333, 337t
  and vision care, clinical practice for 128
  captures 41f
  care 272
    importance of regular 1
  categorized, components of 1t
  causes 306
  chambers of 3fc
  continues, structural development of 313
  coordinate use of both 312
  diseases, common aging 342
  dominance, importance of 45
  fatigue 284
  focus 312
  fogging of 292
  infections 13
  motility 338, 339
  muscle diseases 13
  parts of 3, 3f
  physiological changes in 341
  rubbing of 65, 90, 284
  squeezing 65

squinting of 284
strain 62, 63, 85, 264, 284
    diagnosing 63
    symptoms of 290
structure and function 1
trauma to 13

F

Facultative hypermetropia 88
Fan and Block chart 293*f*, 293, 365
Far point
    concept of 192
    principle 192*f*
Farsightedness, severe 87
Fatigue 35
Field, depth of 54
Filter, red and green 131, 131*f*
Fine-tuning nose pads 364
Fingers, counting 152
Fitting contact lenses 215
Fixation 36
    target 212
Flare 62
Flexible test distance 344
Fluctuating vision 265
Focus, depth of 54
Fogging 230*fc*
    clinical significance of 229
    method 228, 278, 311
        of refraction 229
        of subjective refraction 229, 324
        step-by-step of 231
Forehead wrinkling 284
Fovea 7*f*, 8
Frame, trial 133*f*
Fundus 2
Fusion 40
    implies 40
Fusional vergence dysfunction 35

G

General health awareness 169
Geriatric refraction 332
    routine 341
Glare 62
    recovery time 339
Glaucoma 96, 140, 303, 333, 342
Goblet cells 16
Golden rule, history taking 167
Good vision 32

H

Habitual
    correction 125, 185, 218, 256, 259
        use of 259*fc*
    reading distance 301*f*
    undercorrected patients 264
    visual acuity 158, 184
Halberg trial clip 345*f*
    use of 344
Haloes around light 62
Hand motion 152
Head, trauma to 13
Headache 34, 35, 64, 90, 284, 287, 306
Heine Beta 200 retinoscope 208
Hole in card test 49*f*, 49
Hormonal fluctuations 266
Hunting cylinder 238
Hypermetropia 84, 86, 87, 286, 325, 327, 328
    absolute 88
    age-related correction criteria for 283*t*
    correction of 282
    degree of 87, 282, 285, 287
    high 288
    increases 315
    latent 89, 229
    manifest 89
    optimal correction of 284
    pathological 93
    refraction in 281
    tendency for 87
    total 89
    type of 88, 88*fc*
Hypermetropic 309
    anisometropia 305
    correction, factors affecting 282*fc*
    eye 87*f*
        optical condition of 281
    for red light 131
Hyperopia 284, 315
    adult 263
    latent 227
Hyperopic anisometropia 227
Hypothetical vitreous 230

I

Illumination 151, 239, 244, 246
    changing 344
    room 194, 221

Induced prism, effect of 307
Inferences 137
Iris 4f, 5, 334
Itching 90

J

Jack-in-the-box phenomenon 310
Jackson Cross-cylinder test 237, 292, 292f, 365
    cylinder axis verification using 237f
    hunting cylinder using 238f
    verifying cylinder power using 238f
Jaeger Notation 162
Javal-Schiotz keratometry 216

K

Kay Picture test 146
Keratoconus 158
Keratometer 185
Keratometry 120, 215, 217, 311
    general principle of 215
    measures 215
    of great importance 215
    one-position 216, 216f
    two-position 215, 216, 216f
    types of 215
    uses 217
Krause, glands of 18

L

Lacrimal
    apparatus 10
    canaliculi 11
    puncta 11
    sac 11
    system 334
Landolt 'C' 146
Lazy eye 316
Lea symbol 146
Lens 4f, 6
    altering trial 224
    correcting 201
    holder 180
    plate 180
    power of 174
    set, complete trial 129f
    simulate 129
    stand 180
Lensmeter 174, 177f
    adjusting eyepiece of 176f
    brands of 174
    serves 179
    switching on 176f
    types of targets found in 175f
Lensometry 173
Letter, linear size of linear size of, 149
Levator palpebrae superioris muscle 15, 16f, 16
Lids, twitching of 90
Light
    beam, projecting 194
    flashes of 66
    perception 152
    rays of 71
    room 222
    sensitivity 338, 339
    source 189, 211
    transmitted pinhole 159f
    wavelength of 75f
Limbus 4f, 5
LogMAR 144, 145
    acuity 144t

M

Macula 7f, 8
Macular functioning 132
Maculopathy 333, 342
Maddox rod 132, 132f
    use of 346
Manual
    lensmeter 173, 174f
    phoropter 133f
Meibomian glands 17, 17f
MEM card 209f
Memory 181
    measurement values in 183
Mental
    fortitude 353
    unhappiness 90
Meridional aniseikonic error 290
Mesopic vision 29, 32
Miles test 47, 48f
Minimum angle of resolution 143, 144
Mirror 190
Moll, glands of 18
Monochromatic
    aberrations 76
    light, use of 139
Monocular
    subjective refraction 324
    trial frame, useful 344

vision 42
visual field 50f
Monovision, representation of 46f
Motion
　reflex 193, 198, 199, 199f
　sickness 35
Motor fusion reflex eliminates 39
Multifocal contact lenses 46
　measurement of 183
Multiple tests like bichrome tests 365
Muscle
　balance, assessment of 366
　dilator 15
　imbalance 284
　　ruling out 366
Muscular imbalance, treat secondary 307
Myopia 84, 85, 275, 326, 327, 328
　case of 207
　children typically develop 328
　classification of 276
　degree of 86
　different degrees of 276t
　grades of 276
　higher degree of 278
　low 278
　magnitude of 276
　night 78, 277
　pathological 94, 276
　refraction in 275
　simple 276
　symptoms 85
　treatment of 277
Myopic
　anisometropia, mild to moderate 305
　eye 85f
　refractive errors 354

N

Nasolacrimal duct 11
Near addition 235, 301
　determination of 235
　different ages 235t
　prescription 265
　test for 298, 365
Near duochrome test 298, 300, 366
Near retinoscopy 187, 320
Near test card 134
Near vision 29, 30
　additions, prescription for 302
　intermittent blurring in 34

Near visual acuity 159
　unit measure of 161t
Neurological conditions 13
Neuronal alteration 332
Neutralization 201
Nodal point, angle subtended 54
Nonadaptation re-evaluating refraction 360
Non-presbyope, case of 234

O

Objective autorefractometer, limitations of 213
Objective refraction 120, 173, 185, 187, 364
　methods of 120
Oblique astigmatism 79, 92f
　retinal image 79f
　visual quality 79f
　wavefront map 79f
Observation system 191, 191f
Occlude left eye 239
Occluder 132, 132f
Occupation and lifestyle, understanding 169
Ocular
　and visual condition 169
　discomfort 35, 287
　diseases 342t
　　increased incidence of 265
　dominancy
　　subcategories of 43fc
　　tests for 47
　factors 58
　　encompass conditions 58
　glands 16
　health, indicator of 157
　media opacities 140
　muscles 11, 62fc
　　internal and external 12fc
　pain 64, 284
　structure
　　aging changes in 337
　　physiological changes in 340
　surface issues 367
　system, neuromuscular mechanisms of 254
Oculomotor
　balance 356
　dominance 44

Index

Operation switch 179
Ophthalmic lenses 270
Optic
    aberrations 74, 74*fc*
    alteration 332
    disc 7*f*, 8
    nerve 8, 140
    phenomena 192
Optimal
    near vision, prescription for 366
    visual performance, cornerstone of 353
Optometer 212
Optotypes 147
Orbit 9

P

Pantascopic angle 307
Pantoscopic tilt 134
Perception, depth 25
Peripheral
    light rays 151
    rays 78
    vision 31
        loss of 66
    visual field 51
Phenomena
    intensity 204
    skew 204, 205*f*
    thickness 204, 204*f*
Phoria
    high 353
    vertical 35
Phoropters 133
Photopic vision 29, 31
Photostress test, use of 346
Physical
    changes in crystalline lens 95, 295
    training 353
Pilot lamp 180
Pinhole
    acuity 158
    disc 130, 130*f*
        multiple 130
    test, use of 347
Pistol shooters 355
Place cross grid 299
Platform, placing spectacle lens onto 177*f*
Plus 1.00 D blur test 50

Pointing test 49, 49*f*
Poor binocularity, signs of 282
Porta test 48, 48*f*
Posture, practitioner and patient 195*f*
Power
    reading scale 177*f*
    supply 190
Practice protocol 267
Pray's astigmatic letters' 293
Preferential looking technique 319
Presbyopes
    case of 234
    undercorrected 300
Presbyopia 95
    correction of 297
    failure of accommodation in 296*fc*
    onset of 265, 303
    premature onset of 96, 303
    refraction in 295
    symptoms 96
Presbyopic 95*f*, 295*f*
    correction, final prescription for 303
Prescribing 115, 249
    astigmatic correction 291
    correction 347, 356
        criteria 283
        fundamental rule for 261
    decision, factors influence 256
Printed panel charts 154
Prism 129, 129*f*, 179*f*, 182
    dissociated test, procedure of 247
    lenses, use of 346
Progressive addition lens, measurement of 184
Projection system 189, 190*f*
Projector test charts 155, 156*f*
Pseudomyopia 227, 277
Pseudoneutrality 202
Psychotherapy 267
Pupil 5, 94, 201*f*, 335
    dilated 202
    size of 15, 73, 139
Pupillae, dilator 15, 15*f*
Purkinje image 215

R

Reading
    addition 235
    multiple 210
Refinement tests 120, 243

Index

Reflex 196
  band 197
  brilliance of 196
  confusing 200
  movement 198
    speed of 196
  triangular 200, 200*f*
  types of movement of 198*fc*
Refraction 320, 322, 323
  completed, assessment of 217
  correction, refinement of 244*fc*
  flow of re-evaluating 361
  fogging method of 232*fc*
  manifest 118
  objective method of 187, 188*f*
  placing slit for 240*f*
  post-cycloplegic 119
  process 229, 340
  scripting effective case history for 168
  skillful static 324
  subjective methods of 220
  temporary changes in 265
  using stenopeic slit 239
Refractive amblyopia 316
Refractive components 1
  changes in 315
Refractive correction 124, 213, 260, 263
  changes in 253
  prescribing 250*fc*, 257*fc*, 325
  prescription for 261, 268
Refractive error 61, 84, 140, 275, 314
  amount of 356
  assessment 341
  average 320
  calculation of 212
  changes 340
  correction of 122, 355
  degree of 354
  examination of 67
  like myopia 315
  measurement of 243, 249, 256, 318, 340, 341
  minor uncorrected 352
  uncorrected 333
  using appropriate tests 108
Regular astigmatism 84
Resolution
  logarithm of minimum angle of 143
  minimum angle of 144*t*

Retina 2, 7*f*, 7, 52, 335
  intact 140
  light focuses on 72*f*
Retinal
  adaptation 222
  image 71, 79*f*
    foundation of vision 71
    quality of 72
Retinopathy 333, 342
  of prematurity 317
Retinoscope 185, 208
  components of projection system of 190*fc*
  parts of 189
  practitioner posture with 195*f*
  principle of 192
  types of 191
Retinoscopic principle 212
Retinoscopy 120, 187, 209, 311, 365
  accuracy of 324
  concept of 198
  cylinder axis 203*fc*
  dynamic 187, 188
  nonrefractive uses of 207
  reflex 196*f*
  results 205
    compensated values of 206*f*
    cross chart for recording 206*f*
  static 187, 324
  step-by-step procedure for 208*fc*
Rods and cones 8
Roving ring scotoma 310

S

Saccade 37
Scheiner disc principle 212
Scissors-like movement 199, 200*f*
Sclera 3, 4*f*, 336
Scotopic vision 29, 31
Segment abnormalities
  anterior 214
  resulting, posterior 214
Sensory dominance 44
Sheridan gardiner 146
Sighting dominance 44
Simultaneous macular perception 40
Single control ring 208
Single vision lens measurement
  framed 183
  screen 182*f*

Index

Sleeve, focusing 190
Slit 131
   removing 240*f*
Sloan and Habel's M units 160
Smooth pursuit 37
Snellen's
   acuity, reduced 162
   chart 223, 233
   fraction 122, 141
      20 feet 143
      4 meters 143
      6 meters 143
      expresses 141
      in feet 143, 144, 145, 146
      in meter 143, 144, 146
   notations
      equivalent 162
      recorded test distance 143*t*
   optotype, dimension of 148*f*
   test chart 146, 147, 149, 226
      design 150
      letter size 149*t*
      linear size of letters used in 54*t*
      normal values 153
      optotypes 147
      principle 147
      test distance 150
      testing procedure 153
   visual acuity test chart letters 54
      size 149
Spatial
   distortions 306
   perception 25
   relationships 259
   resolution, essential for 139
Spectacle
   correction 307
   frame fitting, re-checking 363
   lens, rechecking 361, 363
   using brow rest with 195*f*
Spherical
   aberration 77, 77*f*, 78
      effect of 78
      retinal image 78*f*
      visual quality 78*f*
      wavefront map 78*f*
   and astigmatic reflex 197
   and cylinder trial lenses 128
   correction 232, 365
      modification in 258
      change in 251

   lens 128
   used to correct meridian values 240*f*
Spherocylinder
   form, transforming meridian values into 241*f*
   lens 178
Sphincter pupillae 15*f*, 15
Sports
   athletes, refraction for 352
   good refraction in 353
   retinoscope 191
Stable tear film 140
Stamina, decreased reading 306
Standard test distance 142
Stenopeic slit 130, 130*f*, 293, 311, 345, 365
   refraction 241
Stereopsis 41
   reduced 284
Stimulus
   changes 341
   contrast of 139
Strabismic amblyopia 316
Strabismus 305, 316
Straddling axis 204
Streak
   horizontal 195*f*
   narrow 197*f*
   projecting 194, 195*f*
   retinoscope 189*f*, 191
   vertical 195*f*
   wide 197*f*
Stress 266
Stycar visual acuity test 146
Subjective method 365
Subjective refraction 120, 220, 364
   challenges faced during 222
   delayed 233, 234
   four methods of 224*f*
   in hypermetropia 288
   manifest monocular 224, 226*fc*
   methods of 224
   near 300, 366
Supportive components 1

T

Target
   static and dynamic states of 260
   types of 175*f*
   use of internal fixating 214

Index

Task, loss of concentration 35
Thumb, rule of 251
Thyroid disorders 265
Tiring, early 90
Total corneal power, estimation of 217
Transduction 23
Trauma-induced corneal edema 277
Trial and error method 231, 298
Trial framing 124, 133, 367
Trial lens set 128
Tumbling 'E' 146

U

Uncut single vision lens, measurement of 181

V

Vergence 34, 37, 337, 339
    function disorder, implications of 35*t*
Versions 38*f*
Vertigo 284
Vestibular-ocular movement 38*f*, 38
Vigilant 59
Vision 250
    and visual
        function 22
        perception 22
        responses 261
    blurring of 33
    care, realm of 271
    cause blurring of 60
    central 30
    chart 225*f*
    classification of 29
    components of 32, 32*fc*
    correction
        for sports athletes diverges 353
        mode of 171
        options for 269
    development of 313
    distorted 61
    important foundation of 71
    in anisometropia 306
    in aphakia 309
    in astigmatism 92, 251
    in sports, role of 353
    process of 22, 22*fc*, 250
    with habitual correction 173
Visual acuity 32, 33, 43, 136, 137, 139, 140, 141, 142, 151, 157, 185, 285, 313, 336, 339, 347
    assessing 185
    chart 151
    clinical assessment of 157
    designation of 141, 141*fc*
    estimation of 320
    factors affecting 137, 138*fc*
    for preschool children 146
    impaired 342
    in astigmatism 92
    in different degree of
        myopia 86*t*
        hypermetropia 285*t*
    in hypermetropia 89
    in myopia 86
    legally measuring 137
    measuring 33, 136, 137, 137*t*, 142, 158, 319, 322
        with spectacle 361, 362
    principal measures of 157*fc*
    rating 144, 145*t*
    recording 151
    test 136, 137, 141
        chart formats 146, 154, 154*fc*
        implications of 140
        limitations of 140
        objectives of 136
    uncorrected 157, 173, 184, 218
    with habitual correction 218
Visual adaptation 254
Visual angle 52
    concept of 53
    formed point n 53*f*
Visual apparatus 58
Visual attention 28
Visual comfort 252
Visual efficiency 145, 146*t*
Visual field 50, 338, 339
    restrictions of 310
Visual functions 339
    age-related development of 313
    aging changes in 336, 339, 339*t*
Visual impairment reduces 332
Visual issues 170
Visual pathway 140
Visual perception 23, 24, 27, 257
    different facets of 25
    environment 24*fc*
    facets of 25
    presence of 140
    stages of 23*fc*

Visual quality 79*f*
Visual satisfaction 255, 256, 256*fc*
    triad 255*f*
Visual stimuli, rapidly changing 353
Visual symptoms 57, 59, 60
    causes of 57
    manifestation of 57
    optical correction of 66
    reasons for 58*fc*
Visual system 26
Visually evoked potentials, utilizing 319
Visually impaired, refraction in 342
Vitreous 1, 335
    humor 8

W

Wavefront
    data 81
    map 79*f*
Weariness, sensation of 57
Wolfring, glands of 18
Working distance 193, 193*f*

Z

Zeis, glands of 18
Zernike mode 80
Zonule of Zinn 6